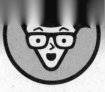

Getting
Pregnant

by John S. Rinehart, MD, PhD, JD;
Lisa A. Rinehart, RN, BSN, JD;
Jackie Meyers-Thompson, BA;
Sharon Perkins, RN

for
dummies®
A Wiley Brand

Getting Pregnant For Dummies®

Published by: **John Wiley & Sons, Inc.**, 111 River Street, Hoboken, NJ 07030-5774, www.wiley.com

Copyright © 2020 by John Wiley & Sons, Inc., Hoboken, New Jersey

Published simultaneously in Canada

For general information on our other products and services, please contact our Customer Care Department within the U.S. at 877-762-2974, outside the U.S. at 317-572-3993, or fax 317-572-4002. For technical support, please visit https://hub.wiley.com/community/support/dummies.

Wiley publishes in a variety of print and electronic formats and by print-on-demand. Some material included with standard print versions of this book may not be included in e-books or in print-on-demand. If this book refers to media such as a CD or DVD that is not included in the version you purchased, you may download this material at http://booksupport.wiley.com. For more information about Wiley products, visit www.wiley.com.

Library of Congress Control Number: 2020930130

ISBN 978-1-119-60115-9 (pbk); ISBN 978-1-119-60119-7 (ebk); ISBN 978-1-119-60123-4 (ebk)

Manufactured in the United States of America

V10017238_013020

Contents at a Glance

Table of Contents

PART 3: SEEKING ANSWERS, IDENTIFYING CAUSES, AND DEALING WITH DISAPPOINTMENTS

Introduction

I f you're dealing with infertility, you may feel alone, confused, and depressed over the potential loss of the dream you've cherished since childhood: the dream of having a baby of your own.

Infertility is a medical problem for 6–8 million Americans. Deemed a disease by the World Health Organization but debated as a symptom by many professional organizations, insurance companies often deny coverage for its diagnosis and treatment. Many people (the "just relax and you'll get pregnant" crowd) don't understand its biological origins, and a few (the "take this magic pill and you'll get pregnant, guaranteed!" group) even exploit those suffering from it. There is good news on the infertility front, however; not only are medical treatments for infertility making great gains, but there's also more awareness of the emotional and social effects of infertility. In fact, most reproductive medicine centers like to call themselves *fertility* centers now.

Getting Pregnant For Dummies was conceived by combining Jackie Thompson's knowledge of infertility from a patient's viewpoint, Lisa Rinehart's wealth of information as an infertility nurse and reproductive law attorney, and Dr. John Rinehart's 40 years of clinical practice in reproductive medicine. We wrote this book so that patients dealing with infertility will know that they're not alone and what they may be up against. We hope it finds its way to the bookshelves and nightstands of all the patients who need it to help find the road to their baby.

About This Book

This book is our attempt to help those of you who want to walk into the doctor's office and not walk out feeling out of control of your own fertility. Our vision is to provide fertility patients — both those at the starting line and those closer to the finish — and the people who love them with as much information as we can on the options available to them. We discuss topics ranging from the scientific to the spiritual.

You can read through this book from front to back and feel confident that you can find the answer to just about any fertility issue, from natural family planning to cloning. But if you're like most people, you'll probably look through the table of contents, zero in on the chapters that affect you, and jump directly to them. This book is meant as a resource, which means that you can go back to it whenever a new issue or question arises and find the answer you need without reading through everything that comes before.

This book is meant for people with every degree of fertility expertise, from the novice to the jaded, been-there-done-that patient. The no-tech and low-tech fertility chapters come first, so you can skip them if you're already a veteran and move right into high-tech and *really* high-tech stuff found in the second half of the book.

We intersperse personal stories throughout the book; these (we hope!) make interesting reading from the viewpoint of either Lisa (an infertility nurse/attorney), Jackie (an infertility patient), or Dr. R (the IVF doctor). If you skip them, you won't miss any essential information, although you may miss a few humorous sidelines or "I did it, so you can too" stories.

To help you pick out information from a page, we use the following conventions throughout the text to make elements consistent and easy to understand; the last thing we want to do is confuse you!

>> New terms appear in *italics* and are closely preceded or followed by an easy-to-understand definition. *Italics* are also used for emphasis.

>> **Bold** highlights the keywords in bulleted lists.

We think every word in this book is interesting and educational, but we understand that sometimes you just need a quick answer to a burning question. Other times you want to discover everything possible about infertility, even the technical stuff. We've designated some information as interesting-but-not-essential-to-read. Feel free to read it, but if you skip it, you're not missing anything vital. Optional sections are

>> **Text in sidebars:** Shaded boxes that appear throughout the book. The information they contain may be anything from personal stories to technical information.

>> **Anything with a Technical Stuff icon attached:** This information is interesting but not essential. It simply enhances your understanding of a particular topic.

Note: The information provided in this book is based upon the best evidence available today. The authors used practice guidelines from both The American College of Obstetricians and Gynecologists and The American Society for

Reproductive Medicine, systematic reviews, and meta-analyses when they were available. Science is always discovering new things, so by the time you read this, some of these sources may have been revised.

Foolish Assumptions

We assume that you're reading this book because you want to know more about infertility and because, despite your hopes to the contrary, you and/or a loved one, are dealing with infertility on one level or another, be it your first child or your fifth. We also assume that you want to

>> Understand the biologic causes of infertility

>> Discover what you can do to overcome infertility, from proper timing to changing your diet

>> Be up to date on the latest medical and surgical treatments for infertility

>> Find out about the newest genetic testing for you and your embryos

>> Pursue options for parenthood if the traditional roads fail you, from donor egg to use of a surrogate

Infertility is not the end of the road or the end of your dream of parenthood. There is help available, and we're here to help you find the resources you need, whether your fertility issues are simple to solve or complex.

Icons Used in This Book

Icons are the little images that appear occasionally in the margins next to the text. We use them to let you know that a topic or piece of information is special in some way. *Getting Pregnant For Dummies* includes the following icons:

TIP

This icon identifies information that's helpful and can save you time or trouble.

REMEMBER

This icon highlights key points in the section you're reading.

WARNING

This icon stresses information that describes potentially serious issues, such as side effects to medication or other dangerous problems. Pay attention to warnings — they can keep you out of trouble!

TECHNICAL STUFF

This icon signals information that's interesting but not essential.

PERSONAL STORY

If any of us has a personal story that is funny, informative, inspirational, or otherwise interesting, we identify it with the Personal Story icon. These anecdotes are never essential reading, but they're usually entertaining!

Beyond the Book

This book is already full of information, but we've also provided a handy online Cheat Sheet of some of the most important or most helpful tidbits on the topic of fertility and getting pregnant such as the most important fertility tests, notes about medications and what questions our fertility doctor will ask you. Simply go to www.dummies.com and type "Getting Pregnant For Dummies Cheat Sheet" in the search box.

Where to Go from Here

This book is set up so that you can open it at any point and be able to understand the information right in front of you.

The early chapters of this book deal with infertility issues that can be solved fairly easily, like timing. If you don't have a basic understanding of human biology, Chapter 2 can help you understand the complexity of the human reproductive system.

On the other hand, if the emotional aspects of infertility are impacting your relationships, Chapter 10 may be more what you need to read.

The point is that you don't have to read everything (although you certainly can, and you may discover something you never knew before)! Just flip to the table of contents or index, find a subject that interests you, and turn to that chapter.

However you choose to use this book, we hope it's helpful.

1

Are We There Yet? Wondering Why You're Not Pregnant

Chapter **1**

Where, Oh Where, Can My Baby Be?

I f you're reading this book, the odds are good that you want to have a baby. You may actually have been trying to have a baby for a while without success, and maybe you're becoming frustrated, annoyed, and a little scared — are you *ever* going to have the family you've dreamed of?

We want to help make this process easier for you — less stressful and more successful. In this chapter, we tell you the official definition of infertility (it may surprise you!), give you statistics on infertility today, show you how to shake your family tree for genetic problems, and talk about the cost of infertility — the emotional cost as well as the monetary cost. Where possible, the authors have relied upon the principles of evidence based medicine and The American Society for Reproductive Medicine guidelines. The authors have also used their extensive clinical experience to bring some practical advice. In the end, there is no *one* way to address a person's fertility issues. Furthermore, things change rapidly, so an initial game plan may need modification as the process develops.

Defining Infertility

Infertility as defined by the experts may surprise you. According to guidelines established by infertility specialists, you're not considered to be infertile until you've been trying to get pregnant for one year if you're under age 35. That means that trying to get pregnant last week and not having signs of pregnancy this week does *not* mean that you're infertile. If you are over the age of 35, you can breathe a sigh of relief in that you *only* have to try actively for six months before an investigation as to why you haven't conceived can begin — and may be covered by insurance. However, some states that mandate insurance coverage use the one-year rule (especially for certain age groups) and will not provide benefits until you hit the one-year mark.

However, since the modern world is one of immediate gratification and answers that seem to appear at the speed of Google, it can be hard — if not downright impossible — to try to get pregnant for a full year without getting impatient, discouraged, or just plain panicked. There's nothing wrong with going to see your gynecologist to talk about why you're not getting pregnant after just a few months; in fact, your coauthors, being fairly impatient people themselves, would consider you to be a candidate for sainthood if you could wait a year — or even six months! — without talking to your doctor.

Looking at Infertility Statistics

Most women know that the older you get, the harder it is to get pregnant. But what about race, socioeconomic status, geography, and heredity as fertility factors? In the next sections we look at how infertility affects different groups.

Making babies: An inefficient process at best

You may think of Mother Nature as a pretty efficient woman, and for many women that is true. One common misperception is that a woman has a 20 percent chance of conceiving each month she tries. That is simply not true. The chance of conceiving depends upon a woman's age and how long the woman has been trying to get pregnant.

Unfortunately, as you go through this book, you will hear way too much about how age reduces a woman's chance of conceiving. We all wish this weren't true, but aging is an inevitability of life. Common sense should tell you that a 44-year-old woman has less of a chance of conceiving than a 24-year-old woman. But a subtlety of infertility is that there are actually three sub-groups within any group of people who start to try to achieve a pregnancy. The majority do not have a problem achieving a pregnancy, a small group are sterile, and an intermediate group are *subfertile*, meaning they will conceive, just not within the one-year time frame or without technology helping.

Women with normal fertility will conceive quickly. Some estimates place the chance of conceiving in the first month of trying as high as 40 percent. After three months, 65 percent of women who conceive naturally are pregnant, and by six months, 85 percent are pregnant. After that the chance of achieving a pregnancy gets less and less each month because those not getting pregnant easily have a greater chance of being subfertile or sterile. This is true regardless of age. So a 40-year-old female with normal fertility will get pregnant quickly. It's just that by age 40 as many as 40 percent are functionally sterile. Looking at 100 women under age 35 trying to get pregnant, the breakdown looks like this:

>> Eighty-five will be pregnant within one year.

>> Ten more will be pregnant after two years of trying without medical intervention.

>> Five won't get pregnant without some help from the medicine man or maybe not at all.

High-tech infertility treatments, such as in vitro fertilization (IVF), claim a success rate of about 50 percent for those under age 35. But people using IVF have the diagnosis of infertility, and even if they use IVF multiple times, some will never achieve a pregnancy. Estimates of the cumulative live birth rate for women under the age of 35 is about 85 percent, meaning that if women under the age of 35 try multiple cycles of IVF, 15 percent will never conceive and have a child that is genetically theirs.

Age and infertility

If you're over 35, you're in good company; 26 percent of all first-time moms in the United States are over 35! Despite this, Mother Nature doesn't make it easy to get pregnant past age 35. There is also an exceedingly higher rate of women who begin having children in their 40s and even 50s, but keep in mind, unlike the tabloids would like you to think, many of these women may require the intervention of an donor egg and/or surrogacy . . . but more on this later! However, a number of women *do* begin or continue to have children without help through their early to middle 40s. We discuss the impact of age in greater detail in Chapter 7.

For example:

>> By your late 30s, you have a 10 percent chance of getting pregnant in any given month, and 17 percent of those who do will miscarry.

>> If you're over 40, the pregnancy rate per month slips to 5 percent, with 34 percent of those miscarrying.

>> By age 45, your chance per month of conceiving is less than 1 percent, and 53 percent of those will miscarry.

Race and infertility

Does your racial background affect your chance for pregnancy? There is a slight difference in infertility rates, with Hispanic women under 35 experiencing a 7 percent infertility rate, Caucasians a 6.4 percent infertility rate, and African American women recording a 10.5 percent rate of infertility. These differences may be due to socioeconomic factors, such as poverty, poor nutrition, or lack of physician care, rather than strictly racial issues.

High-tech treatments and infertility

If you're already frantically reading your insurance booklet and shaking the piggy bank in hopes of finding a few spare thousand dollars to pay for high-tech infertility treatments, you may take comfort in the following statistic: Only around 3 percent of infertile couples end up doing high-tech treatment like in vitro fertilization to get pregnant (You can find everything you need to know about IVF in Chapters 15 to 18.)

But IVF has been a boon to those seeking to conceive. Since the first IVF baby (Louise Brown in 1978 in England), over 6 million babies have been born through IVF. That number is expected to explode to 200 million by the end of this century. Considering Dr. John Rinehart's look back to the early days of success, IVF has come a long way: "In the early days of IVF, success was so rare that we would buy a bottle of champagne for each woman who delivered a baby. Today, it would take a vineyard to supply that much champagne."

Shaking Down the Family Tree

It may seem silly to look to your family tree for signs of infertility that could be inherited; after all, *you're* here, so how could your parents have had fertility issues?

Putting together a family birth history

Most of us don't ask our parents about their road to parenthood until we're trying to become parents ourselves. But you may be surprised to find out that it took your parents a number of years to have you or your siblings. It's also possible that people in your family tree may be adopted or the product of artificial insemination, issues that often weren't discussed a few decades ago.

While family lines that are completely infertile tend to die out in a generation (for obvious reasons), some families may be subfertile, with less than average sperm counts or ovulation issues, and still manage to have a child or two.

TIP

Ask the most talkative member of your family for a family "birth history." You may be surprised by what you discover. And remember, sometimes a vehement denial, such as "there's never been any problem in *our* family," may be a clue to dig a little deeper and find out why everyone is so defensive.

Finding out important information

Researching your family history can provide valuable information. For example, you may discover family genetic tendencies that could cause problems on your own reproductive road. Or you may find out that everyone in your family took six months to get pregnant, a fact that may put your mind at ease, particularly around month number five of trying without success.

Before trying to get pregnant, you'll want to know whether any diseases occur more than once on your family tree. If so, the disease may be caused by a dominant gene that you could pass on if you carry it, even if your partner doesn't carry it. Some examples of this can be BRCA 1 and 2 (commonly known as the breast cancer gene, but it can affect men as well with increased predilection toward prostate cancer), muscular dystrophy, Huntington's disease, and more. Depending on how open your family is, finding out this information can be difficult. Many families don't discuss anything related to pregnancy, especially not problems getting pregnant, pregnancy losses, or genetic defects. Just a few generations ago, parents of children with genetic abnormalities were encouraged to put them in a home and tell the relatives the baby had been stillborn.

If your family tree does hold a genetic problem or a birth defect that shows up more than once, you'll probably want to have genetic testing done. A gene map, which can be done from a blood test, will show whether you carry abnormal genes that could cause problems for your child.

Sometimes the only thing you find out from family records is nonspecific, such as "all the Smith boys died young." Try and pin down why they all died young: Did they have hemophilia or muscular dystrophy, or did they all fall out of the same apple tree?

WARNING

If you and your partner are blood relatives, it is especially important to see a genetic counselor before getting pregnant. You may carry more of the same abnormal genes than unrelated partners would, which may make you more likely to have a child with a genetic problem. The risk for serious birth defects is 1 in 20 for second cousins and 1 in 11 for first cousins.

Checking the stats of your race

Even if you're not aware of genetic illnesses in your family, certain populations tend toward specific issues. For example, while sickle cell anemia occurs in 1 of 8 African Americans, cystic fibrosis can be found in 1 of 26 Caucasians and at an even higher percentage among Ashkenazi Jews. Other diseases such as Tay–Sachs and Gaucher are also prevalent among the Jewish population.

Many OB/GYNs suggest screening for the most likely diseases based on your heritage. It doesn't hurt to get this done *before* you become pregnant. While many genetic diseases are recessive, meaning that both parents must carry the gene in order for the baby to develop the disease, should you turn up to be a carrier, your partner can be tested right away. If both you and your partner are carriers, each child from your union holds a 25 percent chance of inheriting both genes and thus the disease. Fifty percent of your children will be carriers of the disease and 25 percent will not have *or* carry the disease.

THE GOOD NEWS ABOUT INHERITED DISEASES

When it comes to inherited diseases, you have options your grandmother and mother never did. You can receive pre-pregnancy genetic counseling or have early pregnancy testing of the fetus for abnormalities. Your grandmother, who may have had children well into her 40s, was more likely to have a baby born with chromosomal abnormalities. Such problems are more common in women over 35, and there was no way to test for them during pregnancy in earlier generations. Your mother may have been afraid to have more than one child if she knew there was a family history of cystic fibrosis or muscular dystrophy. The problem that your aunt had during pregnancy from an inherited bleeding disorder is now a condition that can be diagnosed and treated during pregnancy, increasing your chances of having a healthy, full-term baby. Rh factors may have caused fetal death just two generations ago, but they can now be easily prevented by an injection of RhoGAM, which prevents the growing fetus from having its blood cells attacked in utero.

Remember, these are all statistical numbers. Some families where both parents carry a recessive gene disorder have multiple children in a row who have the disease, despite the 25 percent odds per child. Other families don't. Statistics are based on large numbers of people and the likelihood of any one event occurring. You and your family may or may not fall into the statistical pattern. (We talk a lot more about what your genes do later on in Chapter 3.)

Seeing What Causes Infertility

Infertility has many causes, and figuring out which applies to you may be very simple — or very difficult. Although women used to bear the brunt of blame for infertility, the truth is that male and female factors share equally in infertility. Consider the following statistics:

» One-third of infertility is caused by female factors.

» One-third of infertility is caused by male factors.

» Around 20 percent of infertility is unexplained.

» Around 10 to 15 percent of infertility is caused by a combination of male and female factors.

Among women, the main causes of infertility are

» **Ovulatory disorders:** No ovulation or irregular ovulation

» **Tubal disorders:** Blocked or infected tubes

» **Uterine issues:** Fibroids, polyps, or adhesions

For men the most common causes of infertility are

» Low sperm count

» Decreased sperm motility

» Abnormally shaped sperm

» No sperm at all in the ejaculate

Each of these categories of infertility can be caused by a number of things; for example, a decreased sperm count can be caused by a disease such as diabetes, by a birth defect, or by trauma. A woman can have blocked tubes from endometriosis, pelvic inflammatory disease, or from a congenital malformation. Anovulation can be caused by polycystic ovarian syndrome, premature ovarian failure, or by overexercising. While it may be fairly obvious what the problem is, finding the reason for the problem may be more difficult.

Diagnosing Infertility

You may think this is a no-brainer: If you're not getting pregnant, it seems like you've already diagnosed yourself with infertility! However, diagnosing a lack of pregnancy is the easy part; figuring out why you're not getting pregnant is the hard part.

After reading through Chapter 6, which discusses simple techniques for increasing your pregnancy odds, or Chapters 11 and 12, which explain some of the tests used to diagnose infertility, of this book, you may be able to diagnose the reason for your difficulty in getting pregnant without any help from your doctor. For example, you may be having sex at the wrong time of the month — your "infertility issue" may be solved with a calendar, a thermometer, and an ovulation predictor kit! Or you may not have realized how irregular your periods were — 35 days apart one month, 40 the next, 60 the next — maybe you're not ovulating on a regular basis.

Your gynecologist can run a few simple blood tests to help determine whether or not you're ovulating. Ovulation is, after all, the first step in getting pregnant, and usually blood tests or observation of your own cervical mucus and temperature (see Chapter 6 for ways to figure this out) can help you figure out when you're ovulating so you can time sex accordingly.

If you're still not pregnant after six months of "hitting the mark," it's time for more testing; your doctor may suggest a test to see if your tubes are open and testing on your partner to see if "his boys can swim."

This process of looking for the problem and then seeing if it's fixed can take a few months. Only 20 percent of infertile couples never have a definite answer to why they can't get pregnant, so the odds are in your favor.

Recognizing Why Getting Pregnant Seems Harder Today

Sometimes things seemed easier in Grandma's day. Large families were common, and it appeared that everyone had children. In fact, getting pregnant for some groups of people is more frequent while it seems to have decreased for others.

But for the general population, statistics gathered by the government have shown a rather steady percentage of the population meeting the definition of infertile. This has been near 15 percent since 1965. Some factors that may make it harder to conceive are as follows:

>> **People are having children later in life.** Over age 25, there is a slight but definite decrease in fertility in women. Men are also less fertile at older ages but not for the same reasons as women.

>> **Due to better medical management, people are living longer and getting pregnant (or trying to) despite the presence of serious chronic disease, such as diabetes or lupus.** In the past, just the *presence* of these conditions would have precluded the possibility of pregnancy.

>> **Male infertility, related to decreased sperm counts, has increased.** Many theories circulate as to why this is occurring, with environmental factors being carefully studied. However, caution is needed here since it is not the semen parameters that matter but whether or not a man fathered a child. Lower semen numbers or characteristics do no always translate into lower pregnancy rates.

>> **The incidence of sexually transmitted diseases has increased.** Some of these diseases, such as chlamydia, cause serious damage to the reproductive organs.

>> **More men and women have had either a vasectomy or a tubal ligation at a young age and then decided to have another child.** Needless to say, they immediately face fertility issues due to their previous choices.

>> **It may seem as if everyone had children years ago, but start asking questions and you'll get a different story.** You may find out that Uncle Charlie wasn't really Aunt Jo's son; he was her sister's child, whom she raised after his mother died young, and on and on. Everyone may have been raising children, but many of those children may have been extended family members.

>> **People today talk more.** Just because you never heard about your grandmother's stillborns or your mother's miscarriages doesn't mean they didn't happen. Pregnancy talk today is big business, and everyone in the world seems to be in the news talking about their babies, lack of babies, adopted babies, and how they got pregnant. This focus puts a constant in-your-face emphasis on pregnancy. It also makes you feel, when you're trying to get pregnant, like everyone else is doing it — and doing it better than you are!

REMEMBER

Relax, this is only the beginning for you, and we do our best to help you start baby making with the best of them.

Calculating the Cost of Infertility

Infertility costs a lot. We're not just talking money here; the emotional toll is usually much higher and longer lasting than any hit to your pocketbook. In the next sections, we look at the costs of infertility on your self-esteem, your marriage, and last of all on your wallet. While it may be uncomfortable to talk about the cost of infertility treatments, lack of funds is one of the main reasons people do not pursue fertility treatment.

Preparing for the emotional toll

Infertility is not for the faint of heart. Will it test your mental, physical, and spiritual strength? Um, possibly. Will you come out a better person than before? No guarantee, but as with all of life's challenges, the better prepared you are going in, the more likely your psyche is to survive and thrive.

In this book, we discuss a lot about support, be it your partner, friends, family, professionals, or online networks. It doesn't matter in what shape it comes, everyone needs a little help from their friends, no matter who those friends may be.

You may decide to let just a few close confidantes know of your situation with trying to conceive. You may tell anyone who will listen. Regardless, know that at some point, someone will say something wrong. Set the ground rules now. If you don't want to be asked how *things* are going (secret speak for "Are you pregnant yet?"), tell your network up-front that you will let them know when there is something to know. Their overenthusiasm may annoy you time and again, but they are probably almost as excited as you are to hear about your success.

While you don't want to anticipate a long, arduous battle with your fertility, or lack thereof, don't set yourself up to expect that within a month you'll be shopping online for maternity clothes. Decorating the baby's room at this point is probably not a great idea either. If all goes well and success finds you early, that's great — and we promise you that you'll have plenty of time to find the perfect maternity wardrobe and baby collection. If not, you will only set yourself up for disappointment, and the goal is to keep that to a minimum as best you can, in the areas over which you *do* have control. Your thinking is one of them.

Recognizing how infertility affects your partnership

Whether the infertility issues are yours, your partner's, or something you share, be certain that you most likely will share the ups and downs of baby making.

Infertility is tough on the most resilient of individuals and couples. It will find the weak spots in you and your relationship. Steady yourself and your union for what could be turbulent waters ahead (this includes success *and* a new baby!)

When it comes to baby making, sooner is often better than later, but keep in mind that this is from a biological perspective. And although you may hear the biological clock ticking away, ready-or-not is not the best way to make your decision about when to conceive. The state of your union is an issue we revisit throughout this book, as it is one of the most important aspects in dealing with fertility, infertility, and baby makes three (or more). And although biology is a key issue in deciding if and when you're ready to conceive, maturity, financial security, and stability are equally important, whether your challenge is trying to get pregnant or trying to raise said baby in a difficult and expensive world.

REMEMBER

For people in a partnership relationship, the quality of your partnership is the foundation for your family. Take the time to make sure that it's solid before moving on to the next level. Revisit it often to make sure it's staying secure through the ups and downs of trying to conceive. For people not in a partnership relationship, the status of your support system can be one of your biggest assets in your journey through the fertility process.

TIP

Just keep talking! As with all other areas, communication is key in the decision to add on to your family, whether you're successful right away or not. If you find yourselves at an impasse, enlist the help of an outside party: a member of the clergy, a therapist, or a physician to help you sort out feelings and facts.

Adding up the financial cost

Talk about rubbing salt on a wound. Infertility treatments can be difficult enough, but treating infertility can be costly as well. The rising costs of medical treatment in general is a major problem in the U.S. today. It seems unfair that the limit to having children should come down to money but in many circumstances this is true. Dr. R. suggests that you explore the potential total cost for treatments that are suggested along with the overall chance of having a child (see Chapter 15 to look at dealing with the costs of IVF). Your allocation of resources may be significantly altered if you establish guidelines up front; otherwise, you run the risk of the "Vegas syndrome" (believing that just one more hand will make you a fortune or one more IVF cycle will get you a baby). For example, suppose a 41-year-old woman wants to use IVF to have a child that is biologically hers. One center has estimated that for some women in this situation, the chance to have a child can cost as much as $400,000. And even if a person spent that much, there is no guarantee that a successful pregnancy will occur. Knowing that, a couple may choose to use donor eggs for a much higher chance of success for much less money.

TIP

Just like playing the stock market, be a smart investor. Make a life plan, set limits and goals, and stick to them.

Like everything, infertility costs vary and can depend on where you live, which physician/practice you see, and most importantly, whether your treatment is small, medium, or large.

When you're starting out, expect to pay $20 to $45 for an ovulation predictor kit and about the same for home pregnancy kits. This is the easy stuff. We haven't brought in the professionals yet.

What about insurance, you ask? "What about it?" we answer. Only 16 states have mandated coverage for infertility, meaning that for those who aren't fortunate enough to live in one of these areas, infertility treatments are paid for out-of-pocket — yours, that is. Even if you have insurance coverage, you may be amazed to see how little of your bill is covered. Some insurance plans cover only monitoring, meaning the frequent blood draws and ultrasounds. Because these can run well over $5,000 per cycle, this coverage is a help. Other plans cover only the medications (which can cost between $2000 and $9,000), which is a help, but by no means relief from the total cost.

Many insurance plans, however, will cover the tests and procedures related to diagnosing your particular infertility problem. This can be very helpful as well because many cases of infertility require blood work, ultrasound, and even an exploratory surgical procedure to determine a cause for infertility — a mere start-ing point for treatment. This generally applies to both you and your partner, but double-check this with your insurance company prior to signing up for the "party platter" of tests.

Once diagnosed, and even if you escape diagnosis (20 percent of infertility is unexplained), that's when the real costs can kick in. Should your problem be resolved quickly and easily, you may get by with the cost of a few months' worth of Clomid (a pill that causes super ovulation in order to push your ovaries into producing one or more follicles that can be fertilized), a few ultrasounds (which generally cost anywhere from $200 to $500 depending on where you live and which physician practice you frequent) and approximately $200 per blood draw for the basic tests needed to monitor your cycle. If you need IUI (intrauterine insemination), the cost is generally $600 per insemination.

If you are to be monitored via blood work and ultrasound throughout the month, some clinics offer "package" prices, which can range from $900 to $2,000 for blood work and ultrasounds for one month.

If your cycle requires injectable gonadotropins (Repronex, Follistim, Gonal F, Menopurto, to name a few), you are looking at a cost of $1 per unit. Gonadotropins now come in an injectable form containing between 300 and 900 units. IVF cycles can use between 75 and 600 units per day for 10–12 days. If you are also adding in luteal support (which occurs after the egg has supposedly been fertilized), pro-gesterone and estrogen may run you a few hundred dollars per cycle (a bargain compared to other costs!).

Keep in mind that these are all approximate costs. Later on in the book, we discuss places to purchase medications that may offer better deals and other methods that you can use to cut your costs.

If you move up to the big time, keep in mind that the average IVF cycle costs between $10,000 and $15,000. Of that, about $4,000 to $5,000 is spent on medi-cation, and another $4,000 to $10,000 goes to your clinic.

But, for now, we suggest taking it one step at a time. You've bought this book, and if you get pregnant from the information you find here, consider it a great bargain!

» **Understanding your menstrual cycle**

» **Looking at how sperm works**

» **Sharing the best time for sex and conception**

Chapter **2**

What Does Anatomy Have to Do with It?

You may think that you know how to get pregnant. Doesn't everybody? Not necessarily! In this chapter, we review basic male and female biology, educate you on the inner workings of your menstrual cycle, and explain how sperm is supposed to work. Then we unlock the secrets of conception and how sex is meant to get you to pregnancy!

Reviewing the Female Anatomy

Were you paying attention in Biology 101? You may have taken a quick peek at the film on the miracle of birth and announced loudly to all your friends, "Eww, gross, I'm never having kids!" And yet here you are, some undisclosed number of years later, wishing you had paid more attention back then. Don't worry; we're here to fill in the gaps in your reproductive education.

The human body has the basics and the accessories — just like at Macy's! When you buy an outfit, you can be dressed with just the basics, but the accessories really pull your outfit together. When you're trying to have a baby, the parts that you don't see — the "accessories" — determine whether you can get pregnant.

A naked woman is pretty unrevealing from a reproductive viewpoint. You can't see the organs that count in childbearing, so you can't tell at a glance whether yours are present and functioning. Take a look at what should be inside every woman, starting from the outside and working your way "inside." (See Figure 2-1.)

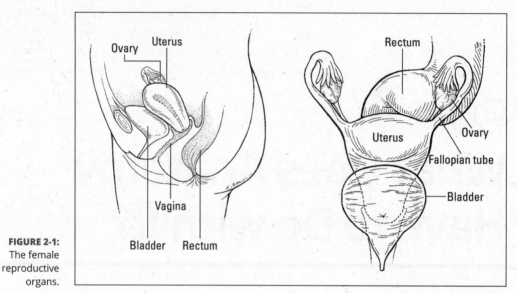

FIGURE 2-1: The female reproductive organs.

The vagina

The vagina mostly serves as a passageway, first for the penis to deliver sperm up near the opening of the uterus, and later for the delivery of the baby. If you have a very small vaginal opening, intercourse may be uncomfortable. If your vaginal opening is large, as it may be after having a baby, sex may be less pleasurable. Neither condition, however, has any effect on your ability to get pregnant.

The vagina secretes fluid during sexual arousal, making it easier — and a lot more enjoyable! — for a penis to enter the vagina. Sometimes (especially when you have to have sex at a particular time), the lubrication function may not work as well as it should. In these cases, you may need a personal lubricant. This is much better for your vagina than trying to have a "dry experience," which causes abrasion of the vagina and will make intercourse that much more uncomfortable the next time.

TIP

There is an entire industry that has grown up over lubricants, intercourse, and fertility. Does it really make that much difference? Maybe. For example, Vaseline is a terrible lubricant because it is too thick. Some lubricants may actually kill sperm. So if you want to spend money on lubricants that have been designed for couples trying to conceive, go ahead. If you want to be practical, plain old vegetable oil, the kind you cook with, is just as good.

TECHNICAL STUFF

In very rare cases, the uterus and vagina of some women do not develop normally and may be missing, even though the ovaries function properly and external genitalia are normal. The formal name of this syndrome is Mayer-Rokitansky-Küster-Hauser, a condition that is usually diagnosed when you don't start your periods by age 16.

Found at the entrance to the vagina, the *hymen* is a nonfunctional piece of circular tissue that has no physiologic function and very few nerve endings. This donut-shaped piece of tissue generally has one or more small opening(s) at birth and, as the baby girl grows, the tissue thins and stretches. While bleeding during a woman's first act of intercourse is often described as "tearing the hymen," in truth, by the time a girl reaches adolescence, the hymen is not usually a barrier to tampons or an erection. An *imperforate hymen*, one that has no holes, occurs in less than ½ percent of the female population and can be corrected with a very simple procedure to snip open the hymen. Women with an imperforate hymen will not have periods (amenorrhea), as the hymen can cause blood to back up behind the small opening. This blood can be forced back up into the fallopian tubes. Women with an imperforate hymen have a higher incidence of endometriosis, a disease that can affect your ability to get pregnant in several ways. (See Chapter 7 for more on endometriosis.)

The cervix

The *cervix* is the lower part of the uterus. It keeps the baby from falling out of the uterus when you're pregnant because it's a tight, muscle-like tissue. The cervix also guards against infection because it's filled with mucus that forms a barrier between your vagina and the inside of the uterus. If you have an *incompetent cervix*, it means that the cervix doesn't stay tight and closed when you're pregnant but starts to open up from the expansion of the uterus and the weight of the growing baby. The hallmark of an incompetent cervix is painless, cervical dilation in the second trimester of pregnancy. An incompetent cervix is usually stitched with a suture called a *cerclage*. Issues with an incompetent cervix do not appear until the second trimester when the baby is larger, so a cerclage is not placed until the early second trimester at around 16–18 weeks.

The uterus

The *uterus*, or womb, is a pear-shaped organ designed to hold and nourish a baby for nine months. The uterus acts as an incubator for the pregnancy, allowing the child to develop to a stage that it can exist in the environment on its own. But the uterus also has to be structured for labor, which allows delivery of the child. So it has two functional layers: an interior lining for implantation and growth of the pregnancy (endometrium) and a muscular layer for labor (myometrium). Every month the lining of the uterus, called the *endometrium*, thickens to make a nourishing bed for an embryo. If you don't get pregnant that month, the lining breaks down and is shed as your *menstrual flow*, or *period*.

Nonconformity is (usually) okay

Many women have a uterus that doesn't conform to the standard upside-down pear shape you've probably seen in pictures marked "this is your uterus." Much has been said about the position of the uterus, but in reality, it makes no difference. Most women have a uterus that points to the pubic bone, which is considered the normal position (also called an anteverted uterus). Twenty percent of women have a uterus that points toward their back (called a "tipped" or retroverted uterus), which, contrary to what many women believe, does not cause problems getting pregnant. However, the real situation is that when a woman is in the upright position, the uterus is parallel to the floor. Since primitive humans were upright most of the time, this is the natural opposition of the uterus and only when gynecologists started examining women lying down did this become an issue. Mother nature probably could care less which way the uterus faces.

Abnormalities that can affect fertility

**TECHNICAL
STUFF**

Around 2 to 3 percent of women have a uterus that is abnormal in its size, shape, or structure. The uterus starts as two separate tubes, which should then join. Once joined, the wall separating the two tubes is dissolved. Sometimes errors in the shape of the uterus occur because there was a failed joining of the tubes (fusion defects) or because the wall does not dissolve (canalization defects). It's hard to know how many women have uterine anomalies because most women do not have tests to determine the shape of their uterus, so the occurrence will be different for women without infertility and infertile patients who undergo testing. The most common uterine anomaly is the *arcuate* uterus, which is a very mild fusion problem. The very last part of the tubes fails to join, leaving a somewhat heart-shaped uterus. This type of uterine anomaly does not impact fertility or miscarriage, but it is reported whenever imaging of the uterus (usually using ultrasound) is done — which can cause concern if no one tells you that this is not an important finding. It's like distinguishing brown eyes from blue eyes; interesting but not predictive of infertility.

The most common variation in the shape of the uterus that can impact fertility and miscarriage rate is caused by a canalization defect and called a *septate uterus*, which means that a band of tissue *(septum)* partially or completely divides the inside of the uterus. This is a congenital condition that occurs while a female fetus is developing in utero when the wall is not properly dissolved. It can affect all or part of the wall so there are many variations on how much of a septum occurs. Septate uterus occurs in multiple forms in less than 3 percent of all women. Fusion defects can create a uterus with two horns (bicornuate) or two separate uteri or even two cervices and two vaginas. Sometimes only one tube forms and thus only one side of the uterus develops, and there is no fallopian tube on that side since the fallopian tubes also develop from the initial tube. This is called a *unicornuate* (one horn). Depending upon the extent of the abnormality, women who have bicornuate and unicornuate uteri usually do not have problems conceiving or keeping a pregnancy. Fusion defects may result in pregnancy complications such as premature labor or malpresentation of the fetus such as a breech. Treatment for uterine defects depends upon which defect is present, the pregnancy history of the woman, and how severe the defect is. In general, only canalization defects are treated, and these require surgery.

Even if the shape of your uterus is normal, it may contain some unwanted "accessories" — growths such as polyps and fibroids — which may decrease the chance that an embryo can implant and grow in your uterus. These are easily diagnosed by a transvaginal ultrasound and/or an MRI and are not always an issue depending upon where they are located in the uterus. If placement is a problem for an implanting embryo, they can be removed before trying to get pregnant. Polyps are easily removed and don't cause any complications after they're gone. Removing fibroids may be more complex. Small ones may be removed through the vagina by entering the uterus through the cervix in an outpatient surgicenter, but large ones may require an abdominal incision and a hospital stay of a couple of days. Removing fibroids can leave scar tissue in the cavity that can make it harder to get pregnant because the fetus won't be able to implant in the scarred area. In rare cases, you may also need a cesarean section after fibroid removal.

Scar tissue can also form in your uterus after a dilation and curettage (D&C for short) for problems like retained tissue after a delivery or miscarriage. If there's a lot of scar tissue, nearly filling the uterus, it's called *Asherman's syndrome*. Obviously, the more scar tissue, the harder it becomes to achieve a pregnancy. The scar tissue can be removed surgically, which may increase your chance of achieving a pregnancy. Commonly, the surgery will need to be repeated until enough of the scars have been removed.

The ovaries

Most women have two ovaries, which contain the most important accessory of all — eggs! How many eggs? Less every year, since every day of your life, eggs are lost through *atresia*, which means that they die off because they're not being stimulated to mature. For example:

>> Before birth, a girl fetus's ovaries contain around 6 to 7 million eggs. The production of eggs stops when the fetus is near five months.

>> A newborn baby girl's ovaries contain about 2 to 3 million eggs.

>> By puberty, only 300,000 to 400,000 eggs remain.

>> Every month, 500 to 1,000 eggs are recruited from the resting pool and start down the path to maturity where they are capable of creating a normal embryo. This path takes over five months, and many eggs are killed by the ovary along the way. When a woman starts her period only about 20 to 30 remain, and in the next two weeks only one will emerge as the best egg. This egg is the one that is ovulated.

>> By a woman's late 30s, only 25,000 or so eggs remain.

>> By age 50, only 1,000 or so eggs remain, and many are chromosomally abnormal because of the impact of aging on egg quality.

The eggs

You may wonder what eggs contain to make them into your potential screaming newborn. The answer is chromosomes — 23 chromosomes, to be exact. Each chromosome contains the genes that determine whether your baby is tall or short, blond or brunette, and, to some extent, fat or thin. The egg also contains considerable machinery necessary to mix the male and female chromosomes and then divide the chromosomes into the correct number for each daughter cell that results from the first cell division that the fertilized egg undergoes.

TECHNICAL STUFF

Of course, there's more to an egg than chromosomes. Three protective layers surround the egg, starting with the *cumulus layer.* That's the nourishing and protecting fluffy layers of cells that completely surround the egg. Moving inward, you'll see the *corona radiate,* the protective single layer of cells covering the *zona pellucida,* the "shell" of the egg. A mature, ready-for-fertilization oocyte, or egg, has a small attachment called a *polar body,* which is the remnant left after the egg divides (a process called *meiosis*) so that it contains only 23 chromosomes. The polar body also contains 23 chromosomes.

REMEMBER

All cells in the human body besides eggs and sperm have 46 chromosomes. Eggs and sperm each have 23, so the baby they create has 46.

Each month, one egg is released from one of your ovaries. The decision about which one ovulates (right or left) is random; they do not necessarily alternate. If you have only one ovary, either because you were born that way or because one was surgically removed, your one ovary generally takes over egg making each month so that you still ovulate each month.

The fallopian tubes

You should have two fallopian tubes, one near each ovary. Tubes are kind of like a pickup bar — a place where sperm and egg should meet and, it is hoped, go on to create something bigger and better: a baby! When an egg is released from the ovary, little projections called *fimbriae* on the end of the tube move back and forth to "entice" the egg into the tube. Once in the fallopian tube, the egg needs a few days to shimmy down to the uterus. One hopes along the way it meets Mr. Sperm and fertilizes, thereby transforming into an embryo by the time it reaches the uterus. Damaged tubes, usually damaged from infection but sometimes from endometriosis or surgery, are a very common cause of infertility. We talk about this in depth in Chapter 11.

REMEMBER

The egg does not have to be picked up by the fallopian tube nearest the ovary. As much as 15-20 percent of the time, the opposite tube can do the job. So if you only have one open tube, and you ovulate from the opposite ovary, pregnancy can still occur.

The breasts

Breasts aren't necessary for getting pregnant; women who have had breasts removed can get pregnant. The normal number of breasts, of course, is two. Nipples are a different matter. As many as 1 in 20 people have more than two nipples. The extras may be nothing more than reddish brown, rough pieces of skin, often found in line with the main nipples. Check yourself out!

Controlling your hormones

You can have all the reproductive organs you need, all in perfect order, and still have no chance of getting pregnant. You can't get pregnant unless your organs are all synchronized to produce an egg and prepare a proper "landing spot" for it in the uterus at the proper time. What you need to orchestrate the process are *hormones*, which are chemical substances released from one part of the body that cause a reaction in another part of the body.

The three female hormone-control systems that work together to orchestrate your menstrual cycle are

>> **The hypothalamus:** The small structure in the middle of the brain that regulates the nervous and endocrine systems, as well as body weight and temperature.

>> **The pituitary:** An endocrine gland at the base of the brain below the hypothalamus that secretes several hormones, including follicle stimulating hormone (FSH) and luteinizing hormone (LH), which are critical for reproduction. The pituitary gland used to be called the "master gland" as it plays a large role in controlling functions of the endocrine systems, adrenal glands, ovaries, and testes.

>> **The ovary:** The female reproductive organ that produces estrogen, progesterone, and eggs.

These three hormone systems work together in a feedback system called the hypothalamus-pituitary-ovarian axis, which simply means that they function together to produce a seamless masterpiece — your menstrual cycle.

The main female hormones are:

>> Estrogen (E2)

>> Luteinizing hormone (LH)

>> Follicle-stimulating hormone (FSH)

>> Progesterone (P4)

In Sync: How Female Reproductive Parts Work Together

All the components of your reproductive tract — the vagina, uterus, ovaries, fallopian tubes, and the glands that orchestrate your hormones — have to work together perfectly for you to be able to get pregnant. (Yes, you need sperm, too, but we get to that in a later section, "Hanging Out with the Guys.")

Although your menstrual cycle seems simple enough, a lot of things, unfortunately, can go wrong. We not only address how your cycle works but also how it may not work in the next few sections.

Taking a spin on the menstrual cycle

The hormone-secreting systems work to create your menstrual cycle like this:

1. **Menstrual Phase:** During menstruation, the old uterine lining breaks down and passes through the vagina as menstrual flow. This process takes three to seven days and is commonly called a "period."

2. **Follicular/Proliferative Phase:** On Day 1 of bleeding, the pituitary gland, under influence from the hypothalamus, releases *follicle-stimulating hormone (FSH)*. The rising FSH levels cause the ovaries to rescue the 10 to 20 remaining follicles, called antral follicles, which begin to grow. The cells surrounding each egg secrete a liquid, forming a follicle, a fluid-filled sac. Each follicle contains one immature egg. During the *follicular phase,* one follicle continues to develop, and the others die. In the ovary, the one egg-containing follicle is growing (in response to FSH and *luteinizing hormone (LH),* which is also produced by the pituitary), and this growing follicle begins producing estrogen. The estrogen produced by the ovary causes the uterine lining to thicken or proliferate. This is called the *proliferative phase* of the uterus. The follicular phase and the proliferative phase occur in the first half of the menstrual cycle. One refers to what's happening in the ovary (follicular phase), and the other refers to what's happening in the uterus (proliferative phase).

   One follicle becomes dominant, growing faster than the others. As the dominant follicle grows, it produces more estrogen, which also increases the lining of the uterus. The amount of FSH released decreases, and the smaller follicles stop growing and are reabsorbed.

   A large amount of LH, called an *LH surge,* is released from the pituitary gland as the estrogen rises. This makes the egg inside the dominant follicle mature.

3. **Ovulation:** The follicleopens; the egg is released *(ovulation)* and is picked up by one of the fallopian tubes. If the egg is joined by sperm, it will continue to travel through the fallopian tube to the uterus. The uterine lining has now developed enough to support embryo implantation, and the endometrial glands of the uterine lining secrete proteins that help guide the embryo to the correct spot.

4. **Luteal phase:** The leftover part of the follicle, now called the *corpus luteum,* produces *progesterone* and some estrogen, which help an embryo implant. If you are not pregnant, the corpus luteum collapses, progesterone and estrogen levels decline, the uterine lining begins to break down, and menstruation begins roughly two weeks after ovulation.

Recognizing the importance of regular periods

Do your periods always come every 28 days like clockwork? If they do, you're a rarity; only one in ten women fall into what we've been conditioned to think of as a "normal" menstrual pattern. Most women have cycles 25 to 31 days apart.

When your doctor asks you how long your cycles are, he's asking how many days are between Day 1 of one period and Day 1 of the next period. When he asks how long your period is, he's asking how many days you bleed. Day 1 of your period is the first day of normal (for you) flow, not the day when you have light or irregular spotting before your wonder period starts.

If you are on, or have been on, birth control pills, be sure to note that in charting your menstrual pattern. The pill chemically coordinates your cycle to come at the same time each month (provided you take the pill correctly!).

What's regular for you may not be regular for someone else but having some sort of pattern to your periods is important because it indicates that you're producing and releasing eggs on a regular basis. But just because a woman is having periods does not give us any further information about egg quality or whether her uterus can support a pregnancy.

If your cycles are very long or very irregular, you may not be maturing eggs, you may not have sufficient hormone levels, or there may be other underlying medical issues. See the next section, "Understanding the causes of malfunctioning menstrual cycles" for more on how irregular cycles affect your chance of getting pregnant.

Understanding the causes of malfunctioning menstrual cycles

Although it may seem like your menstrual cycle runs like clockwork, always appearing on the expected day, the likelihood is that at least part of the time, your cycle is out of sync, showing up too early, too late, or not at all, even though you're not pregnant. Irregular periods not only make it hard to determine when you ovulate, but they can also indicate that your reproductive system is in need of fine-tuning. In this section, we discuss all the ways cycles can get out of sync, what it can mean, and how your doctor may suggest fixing them.

Menstrual cycles that don't fall into the norm can indicate that you're not ovulating at all or that you're only ovulating occasionally. An occasional irregular cycle can be brought about by stress; a change in routine, exercise, or eating patterns;

or illness, but periods that are "never the same length twice," consistently shorter than normal or longer than normal, should be evaluated by your doctor.

Bleeding too often — short cycles

If your cycles are very short — less than 25 days apart on a regular basis, you may be ovulating too soon. Since the period between ovulation and the start of your period should consistently be 14 days, if your periods are short, it usually (but not always — we discuss the alternative in this section) means that you have a short follicular phase, the time between your period and your ovulation.

A short follicular phase can mean that the egg is developing in the incorrect time frame. Short follicular phases can occur when your ovarian reserve, the number of eggs you still have in your ovaries, is starting to decrease. It occurs because there is an elevation of the FSH level in the previous cycle, which accelerates the development of the egg. So, a clinical pearl is that short cycles may raise red flags about reduced ovarian reserve. A woman who has traditionally had cycles ranging from 28–32 days and then notices that they have shortened to 26–27 days may be showing signs of reduced ovarian reserve. This is especially true if she is over the age of 35.

For quite some time, a lot of emphasis was placed on the second half of the cycle or the luteal phase. If this was shorter than ten days, a diagnosis of luteal phase defect was made and sometimes progesterone was used to try to correct for this. While there may be some controversy about this, recent understanding of how the cycle works has suggested that there may not be a luteal phase defect. The luteal phase is dependent upon the first half of the cycle, the follicular phase. The follicular phase is dependent upon the quality of the egg. So short luteal phases are a product of poor egg quality.

Bleeding too infrequently or skipping periods

Cycles that are very long, over 35 days apart, can indicate that you're not ovulating regularly. This can be a factor of excessive exercise, weight change, or other factors, but it can also be caused by polycystic ovary syndrome, or PCOS. PCOS can cause changes in hormone ratios that can be diagnosed by your doctor, as well as physical changes such as excessive hair, weight gain, and acne. (See Chapter 7 for more on PCOS.)

Endometriosis, premature ovarian insufficiency (see Chapter 7 for more on both of these), abnormal thyroid levels, or high prolactin levels (see Chapter 11 for the details on diagnosing infertility causes through blood tests) can also cause irregular or absent periods.

Bleeding between periods

Bleeding between periods can indicate that something is wrong inside your uterus or that your hormones are out of balance. Some of the things that can go wrong with your uterus to cause irregular bleeding are

>> **Cervical irritations or infections:** Possible causes of cervical bleeding especially if this occurs after intercourse

>> **Fibroids:** Benign growths found in the uterine wall

>> **Polyps:** Small fleshy growths found on the endometrium, the lining of the uterus, or the cervix

Bleeding too heavily (menorrhagia)

Bleeding too heavily and passing clots can be "normal" for some women, especially in women who are overweight. Fibroids, PCOS, and irregular periods can be related to heavier-than-normal bleeding. Heavy bleeding can also be a sign of recurrent early miscarriage (see Chapter 13).

Women who bleed heavily every month are at risk for becoming *anemic* (having a decreased number of red blood cells). Anemia can lead to fatigue and weakness, so heavy periods should be checked out with your doctor. A simple blood test can diagnose anemia.

Having scant periods

If your period is very light, it could be a normal variant (in which case, lucky you!), or it could be a sign that your uterine lining isn't getting as thick as it should. Scant periods are typical if you're using birth control pills or have just stopped using them, or if your periods have just started. If your lining isn't thickening properly, you may not be ovulating normally, so seeing your doctor is a good idea.

Experiencing painful periods (dysmenorrhea)

Up to 40 percent of women experience pain with their periods, called *dysmenorrhea*. Dysmenorrhea falls into two categories:

>> **Primary dysmenorrhea** has no other underlying cause besides the release of *prostaglandins* (chemicals made by cells that have specific functions such as controlling body temperature, stimulating smooth muscle, and influencing heat cycles) in the uterus, which cause uterine contractions.

>> **Secondary dysmenorrhea** is caused by disease present in addition to the normal release of prostaglandins, such as endometriosis, fibroids, or infection.

REMEMBER

Because painful periods can be caused by diseases that can interfere with getting pregnant, such as endometriosis, you should always see your doctor if you have painful periods. Dysmenorrhea is the most common symptom of endometriosis, which affects over 5 million women in North America and may cause infertility in up to 30 to 40 percent of its sufferers.

The release of prostaglandins that cause cramping can also cause nausea, diarrhea, and exhaustion, just to make you feel really terrible during your periods. Taking anti-inflammatory medications such as ibuprofen can help with the symptoms.

Hanging Out with the Guys

Compared to women, guys let it all hang out, reproductively speaking. The external male reproductive organs include the penis, scrotum, and the testicles. Take a look at what every guy should have. See Figure 2-2 for a graphic portrayal of your average man.

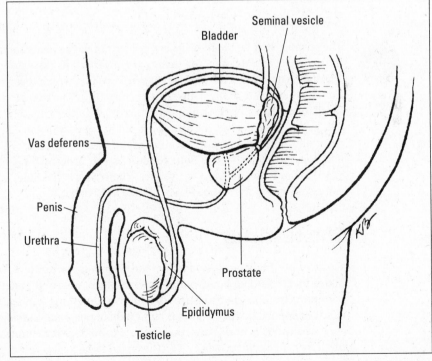

FIGURE 2-2: The male reproductive organs.

Illustration by Kathryn Born

The penis

The number-one guy concern is probably related to penis size: How do I compare to everyone else? For those obsessed, here are the standards: normal length when flaccid, or limp, 3.9 inches; stretched (still limp), 4.8 inches; erect, 5 to 7 inches, with an average erect size of 5.1 inches. We hope that bit of info made most of you fellows feel better. A small penis, less than 1.9 inches limp, is usually able to impregnate as long as it can get the sperm into the vagina, up toward the cervix. Size is rarely an issue in infertility.

Size may not matter, but function does. If you have seen commercials for *erectile dysfunction* (ED), you may be comforted to know that even athletes and famous men have problems with erectile dysfunction (ED), also known as *impotence*. As nice as it is to know that you're not alone, this condition can be an embarrassing detriment to getting pregnant. Impotence, the inability to have or sustain an erection, is more common as men get older; as many as 50 percent of men between the ages of 40 and 70 have had problems with impotence. Impotence can be caused by diseases such as diabetes or by chronic conditions, such as alcohol abuse, or it can be a side effect of medications. (We discuss impotence in Chapter 12.) ED can be a problem that occurs as patients move through treatment for infertility. Performance anxiety and the sterile nature of fertility treatments may cause ED. Adjusting the environment or using frozen sperm specimens collected under less stressful conditions can help reduce ED.

TECHNICAL STUFF

The opening that lets both urine and sperm out of the penis should be at the tip of the penis, located dead center. Two types of variations can cause problems getting pregnant. One in around 300 men has *hypospadias*, which means that the opening is on the underside of the penis. In 20 percent of cases, this problem is hereditary. Epispadias occurs far less frequently; only 1 in approximately 100,000 men has epispadias. In *epispadias*, the opening is on the top of the penis. Both conditions are associated with an unusual curvature of the erect penis; it curves up in epispadias and down in hypospadias. Both conditions can prevent the sperm from getting exactly where they need to be. Surgical correction is possible, and inseminations can also help get the sperm to where they need to go.

The testicles

Testicles are the sperm production and warehouse site. Here, as in many other places on the human body, nature has been generous and given two of the same body part (testicles, in this instance), in case something happens to one. Testicles first develop inside the abdomen and gradually descend outside the body by the time a baby boy is born. At birth, about 4 in 100 boys have undescended testicles, properly called *cryptorchidism.* Testicles need to be kept a few degrees cooler than

98 degrees for sperm to develop properly, so to prevent future infertility, doctors usually recommend surgery to lower the testicles outside the body as soon as the baby is a year old.

The testicles are contained in a pouch of skin called the *scrotum*. In about 80 percent of men, the left testicle is bigger and hangs lower. Sometimes the scrotum is abnormally large, which can be caused by a *hydrocele* (a collection of fluid inside the scrotum), or by a *varicocele* (dilated or varicose veins in the scrotum). These conditions can be surgically corrected. If left alone, they can raise the temperature of the testes and may cause infertility.

TECHNICAL STUFF

Sperm are produced every day, but it takes about 70 days for the new sperm to fully mature. Sperm production starts in the testes. FSH and LH, the same hormones that develop eggs, are needed to begin sperm production. LH stimulates production of testosterone, another male hormone. The sperm mature in the epididymis and travel through the vas deferens up to the seminal vesicle and the prostate, where they're bathed in the fluid known as semen. They're then ejaculated through the urethra during male orgasm.

Sperm — 200 million of them!

Nature designed women to have one child at a time — which is why most women will release a single egg every month. The eggs enter the fallopian tube. The tube has a very special environment designed to meet the metabolic needs of the egg and the early developing embryo. The tube also has cells with hair-like projections so that the egg and then the embryo can be transported to the uterus. Sperm fertilize the egg in the fallopian tube. A normal ejaculate may contain over 100 million sperm, but only about 100–1,000 actually make it to the egg. The sperm have proteins on their surface that match proteins on the shell of the egg and allow the sperm to bind to the shell of the egg. The sperm do not mechanically pierce the egg; they release proteins that biochemically digest a pathway through the shell, and once near the egg, bind to the egg. The egg then brings the sperm inside. There are packages of proteins just inside the wall of the egg that are released once a sperm enters. They harden the shell and prevent fertilization by more than one sperm. The fertilized egg is now called an embryo and will grow to an 8-32 cell embryo in the fallopian tube before being transported to the uterus.

Why are there so many more sperm than eggs? Because it's a *long* way through the uterus and up the tubes, and because only 50 percent (of a *good* sperm sample) of the sperm know how to swim forward, *and* because some of them are barely moving, a tremendous number of sperm are needed to ensure that a few hundred will get through to the egg. Their journey is like one of you trying to swim across the Pacific Ocean. If there were 200 million of you, maybe a few hundred would make it. Imagine if you had to fertilize an egg when you finally got there! (We talk about sperm and male factor issues much more in Chapter 12.)

Putting Male and Female Parts Together

Now that you know how all your parts work, are you ready to have a baby? Yes? Then it's time to have sex. No, not right now. (Well, okay, if you must, but proper timing will enhance the chance for pregnancy.) So it is important to have sex when the timing is right. How do you know when the timing is right? This is more than just mood lighting and foreplay. To get pregnant, you need to be close to ovulation.

Recognizing signs of ovulation

It normally takes between 10 and 14 days to mature a good egg and release it, so if you have 28- to 30-day cycles, you may ovulate sometime between day 14 and day 16 of your cycle. Shorter cycles have an earlier ovulation day, and longer cycles a later ovulation day. How do you know if you've ovulated? Some women experience a sharp pain when they ovulate, called *mittelschmertz*, or have a vaginal discharge; however, these symptoms are very subjective and are not reliable indicators of ovulation. A more reliable method is correctly using an ovulation predictor kit. That said, you may be able to tell that you're ovulating in a few simple ways, just by watching the calendar and being observant about your bodily functions.

REMEMBER

Usually the mucus from your cervix increases around the time of ovulation. It also becomes very thin, clear, and stretchy; you can easily stretch it out a couple of inches. Rising estrogen levels from a developing follicle create this mucus, which is easier for sperm to swim through than your usual thicker mucus and also has an alkaline pH, which helps the sperm live longer. At other times of the month, cervical mucus is acidic. Be sure that you're not confusing cervical mucus with semen from previous sex or increased secretions from sexual arousal.

If you have no objection to feeling around inside your vagina, you'll also notice that your cervix becomes softer, slightly open, and easier to locate with your fingers when you're about to ovulate. At other times of the month, the cervix is found farther back in the uterus, feels firmer to the touch, and is tightly closed.

About 20 percent of women have pain called *mittelschmertz* (German for "middle pain") when they ovulate. The pain seems to be caused by blood and fluid released from the ruptured follicle irritating the tissues around the ovary. Sometimes a small amount of vaginal bleeding occurs with ovulation, too.

Some women have headaches around the time of ovulation, and others complain of bloating or breast pain. You're probably already aware of your personal ovulation indicators, but you may have just never paid much attention to them; just don't be disappointed if you don't have these symptoms — that doesn't mean you are not ovulating!

Paying attention to when you ovulate is okay but unnecessary. If a woman has regular cycles every 28–32 days, she will ovulate around midcycle. If the goal is to get pregnant through intercourse, then having intercourse every other day around mid-cycle will maximize the chance of getting pregnant. You can have intercourse more frequently if you want. You do not need to worry that you are having too much intercourse. Men do not improve their chances for conception by storing sperm. They aren't stored in the man's body — in fact they die and are removed.

Timing and fertility

Timing is everything when it comes to getting pregnant. Many women miss the mark month after month because of mistaken ideas about the best time to get pregnant.

TIP

Sperm and eggs both have a short shelf life; eggs are capable of being fertilized for around 24 hours, and sperm can live up to four days in the proper environment, such as the fluid that fills the fallopian tubes. That means that if you don't have sex within a few days before ovulation, you're not going to get pregnant.

Many women have been conditioned to believe that ovulation occurs on day 14; they have sex on days 12, 13, or 14 in hopes of hitting the right time. But the most consistent thing about your menstrual cycle should be that ovulation occurs 14 days before your period begins. So, if your cycles are 28 days, you ovulate on day 14. But if your cycles are short, say 25 days, you're actually ovulating on day 11, and having sex starting on day 12 will be too late to achieve a pregnancy.

On the other hand, if your cycles are long, say 34 days, you don't ovulate until day 20. Having sex on day 14 will be way too early, since sperm don't live for a week.

So, timing sex correctly when you want to get pregnant is dependent on a solid knowledge of when you're ovulating. We discuss the ways ovulation can be most accurately predicted in Chapter 6.

TIP Sperm live longer in your body than the egg, so err on the early side when deciding when to start having sex. Every other day is enough, and there is no harm in having extra sperm around. When in doubt, just do it!

Conceiving a Baby: How Sex Should Work

The time is right, the moon is bright, and it's time to get pregnant. Here's what needs to happen:

1. It's near ovulation; an egg is about to release from its follicle.

2. You and your partner become aroused. Your vagina produces secretions that make it easier for the now erect penis to enter the vagina.

3. During the man's orgasm, several million sperm are forcefully ejaculated into the vagina. As they pass through the cervix into the uterus, the cervical mucus "filters" the sperm so that they're ready to penetrate an egg.

4. Your egg releases from the follicle and enters one of your fallopian tubes.

5. The sperm swim through the uterus up to the fallopian tubes.

6. The next day your egg meets up with several hundred sperm in the fallopian tube, and the sperm all attach themselves to the egg.

7. One sperm breaks through the outer layer of the egg causing a chemical reaction that makes the egg immediately impenetrable to the rest of the sperm.

8. The genetic material of the egg and sperm combine, and the newly created embryo is moved down the fallopian tube to the uterus. Cells which line the inside of the tube have hair-like projections and create a wave, much like moving a beach ball in the crowd at a football game. The embryo remains in the tube for a couple of days where is develops and then is moved into the uterus. So the tube is both a transporter and an incubator for the developing embryo.

9. The embryo implants in the uterine wall and grows, and you miss your period.

10. You're pregnant! Congratulations.

TIP

There is no "best" position for making babies.While some "helpful" books, articles, blogs, and even healthcare providers may tell you that lying on your back for a while or elevating your hips after sex will help you get pregnant, doing so isn't necessary. Similarly, you may have heard that certain sexual positions may work better than others — not so much. You can choose whatever position during or after sex that is right for you and your partner.

Figuring Out How Often to Have Sex

When you're trying to get pregnant, it is important to have intercourse every other day. It is a myth that you can have too much sex. Increased ejaculation may make the sperm count lower, but it does not decrease pregnancy rates. In fact, some men with low counts actually increase the amount of sperm they ejaculate with more frequent ejaculations.

When you're close to ovulating, have sex at least every other day; every day is okay. Most doctors recommend the two days before and the day you ovulate as the best time for conception. Other than that, timing should remain routine so that there are no prolonged periods of abstinence. Infertility can severely decrease the joy of sex and the intimacy that usually accompanies intercourse. Don't drive yourself crazy with things that don't matter.

Chapter 3

Blame It on My Genes! The Role of Genetics and Family History

Nothing is more popular around the dinner table than crediting or blaming your family for who you are. You are so good at math — just like your dad. You sing like a dream — just like your mom. Always late like your Aunt Ellen! Grandma's eyes, Grandpa's hair, Aunt Susie's wit, Uncle Bert's moods . . . and your sister's funny little toe can all be found in you, and it must be because of your genes. But how exactly do genes work, and why are they important if you are trying to have a baby?

Grasping Genetics Basics

Genetics has become a very popular word. With that popularity has come myth and misunderstanding. But the concept of the field of genetics is really quite simple. Genetics deals with the instruction manual on how to build a human. To be exact, a Google search gave the definition of genetics as "the study of heredity and the variation of inherited characteristics."

TIP

One analogy is to view the instructions on how to build a human as a book, passed on from generation to generation, which is called *inherited.* The book is divided into chapters called *chromosomes.* The chapters have paragraphs called *genes,* and the words are made from a very simple alphabet. And just in case you are feeling special, the majority of the book, (99 percent) has the same chapters as the manual for building a chimpanzee. Also, the person you think is, well, "different," actually has the same 99.9 percent of your genetic code. Reassuringly, given the size of the genetic code, that is still over three million differences.

TECHNICAL
STUFF

The estimate is that the human genetic code has over 3 billion units, which is huge, but the lowly *Amoeba dubia* has over 670 billion units. So, it really is not how you say it but what you say that matters.

What are genes and chromosomes?

Genes are a long string of four chemicals called *nucleotides* and lettered as A (adenine), C (cytosine), G (guanine), and T (thymine). Words in the code are made from just these four chemicals, and the alphabet has only four letters. That's really a small alphabet to create a person. The English alphabet has 26 letters, and if you limit the number of syllables a word could have to 14, over 2.75963×10^7 words are possible. Fortunately for those spelling whizzes, the English language has *only* a little over 200,000 words.

The genetic code has only four letters, and the words (*codons*) can be only three letters long, so at most 64 possible combinations are used for the genetic code. The directions for building a human, the genetic code, is a string of three-letter words. However, the string is not one continuous string but rather 23 strings of code. These 23 separated strings are called *chromosomes* (see Figure 3-1). Each time a cell wants to divide, it must accurately create two copies of the genetic code, and it does this one word (codon) at a time.

To complicate this even further, a person inherits one set of chromosomes from each parent so that each cell has two copies of each chromosome. Thus, inheritance is a demanding task of accurately repeating the copying of the code over and over to create the 37 trillion or so cells that make a human.

What do genes do?

Genes are used to direct a cell to make proteins. Proteins are strings of molecules called *amino acids,* and there are 20 that are used to make proteins. Proteins are the workhorse of constructing a human. The DNA uses a different type of genetic material called RNA to assemble proteins from the amino acids. Each gene determines which amino acids are to be used and in what sequence. The way in which the amino acids are strung together determines the three-dimensional structure of the protein.

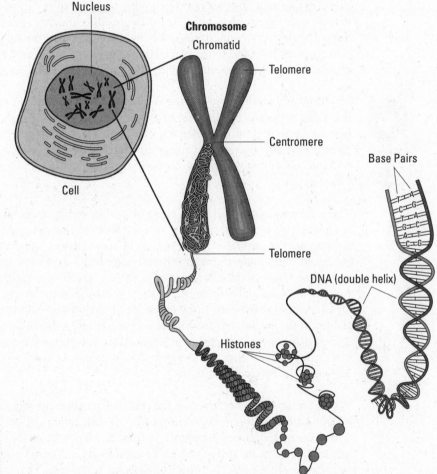

FIGURE 3-1:
Diagram of a chromosome.

REMEMBER

The structure of protein is critical for it to do its job properly. Any error in the sequence of the amino acids may reduce the efficiency of how the protein works or make it completely nonfunctional.

Inheriting Infertility — Really?

The construction of a human is immensely complicated. For proper functioning, all of the various parts need to work together. Any part that does not do its job properly can throw the person out of balance and thus create disease. So normal human functioning means that the systems are in equilibrium and working properly together. Any part not functioning in equilibrium causes the disease. The genetic code determines the basis for the equilibrium; any error in the code can cause the person's equilibrium to be disturbed, and disease follows. For people having problems conceiving, a question that needs to be answered is whether errors in the genetic code are causing the problem of getting pregnant.

REMEMBER

Infertility and sterility are not the same. *Infertility* implies that pregnancy is not occurring in the normal time frame. *Sterility* means that the person will never have her own genetic child. So, when a group of people are diagnosed with infertility, there are actually two groups: one group is sterile, and the other group is *subfertile* and may achieve a pregnancy on their own or may need help with infertility treatments.

There are a number of different types of genetic errors. Sometimes entire chromosomes may be missing or duplicated. There may be deletions of parts of the chromosome or parts that are misplaced or turned around. There can be errors in the letters of the code, thus causing the wrong amino acid to be used. These errors are called *single-nucleotide polymorphisms* (SNPs). SNPs are the most common form of variation among people. The error is the use of the wrong letter such that an A (adenine) is switched to a T (thymine). Most of these will not alter the functioning of the person, but some can cause severe disease such a sickle cell anemia. There are many types of sickle cell disease depending upon the gene mutation, but one form is caused when the sequence GAG is changed to GTG — one single letter can cause the destructive disease.

The two most common chromosomal problems causing sterility in females are 47 XXX and 45 XO (Turner's syndrome). The 47 XXX syndrome occurs in 1 in 1,000 female births and causes premature ovarian deficiency. Turner's syndrome occurs in 1 in 2,000 female births. Turner's syndrome is a disease caused by an entire chromosome being absent. Turner's syndrome results when a person has only one sex chromosome — an X chromosome. This person develops as a female with characteristics such as short stature, a web neck, and a low hairline, and about one-third will have heart defects. These people do not make eggs, so they are menopausal from birth and thus are sterile. However, some people with this problem have a mixture of cells with some having only one but some having two X chromosomes. This condition is called *mosaicism*. Depending upon how many cells are normal, this person may display the signs of a person with Turner's but actually have some eggs. She may be able to have child, which is rare. Or she may have early normal egg development but run out of eggs very early in life and thus lose the ability to have her own child. If this condition is established early, it is possible to harvest some of the eggs and freeze them for later use.

A second example of a chromosomal cause of sterility occurs in males. Being a male is determined by the Y-chromosome. A gene on the Y-chromosome directs a man to make sperm. The gene is called the *sex-determining region* (SRY) and is located on the long arm of the Y chromosome. It is passed unmodified from father to son, and thus any abnormality of the gene will be transmitted to a son.

One region of the SRY gene is called the *azospermic factor* (AZF), and this has three sections termed the a, b, and c regions. Some men with very low sperm counts or with no sperm in the ejaculate have deletions in this region. If a man had a deletion in the "a" region, he will not have sperm and has what is termed Sertoli-only syndrome. That man will not be able to have children that are genetically his. Thus, this type of mutation cannot be inherited. However, if the man has deletions in the "b" or "c" regions, his count may be low or zero but there may be regions of the testes that do make sperm. This man can undergo a testicular biopsy where a very small amount of testicular tissue is removed and tested to see whether sperm are present. If they are, then these can be used in IVF and the man has the possibility for having genetically his own children. If he has a male child, the child will inherit the same deletion as the father, and thus this type of infertility can be inherited.

Males can also have impaired fertility or even be sterile if they have too many Y chromosomes. The person is then XYY and has what is called Klinefelter's syndrome. Some men with this problem do have sperm in the ejaculate and others have sperm which must be extracted from the testes. Unfortunately, some will have no sperm and are thus sterile.

Inheriting Diseases that May Impact Fertility — Different Story!

There are genetic causes of infertility that can be passed down from generation to generation, but these usually involve much less of the genetic code. Some are single gene mutations, and some are structural problems with a part of a chromosome being rearranged but not entire chromosome changes.

For males, myotonic dystrophy is an inherited disease that is called an *autosomal dominant.* This means that if the person has the mutation in just one of the chromosomes, he will have the disease. Thus 50 percent of his offspring will also have the disease. The problem is caused by areas of the gene, which produces a protein required for normal functioning, have unwanted repeated sequences of the letters. The general term for this type of problem is *nucleotide repeat diseases,* and women can have a similar problem causing the *fragile X syndrome.* Some of these men have sperm and thus can have children, but some will have no sperm and be sterile. Males can inherit genetic diseases affecting fertility that are single gene defect problems. For these, a mutation of many mutations within a gene causes the gene to malfunction. An example of this is cystic fibrosis. A man with cystic fibrosis will have no sperm in the ejaculate because the tubes that transport the sperm from the testicle to the penis (the *vas deferens*) do not develop. This is called congenital bilateral absences of the vas deferens and can be treated using sperm extraction from the testis and IVF/ICIS.

One problem for females that has some genetic basis is *polycystic ovary syndrome.* No single gene has been identified that causes PCOS. Rather, there are a number of genetic mutations that can cause PCOS. Also, patients with PCOS have DNA that has been modified so that the directions for constructing the human are not read correctly — these modifications are called *epigenetic* factors. Epigenetic modification of DNA helps explain how the environment can alter the way the genetic code is read, and it plays a major role in a number of diseases.

Another type of problem can occur when there are too many copies of a three-letter word, for example egg (a genetic sequence). Fragile X syndrome is an example of this type of genetic error. Fragile X syndrome results when a region of a gene called the FMR1 gene has too many repeated sequences of the genetic word cgg. The FMR1 gene produces a protein that regulates other proteins to make normal nerve connections. The mutation can result in individuals with severe mental compromise. A family with members with severe mental compromise may benefit from genetic testing to determine whether the family has the abnormal FMR1 gene. A normal number of repeats is 5 to 50. If the sequence has more than 200 repeats, then the result is developmental abnormalities in varying degrees. However, where there are 50–200 repeated sequences, the person may have some developmental problems, or a female may have early ovarian failure. So experts often test a woman with premature ovarian failure to determine whether she has too many repeat sequences.

There are a number of single gene defects that affect the fertility of a person. These are being diagnosed more and more so the list is becoming quite long. It is beyond the scope of this chapter to fully explore these diseases.

Shaking the Family Tree for Information

The fact that genetics is playing a larger role in the cause and potential treatment of all diseases makes knowledge about families important. Doctors are now taking a more extensive family history, and if it seems warranted, they construct a genetic diagram (family tree; see Figure 3-2 for an example).

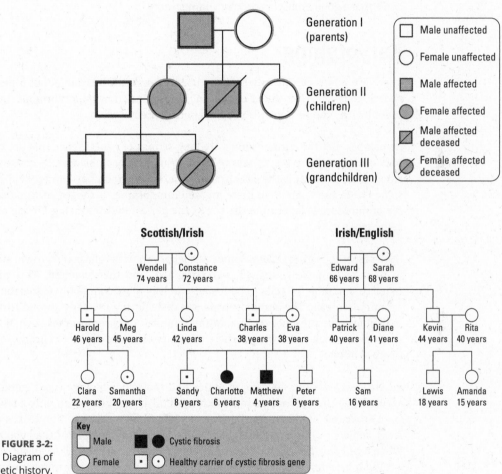

FIGURE 3-2: Diagram of genetic history.

Many people have at least one disease-causing genetic mutation if it occurs on both chromosomes. Fortunately, people have two chromosomes, so the mutation does not cause a clinical problem. But if two people have children and they both have the same mutation, then one out of four children may have the disease. A family tree may show relatives that had symptoms of the diseases which would put the couple on alert to test for the mutation.

Finding Out What's in Your Genes

You may be asking why your fertility doctor would want to know all of the specifics of your genes and your partner's genes (if you are using his sperm). As we explain earlier in this chapter, knowing more about a person's genes provides many more clues about possible diseases. In infertility, knowing about your genes can help explain key questions such as why you are not getting pregnant, why you don't make good embryos, or why you miscarry.

Karyotyping

There are a number of tests that are used to gain information about a person's genetic code. One test, called *karyotyping*, determines how many chromosomes are present. This can be done for people, a fetus, or embryos.

Remember that the chromosomes are long strings of genetic code that are tightly packaged, and there are 23 sets of chromosomes. Chromosomes 1–22 are called autosomes, while 23 is the sex chromosome. Each person has one set of chromosomes from each parent so there are 46 chromosomes arranged in 23 pairs. The sex chromosomes determine the sex of the person with XX being female and XY being male.

Until recently, testing chromosomes was laborious with cells being grown, stopped in their development, stained, photographed, and then counted. This process required a number of cells to be tested and was most commonly associated with an amniocentesis. The amniocentesis was done during the early second trimester to diagnose the presence of an abnormal number of chromosomes such as Down syndrome, which is *trisomy 21*, where the fetus has three copies of chromosome 21 (instead of two).

Recent developments in data analytics and molecular biology (next-generation sequencing) have permitted rapid chromosome determination in only a few cells (4–6) that can be taken from a five-day-old human embryo. The test is called *preimplantation genetic testing for aneuploids.* What's an aneuploid? Glad you asked. When a cell has the correct number of chromosomes, it is called a *euploid cell.* But a cell can have too many chromosomes because it has the wrong number of sets of 23, such as a monoploidy or triploidy. If there is an incorrect number of any single chromosome, such as only one X chromosome (remember Turner's syndrome with 45 XO or trisomy 21 with three number 21 chromosomes so 47, 21 +3), the cell is called an *aneuploid cell.* The value of karyotype testing is that it permits embryo selection such that embryos with the correct number of chromosomes can be transferred. This type of testing cannot correct the number of chromosomes an embryo has, so it does not increase the number of children that can result from an

IVF cycle. But it can permit the transfer of embryos that have the highest chance of creating a pregnancy that can go to term. This reduces the time to conception and reduces the miscarriage rate.

There is controversy as to whether the use of preimplantation genetic testing for screening embryos is indicated, but many physicians and patients are opting for this diagnostic procedure. For some couples, the information from testing for chromosome number can help identify why a person has not conceived and may suggest either doing more cycles of IVF with the woman's own eggs or may identify the need to move on to other options such as stopping treatment, adoption, or using donor eggs.

Spotting single gene defects

A second type of genetic testing can determine if a gene is abnormal. There may be a single nucleotide error, pieces of the gene may be missing or duplicated, or there may be other errors. The advent of next-generation sequencing has permitted easy, cost-effective testing for these errors. Genetic diseases may require that both chromosomes have the same defective gene. These diseases are called recessive. A person may have one defective gene, but the other normal gene compensates for the defective gene. Some genetic diseases require that only one chromosome have the gene defect, and these are call dominant gene diseases. One use of next-gen sequencing is for a family that has a history of a genetic disease. A person, who does not have the genetic disease or an embryo, can be tested for that disease. Since a person receives a chromosome from each parent, there is a double dose of each gene. The person who has a single gene defect is called a carrier for that gene, and the vast majority of these mutations are of the recessive type (requiring both sets of chromosomes to have the gene defect before the disease develops).

Suppose that the gene that is responsible for cystic fibrosis is faulty in the chromosome from one parent but normal in the other. Then the normal gene compensates for the malfunction of the other gene, and the person does not develop cystic fibrosis. The child of these parents may have one abnormal gene and one normal gene and is called a carrier for that gene defect. Sometimes, having one defective gene results in a disease. An example of this is Huntington's chorea (a dominant gene disease), a devastating neurologic disease that does not show up until later in life after the person has reproduced. Huntington's chorea is caused by a gene defect in which too many of the codons exist — similar to the type of problem in fragile X syndrome. The genetic defect for Huntington's and fragile X is not due to an error in the code but rather to too much code. For families with a family history of Huntington's, it is now possible to test embryos and elect not to transfer an embryo that has the defect.

A popular test now is called *carrier screening.* Many people carry a number of gene defects for recessive diseases. For a recessive disease to produce the actual disease, a person has to inherit an abnormal gene form both parents. Thus, many people have unknown gene errors and are disease free, but could have children that develop the genetic disease if the partner also has the gene defect. The advances in genetic testing now permit testing people for many gene defects. Knowing this, a couple can determine whether their children would be at risk for developing the disease. Using IVF and preimplantation genetic diagnosis, the couple can avoid creating a child with the disease.

Looking for other anomalies

As if testing your genes is not enough, scientists are now looking at how we can change your genetic structure, or the genetic structure of your embryos! While it sounds more like science fiction than real medicine, there are some new ideas in the field of genetics that may someday help conquer infertility.

Looking at What's on the Horizon

An expanding area of research for genetic diseases focuses on how the genetic code is actually read. It turns out that while there is a core code, inherited unchanged from generation to generation, the cell is able to modify how the code is read based upon environmental and developmental conditions. Cells do this by adding molecules to the core code, which is called *epigenetics.* For example, one theory of how endometriosis forms is that molecules called *methyl groups* can either be added or removed from the core genetic code, creating new instructions from the genetic code that leads to the formation of endometriosis. Endometriosis is a very complex disease, and this is not the only reason a person develops endometriosis, but the process may add to the risk for developing endometriosis.

A cell requires considerable energy to perform the work it does. The energy is generated by a small structure within the cell called *mitochondria.* Mitochondria are similar to bacteria and have their own set of chromosomes. When errors occur in these genes, the mitochondria do not perform well. This can lead to devastating diseases. One treatment that is being developed is to take normal mitochondria from an embryonic cell and transfer it into the cell from an affected embryo.

A result of more sophisticated chromosome testing of preimplantation embryos is the discovery that not all embryos are either completely euploid or completely aneuploid. Some embryos have cells that have the correct number of chromosomes while other cells in the same embryo have the wrong number of chromosomes. This is called *mosaicism.* Currently, research is attempting to determine what percentage of mosaicism is safe for transfer of a mosaic embryo.

A final advancement is the ability to genetically modify the genetic code of an embryo. The technology uses a procedure called CRISPR (technically CRISPR–Cas9). The use of this for clinical medicine is quite a ways off, but the implications are immense. In theory, it may become possible to actually alter the genetic code. This could provide a way to cure inherited diseases or reduce genetic risk factors for a number of chronic diseases. The use of genetics to improve the human condition is called *eugenics.* The ability to alter the genetic code elevates the field of eugenics to a new level that could challenge both ethics and the legal system. So once again, just as IVF challenged the social environment of reproduction, genetic modification may challenge the social system in very difficult and complex ways.

BENEFITTING FROM THE INSIGHT OF GENETIC COUNSELORS

The field of genetics is extremely complex and fluid. There are people who have advanced training in genetics. They are extremely important for explaining what the results of genetic tests mean and how to use the information from genetic testing to a person's best advantage. Hospitals, fertility practices, and genetic testing companies have genetic counselors available for consultation. The internet is also a source of information. The bottom line is that genetics is an expanding part of medicine. Its role will become even more important as more is discovered about the genetic code and how it works.

Chapter **4**

Before the Baby: Exploring Lifestyle and Behavioral Factors

E ven though you're probably anxious to get started on baby making, take a little time to make sure that you're in the best possible condition for conceiving a healthy baby. This means making sure that you're not carrying an infection that may harm you or your baby and taking a look at your lifestyle habits, good and bad. In this chapter, we tell you how to get in shape physically if you're trying to get pregnant and discuss some behavior that may be decreasing your odds of getting pregnant. We also take a look at how what you eat could influence your chance of conceiving.

Making Healthy Lifestyle Changes

"Everything in moderation" is certainly a good motto for habits, good and bad. Too much exercise can have a less-than-desirable effect, while coffee, drunk in moderation, can be benign. But, before you say yes to things that are better left in the "no" category, consider that some things are best eliminated entirely, particularly when you're trying to conceive.

Giving up smoking

Smoking is bad for you. We all know it. Yet roughly 14 percent of women and 18 percent of men in the United States still smoke. While cigarette warning labels tell you they are addictive, they do not tell you that smoking impacts your reproductive health. Need some good reasons to quit? Here are a few:

>> Women who've smoked more than 100 cigarettes in their lifetime have a 14 percent greater risk of infertility.

>> Smokers take longer to conceive.

>> Smokers increase their relative risk for miscarriage by 1 percent for each cigarette they smoke a day. So, if you are 35 years old, you have a 20 percent chance of miscarriage (in general). If you smoke five cigarettes a day, you now have a 25 percent chance of miscarrying. *But* former smokers have the same risk of miscarriage as those who have never smoked, so quitting can really make a difference!

>> Smokers are two to four times more likely to have an *ectopic* pregnancy (one that implants in the fallopian tube rather than in the uterus, a topic we discuss in detail in Chapter 13) as smoking alters the structure and function of the tubes.

>> Smokers go through menopause earlier because smoking increases free radicals. Free radicals are substances that kill all cells, including eggs, decreasing the number of years pregnancy can occur. Smokers go through menopause three to four years earlier than nonsmokers. This could mean that a 38-year-old smoker is more like a 42-year-old nonsmoker, which, based upon age, would represent a significant decline in fertility.

Smokers also have lower AMH (anti-muellerian hormone) levels than nonsmokers undergoing IVF. AMH is a protein made by egg units (follicles). More egg units means higher AMH, and in terms of eggs, more is always better than fewer. (We talk more about the impact of AMH in Chapter 11.)

>> Smokers' eggs have more genetic abnormalities.

>> Smokers' eggs are prone to *polyspermy*, where two or more sperm enter an egg. The embryos that result are chromosomally abnormal and will not grow.

If you've quit but your partner hasn't, he may want to consider the following:

>> Men who smoke have a lower sperm count.

>> Men who smoke have a 20 percent decrease in sperm motility.

> » Smokers' sperm have more abnormal shapes. Abnormally shaped sperm have a higher rate of chromosomal abnormalities.

> » Secondhand smoke exposure during pregnancy increases miscarriage rates by 11 percent.

WARNING

Many studies have demonstrated that smokers have lower success rates for the treatments for infertility. Bottom line: stop smoking!

I'll drink to that!

A recently published article (Lyhgso, et al. *Human Reproduction* [2019] 34:1334) addressed the issue of mild to moderate alcohol consumption and infertility. The study asked the question: "Does female weekly alcohol intake and binge drinking impact the chance of a successful infertility treatment?" The study gathered information about the alcohol consumption of 1,708 women and their partners undergoing fertility treatment. The outcome was the achievement of a clinical pregnancy and live birth. The study found "low to moderate average weekly alcohol intake was not statistically significantly associated with the chance of achieving a clinical pregnancy or a live birth." The study divided that amount of alcohol consumed per week into none, 1–2 (alcoholic drinks), 3–7, and > 7 drinks. The chance for conception and live birth using either IUI or IVF was the same for all groups. The conclusion from the authors was that the results of their study suggest that it is not necessary to abstain from drinking alcohol when undergoing fertility treatments.

Putting this into perspective, once pregnant, there is ample evidence that heavy alcohol consumption can harm the developing pregnancy. So, the advice to abstain from heavy alcohol consumption while pregnant is appropriate. The American College of Obstetricians and Gynecologists (ACOG) guidelines state that all alcohol types are harmful to an established pregnancy even potentially in the early weeks of pregnancy.

TIP

While all of the preceding information is fascinating, how does it help people trying to conceive? The most important lesson is that total abstinence while in treatment for infertility is unnecessary. There is no harm in having an occasional drink while undergoing infertility treatments. However, once there is a possibility of being pregnant, alcohol consumption should be avoided.

Give me my coffee!

What about coffee? Who doesn't need that morning joe to start the day? Americans drink an average of 2.1 cups of coffee per day. But does that morning cup of coffee decrease the chance for achieving a pregnancy if a person is in treatment for infertility? Remember the alcohol study we talked about in the last section? In a different published study, the same researchers also evaluated the impact of coffee upon the success of infertility treatments. They found that for women undergoing IVF, coffee consumption did not affect the chance of achieving a clinical pregnancy or live birth. *Good news!* Women using IUI and consuming 1–5 cups of coffee a day had an *increased* chance of achieving a clinical pregnancy and live birth. So, if you're suffering a severe morning headache and lethargy, go back to your coffee.

Saying no to drugs

Undoubtedly you know that illegal drugs are taboo when trying to become pregnant! Here are the problems that some common drugs can cause when you're trying to get pregnant.

Cocaine

Cocaine use during pregnancy occurs in over 750,000 pregnancies per year. Cocaine causes constriction of the blood vessels, which can result in early miscarriage, preterm delivery, and problems with the *placenta,* the organ that nourishes the baby. In addition, cocaine can cause menstrual irregularities, possibly making it harder for you to become pregnant.

Marijuana

One of the trending topics of late has been cannabis use and its effects. Marijuana is the most commonly used recreational drug in the United States with an estimated 22 million using the drug in the preceding month and over 117 million lifetime users. Cannabis has been around a long time, but recent changes in legislation and societal attitudes have led to a rise in the use of cannabis. Almost every evil imaginable has at one time or another been linked to the use of cannabis. However, now that so many people are using cannabis — and many legally — efforts are underway to accurately determine the dangers and benefits of cannabis use, including those involving male fertility.

Marijuana lowers sperm count; decreases sperm's motility or sperm's ability to move forward; and lowers the amount of testosterone in males. The problem is that semen study results don't always correlate with pregnancy rates. So while the numbers in the results of a a semen analysis may be worse after marijuana use, the actual chance of conceiving may not be changed. But, does marijuana decrease the chance for males to father a child? The truth is that we just don't know. There is no credible, large study that addresses this issue. That is truly disappointing.

What about women and marijuana? There is some evidence that some women who use marijuana when they are pregnant may have an increase in growth restriction of the fetus and preterm labor. However, there is very little evidence to date about how marijuana affects the ability to conceive. A recent study looked at the use of marijuana and the time it took to conceive for both men and women. The study reported that there was no change in the time it took to conceive based either upon use of marijuana or frequency of use of marijuana.

TIP

So, what is a couple to do? Much like alcohol and cigarette smoking, cannabis may decrease a couple's chance of conceiving. So, until better evidence is obtained, prudence would say to use these substances in moderation, if at all. This would be particularly true for a male, given the reduction in the semen characteristics.

Anabolic steroids

WARNING

Some studies show that as many as 6 to 7 percent of all males have used anabolic steroids before age 18 to build muscle mass. Anabolic steroids are really variations on testosterone. Taking these steroids is like a woman taking a birth control pill. In males, anabolic steroids tell the brain the testis is overworking and thus the brain reduces the release of FSH and LH, both of which are needed for normal sperm production. Extensive and extended use of anabolic steroids can result in permanent loss of sperm production and cause a man to become sterile. Many men will have return of sperm production, but it may take months. So anabolic steroids need to be avoided when a man is trying to father a child.

Understanding Common Infections That Can Cause Uncommon Results

The onset of the sexual revolution in the 1960s caused a lot of fallout, and some of it fell on future fertility. *Sexually transmitted infections*, or STIs, (formerly called STDs or sexually transmitted diseases) have increased dramatically in the last 20 years. More than 13 million Americans each year are affected, and many STDs pack a major anti-fertility wallop for both sexes. The 2017 CDC data on STIs reported that three STIs had a record all-time high. The report stated that gonorrhea rose by 67 percent, syphilis by 76 percent, and chlamydia by 21 percent from the previous year. In 2018, the World Health Organization (WHO) reported an estimated 376 million new cases of STIs each year (namely, chlamydia, gonorrhea, syphilis, or trichomoniasis). One researcher speculated that while people were having less sex, they engaged in riskier sexual habits such as condom-less sex and opioid addicted–related sex.

You may not even know that you have a sexually transmitted disease. Some STDs cause a vaginal or penile discharge, others cause itching or small sores, but some cause no symptoms at all. Most are easily treated with antibiotics. The problem is that many women don't realize they have an infection because most have no clear symptoms. The following sections describe a few of the most damaging STDs and provide some statistics about the diseases in the United States.

HPV: The most common STI

Human papilloma virus (HPV) is the most common STD in the United States, now surpassing chlamydia and gonorrhea. HPV is different from human immunodeficiency virus (HIV). HPV is transmitted through vaginal, oral, or anal sex. Most often, HPV will go away because the immune system eradicates the virus. However, certain variations of HPV can cause genital warts or cancer. The cancers associated with HPV infection include cervical, vaginal, anal, penile, and throat cancers.

Like the situation with many viruses, there is no cure — but there is a vaccine. Beyond that, safe sex limits the risk of transmission. While cancer is the major concern with a positive HPV test, newer studies suggest that HPV may also affect fertility. A recent study evaluated the incidence of HPV in couples undergoing IVF. The study detected HPV in 19 percent of the females and 20 percent of the males. For the males who tested positive, there was a reduction in semen concentration, motility, and shape. The authors did not comment about whether this results in a lower pregnancy rate.

Currently, the gold test standard for HPV in women is the PAP smear (a swab of your cervix), as HPV can cause cervical cancer. Cervical cancer develops slowly in the cells that mark the border between the vagina and the inside of the cervix. The initial infection causes cells to change their appearance, and this can be seen by taking cells from this region of the cervix, staining them, and looking at them under the microscope.

Treatment for PAP smears where a number of cells look abnormal includes further investigating the cervix with a device called a colposcope. This device (and the colposcopy procedure) is just a way to magnify the area of the cervix where cervical cancers start. The areas identified by the colposcope can be biopsied, and potential cervical cancer cells identified through this early detection method can be removed. (The removal procedure is commonly called a LEEP procedure, Loop Electrosurgical Excision Procedure).

Prior to knowing that HPV causes cervical cancer, the PAP was the best way to identify these early precancerous changes. But now, it is known that certain variations of the HPV, called *serotypes*, can identify which people are at risk for developing cervical cancer. So, the more modern PAP is done so that the HPV can be typed and the risk assessed. The use of serotyping has allowed those people who are either HPV negative or have one of the safer variants of HPV to have less frequent PAP smears, such as every three years. Early treatment and more frequent screening can reduce the risk for developing cancer.

There is little data to suggest that HPV has a huge impact on your ability to conceive and, even if you were treated for HPV, the cervical procedures themselves should not increase your infertility risk. So, cancer is a concern with HPV — but impact on fertility, not so much.

TIP

A note about the HPV vaccine: While there is a vaccine for HPV, only about 40 percent of females and 28 percent of males who are in the age range where the vaccine is recommended (ages 11–26) actually have been vaccinated. Optimally, the vaccines should be given to all males and females at age 11–12. There are three different vaccines as of this writing, and for the 9-valent vaccine, the upper age for immunization has been increased to 45 years old for both men and women. As of 2019, the CDC did not recommend vaccinating adults over age 45.

Chlamydia: The most reported STI

Chlamydia is the most reported sexually transmitted infection in the United States — meaning we more often test for it than the other infections. The bacterium *Chlamydia trachomatis* is responsible for the infection. Both men and women can be infected, and both male and female fertility can be damaged. Chlamydia is easily tested by swabbing the penis or vagina and sending the swab to a lab for testing. A new test using urine is also being developed. Chlamydia is easily treated with antibiotics.

Here are some facts about the disease:

>> About 2 million new cases of chlamydia are diagnosed every year.

>> Almost two-thirds of new chlamydia infections occur in 14- to 24-year-olds.

>> Of those women who develop pelvic inflammatory disease (PID), 30 percent will have chlamydia. Each occurrence of PID reduces the chance of achieving a pregnancy by 25 percent due to the damage the infection does to the fallopian tubes.

>> Women with PID are seven to ten times more likely to have an ectopic pregnancy, a pregnancy that grows outside the uterus, usually in the tubes. (For more about ectopic pregnancies, see Chapter 13.)

>> Most women (75 percent) have no symptoms of infection; symptoms include lower abdominal pain, burning with urination, and vaginal irritation.

- » Twenty-five percent of men have no symptoms from chlamydia; the rest may have a discharge from the urethra, or pain and burning on urination.

- » Men with untreated chlamydia can develop *epididymitis,* an infection in the testicles, where sperm are developed. This condition can lead to low sperm counts.

- » Each year, 100,000 women become infertile from chlamydia. With a first episode of PID from chlamydia, 12 percent of women become infertile; a second episode of PID increases infertility to 40 percent. Eighty percent of women who have had PID from chlamydia three or more times are infertile.

- » Chlamydia is largely a silent disease. Only about 10 percent of men become symptomatic, and anywhere from 5–30 percent of women become symptomatic.

It is important to know that symptoms of a chlamydia infection, if any, may not appear until weeks after the person becomes infected. Diagnosis is made using vaginal swabs (for a woman) and penile swabs (for a man).

Chlamydia is treated with oral antibiotics: either a single dose of azithromycin or a seven-day course of doxycycline.

REMEMBER

Having been treated once does not mean you can't get reinfected — in fact reinfection is common. Annual testing for all sexually active women and men is recommended.

WARNING

Untreated chlamydia when you're pregnant can lead to miscarriage, preterm labor, or chlamydial conjunctivitis (eye infections) or chlamydial pneumonia (respiratory infections) in the child. Pregnant women with untreated chlamydia are also at a much higher risk for stillbirth.

Cytomegalovirus (CMV)

Cytomegalovirus (CMV) is caused by a virus — unlike chlamydia, which is caused by a bacterium. The difference is that bacteria do their damage outside of cells while viruses invade cells and do their damage by hijacking part of the DNA machinery. CMV is present in over half of the people by age 40 and one in three children are infected by age 5. Most people have no symptoms when they become infected, but CMV may cause mild symptoms of cough, fatigue, swollen glands, and sore throat. People infected with CMV are infected for life. CMV is spread through human fluids: direct contact through saliva or urine, sexual contact/semen, transplanted organs, blood transfusions, and breast milk (which, along with direct contact, is how many little ones contract the infection).

Most of the time, CMV is inactive (dormant), but it can activate at any time. When the infection activates, it can be spread to other people and babies. Healthy people rarely experience significant problems from CMV, although it can cause mononucleosis. Adults with a compromised immune system are more susceptible to infections that affect the eye, digestive system, and nervous system, and it can cause pneumonia. Infants can be born with congenital CMV, but this is more likely to happen if the mother contracts CMV for the first time when she is pregnant and not from reactivated CMV. Congenital CMV may cause the baby to have loss of vision, neurological problems, hearing loss, seizures, muscle problems and loss of coordination, and impaired intellect. The most common problem for infants with congenital CMV is hearing loss.

There is no cure for CMV, and healthy people generally do not need treatment. However, antiviral medications may be given to babies and people with weakened immune systems.

CMV does not appear to have an impact on fertility, but if it is an active infection, CMV can cause problems in a developing fetus leading to low birth weight, blindness, deafness, mental retardation, small head size, seizures, or damage to the liver or spleen. Testing "positive" for CMV means that you have been infected sometime in your lifetime, but there's no way of knowing when. If your infection is not active, the risks in pregnancy are reduced.

WARNING

If you are CMV negative and are considering using donor sperm, you may want to know if the donor is CMV negative. That way you will not have to worry about getting CMV yourself or it being a factor in any potential pregnancy.

Gonorrhea

Gonorrhea is caused by the bacterium *Neisseria gonorrhoeae*, which can infect the genital tract, mouth, or rectum. Infants can get the disease from an infected mother during childbirth. It can be carried by males and females and can be cured with antibiotics. Here are some other facts about gonorrhea:

>> Each year, 820,000 new cases of gonorrhea are diagnosed.

>> Gonorrhea is the second most reported STI.

>> Gonorrhea can lead to infertility. Like chlamydia, gonorrhea in women can cause PID, leading to tubal damage. Some doctors test for gonorrhea and chlamydia before doing common fertility tests such as a *hysterosalpingogram* (HSG), in which dye is injected into the uterus and fallopian tubes to see whether there are any irregularities. (We discuss HSGs in more detail in Chapter 11.) If you have gonorrhea or chlamydia and push dye into the tubes

and uterus, you may push the infection up also and end up with more tube or uterine damage than you had to begin with.

>> Men with gonorrhea usually have a discharge from the penis and a burning sensation; women may have no symptoms or sometimes pain on urination or an increased vaginal discharge.

Gonorrhea is diagnosed by testing the urine or by taking swabs of the cervix, mouth, or anus. Treatment for uncomplicated gonorrhea involves intramuscular injections of antibiotics (shots!). Lately, drug-resistant forms of gonorrhea have emerged, which makes treatment more difficult, so antibiotic injections are now combined with oral antibiotics when these strains are found.

Syphilis

Syphilis is caused by the bacterium *Treponema pallidum.* The bacterium can be transmitted through genital, oral, or anal contact. The good news is that syphilis is easily cured with penicillin. The bad news is that this infection is on the rise.

>> The number of reported syphilis cases rose over 70 percent from 2013 to 2017.

>> Men, especially men who have sex with other men, are affected the most.

>> Over 100,000 cases of syphilis were reported in 2017, with a rise in syphilis in heterosexual men and women.

>> Syphilis can cause epididymitis in men and can be passed to an unborn child during pregnancy or at birth.

Syphilis frequently starts as a painless sore on such areas as the mouth, genitals, or rectum. The sore is called a *chancre,* and this stage of syphilis is called primary syphilis. The sore may never be noticed and heals without intervention in 3–6 weeks. The next stage of syphilis is called secondary syphilis and is hallmarked by a rash that is frequently painless but can occupy the entire body including the palms of the hands and soles of the feet. This may continue for up to a year. The third stage of syphilis is called tertiary, and 15–30 percent of people infected with syphilis reach tertiary syphilis without treatment. Tertiary syphilis can lead to life-threatening problems with almost every system in the body and may not appear until years after the initial infection. Syphilis was a major cause of death until penicillin was available after World War II. In fact, it's hit some pretty well-known people. Al Capone had tertiary syphilis, which destroyed his brain while he was incarcerated at Alcatraz. Capone was one of the first people to get penicillin, but it was too late. He eventually died at age 48 of heart disease believed to be related to his syphilis infection.

Babies born with syphilis contract the disease through the placenta or during birth. Usually the baby is initially without symptoms but eventually may develop deafness, teeth deformities, or saddle nose (loss of height of the nose.) Syphilis is diagnosed with blood or spinal fluid tests. The initial test is a screening test that does not miss many people who are infected. However, the screening test tells a number of people they do have syphilis when in fact they don't. So, if the first test is positive, a second test is done which accurately identifies the people who truly are infected.

Syphilis is easily treated if diagnosed early. A single injection of penicillin can cure syphilis if diagnosed within a year of exposure, but after that a more extensive treatment with penicillin is needed. Other antibiotics may be used. Contrary to folklore, syphilis can't be caught from a toilet seat.

WARNING

Early detection of syphilis is key, and it can be easily treated with penicillin (or another antibiotic if you are allergic to penicillin). Don't be afraid, embarrassed, or otherwise deterred from talking to your doctor about STIs. Ignoring syphilis can be devastating to you, your partner, and your child.

Genital herpes

Genital herpes is caused by the herpes simplex type 2 virus (HSV). The cold sores some people are prone to on their lips are caused by the herpes simplex type 1 virus (although you can get genital herpes with type 1 and cold sores with type 2 — STIs don't always play by the rules!). Currently, there is no vaccine against genital herpes in the works, but a few scientists are working on one for oral herpes. In the meantime, caution should be exercised when having a sexual relationship with an infected person as it is spread through body fluids. Here's some other information on herpes:

>> Fifty percent of Americans under age 50 are infected with oral herpes.

>> One in eight people in the United States have genital herpes, with 500,000 new cases diagnosed each year.

>> Unlike some of the other STIs, the incidence of genital herpes is decreasing.

>> Once you are infected with the genital herpes virus, it stays in your body forever, even though initial symptoms of flu-like symptoms and chancres may disappear within two to three weeks. Occasional flare-ups can be managed with antiviral medications like acyclovir (Zovirax), famciclovir (Famvir), and valacyclovir (Valtrex).

>> There is no clear link between genital herpes and infertility; however, some researchers have suggested that the virus may cause implantation problems

in women. The bigger issue is if you become infected late in your pregnancy, or you have an outbreak at delivery. Having genital herpes before a pregnancy has a very low risk of transmitting the infection to your baby.

WARNING

» There is a 30–50 percent risk of infecting a fetus if the mother first contracts genital herpes late in her pregnancy.

» If you have an outbreak of genital herpes at the time your baby is ready to be delivered, you'll need to have a cesarean section; if you deliver vaginally without treatment, your baby may suffer from neonatal herpes (leading to central nervous system damage, mental retardation, or even death).

» Antiviral medications are generally safe to take during pregnancy.

HIV

Human immunodeficiency virus (HIV) is a chronic infection that may or may not lead to the disease AIDS (acquired immune deficiency syndrome). At present, there is no cure for HIV or AIDS, although antiviral medications may keep HIV under control for some time. There are over one million people in the U.S. living with HIV, and approximately 15 percent of them are undiagnosed. Just under 40,000 new cases are reported per year.

While some HIV-infected men may have sperm abnormalities (like a lower sperm count), many will see no impact on their ability to father a child. Further, special sperm preparation and IUI or IVF with ICSI can significantly reduce the likelihood of transmitting HIV to their partner or fetus. HIV-infected women do not have fertility issues simply due to their HIV. Pregnancy is another story.

Check out the following facts about HIV and pregnancy:

» Women with HIV can become pregnant and carry the pregnancy to term, but they risk transmitting HIV to the baby or causing birth defects due to the medications they may be on.

» The risk of transmission is about 25 percent if you're untreated but may be reduced dramatically if you receive antiviral drug regimens while you're pregnant.

» You can reduce the chance of infecting a newborn to approximately 2 percent by using antiretroviral meds and not breastfeeding.

» You may reduce the risk of transmission of the disease to your baby if you have a cesarean section rather than a vaginal delivery.

>> You must wait 3 to 18 months after delivery to find out whether your baby is HIV positive, because during pregnancy your antibodies are passed to the baby. This means that all babies of HIV-infected moms will test positive at birth. It can take as long as 18 months for all your antibodies to disappear from your baby's blood. After your antibodies are all gone, if the baby tests positive, it means he or she is infected with the virus.

REMEMBER

You can be tested for sexually transmitted diseases, including HIV, before trying to conceive. If you are using any third-party reproductive techniques, you will be required to have many of these tests (we talk more about this in Chapter 20). If you suspect that you may have an STD, or have been exposed to one, you need to rule out this potential danger to your fertility and your unborn child.

Trichomoniasis

Trichomoniasis (commonly known as "Trich") is a sexually transmitted disease cause by the parasite *Trichomonas vaginalis*. Trich is the most common curable STI, and one estimate reports that 3 percent of all women in the reproductive age are infected. The disease is largely without symptoms in both men and women, with over 80 percent of those infected without symptoms. Symptoms, when they occur, include a vaginal discharge, itching of the perineum, odor, and irritation. There are tests that can be done in your doctor's office from vaginal swabs, but no test is approved for testing males. The treatment is most commonly metronidazole (Flagyl). There is no agreement about the influence of Trich on fertility for males, but it may contribute to male factor infertility. There is, however, some evidence that Trich can affect a pregnancy causing low birth weight, premature rupture of membranes, or prematurity. Some studies have found an association between Trich and infertility, but overall, there is no strong evidence that Trich causes infertility.

Ureaplasma and mycoplasma

Ureaplasma and mycoplasma are microorganisms that can affect different parts of the body, depending on the strain. The genital tracts of both sexes can carry mycoplasma or ureaplasma. The following list gives some other information about the diseases:

>> As many as 40 percent of women and men are carriers of bacteria called *ureaplasma* or *mycoplasma*.

>> Some controversy exists about whether certain strains of ureaplasma and mycoplasma cause problems in getting pregnant; some studies show that they increase the incidence of miscarriage and/or problems with the embryo

implanting in the uterus. This seems to be related to either partner having the infection, which is easily passed between partners.

>> Scientific studies have failed to demonstrate statistically that either ureaplasma or mycoplasma reduces fertility.

TIP

As with other STDs, both partners are easily treated with a 14-day course of an antibiotic, such as doxycycline. Both partners must take the drug, or they'll probably continue to reinfect each other.

A new kid on the block: Zika

Zika is a virus which can cause severe problems for infants if their mother becomes infected while pregnant.

The American College of Obstetricians and Gynecology (ACOG) issued a committee opinion in April of 2019 recommending that healthcare providers continue to caution patients about potential exposure to Zika even though the rate of infection seems to be decreasing.

Infectious agents come in basically four flavors: bacteria, yeast, parasites, and virus. The first three organisms all stay outside of the cell, but the virus enters the cell and hijacks the cell's genetic machinery to turn out more virus — nice Trojan horse! Zika is spread to humans by mosquitos (Aedes species). Transmission of the virus has been reported to occur through sexual contact, blood transfusion, and to a fetus.

Since the virus is spread by mosquitos, which have defined habitats, areas where the mosquitoes reside are consider areas for possible exposure. The virus can also be contracted by having sex with an infected partner without the use of a condom. The signs of being infected include fever, rash, muscle aches, and inflammation of the eye. Symptoms usually occur within the first 3–14 days after exposure.

Zika has been classified as a fetal teratogen (something which causes a malformation of a fetus). If a fetus becomes infected, the fetus may develop a distinct pattern of birth defects which affect the nervous system, the brain, and the skull. Other problems have been reported as a result of a Zika infection such as heart abnormalities, miscarriage, preterm birth, and stillbirth. Women can transmit the virus to a fetus throughout a pregnancy, and the risk of a congenital birth syndrome is 5–10 percent.

As of 2019, there was no vaccine for Zika. Because the infection is from a virus, antibiotics do not work and there is no cure for the infection. That means that the only way to limit the risk of being infected is to avoid those areas where Zika lives.

Thus, ACOG has made recommendations that include avoiding travel to areas where Zika outbreaks occur. Make sure to check before planning your next trip, even in you are in the preconception phase. Sorry, folks! Many of these Zika hot spots are in tropical oases (think Hawaii, the Caribbean, and so on). Keep in mind that skipping this babymoon may be the best gift you give to your future family.

Also, if a woman has been subject to the risk of Zika and is considering conceiving, she should wait at least eight weeks either from having Zika-like symptoms or exposure to try to conceive. If a male partner is at risk either from exposure or symptoms, then the couple should wait at least three months before trying to conceive. ACOG recommends that people with possible exposure or people who are considering traveling to Zika risk areas should consult their obstetrician for advice. The Zika recommendations will change as new information occurs and as possible vaccines are commercially available, so consultation with an OB should provide the latest methods for managing Zika.

STIs May Cause PID: More Than Just a "Pain in the Derriere"

Even though many of the infections discussed earlier in this chapter can be taken care of with appropriate antibiotic treatment, in some cases, there may be lingering effects.

WARNING

Severe abdominal pain with a fever should be immediately evaluated.

Pelvic inflammatory disease (PID) is an infection of the upper female reproductive system, which includes the uterus, tubes, and ovaries. PID is most commonly associated with sexually transmitted diseases and as such, starts in the vagina and moves up into the upper reproductive organs. PID classically shows itself as severe pain in the entire lower abdomen and can include a *fever* (a body temperature of ≥101 degrees Fahrenheit taken twice, six hours apart), a general feeling of being sick, and nausea. PID is most commonly caused by gonorrhoeae or Chlamydia trachomatis.

It has been estimated that about 10 percent of women with these infections develop PID, and PID from gonorrhoeae seems to be more severe. Frequently, other bacteria contribute to the infection. The CDC reports that the rate of PID has been decreasing. In 2006, about 0.8 percent of women between the ages of 15 and 29 contracted PID, but by 2013, this was down to about 0.6 percent, which is a 25 percent decrease. PID can cause damage to the fallopian tubes in the form of scarring or damage to the transport function of the tubes. PID can also cause general pelvic scarring and chronic pain. Estimates have reported that for young women with PID, about 20 percent develop chronic pain, 8 percent have an ectopic pregnancy, and about 15 percent have infertility. PID is treated with antibiotics, and early diagnosis and treatment decrease the long-term complications.

Exploring Specific Lifestyle Choices and Busting Some Common Myths

Most everyone knows about drinking, smoking, and drugs being bad for you when you're trying to get pregnant. In this section, we talk about a few things that affect getting pregnant of which you may not be aware.

Gauging the truth about hot tubs — and other "short" stories

WARNING

Anything that raises the temperature of a man's testicles can decrease sperm production and motility. Hot tubs, saunas, steam rooms, and tight underwear are out for men! Well . . . maybe not out altogether.

It seems that the evidence for this belief is derived from a study published in 2007. Searching for other studies failed to identify any. Even the study authors cautioned that their study was a pilot study and suggested further research, but none was ever reported in searchable databases. The study looked at 11 males, asked them to stop using the hot tub, and found that 5 out of the 6 who did stop had an improvement in the motility of the semen analysis. The study did not attempt to determine whether this change increased the chance for conception. Based upon this extraordinarily weak evidence, it is hard to make a recommendation about hot tubs and fertility. A 1996 study looked at using a scrotal cooling device and infertility. The study had 25 subjects, and 16 of the 25 men had an improvement in the semen while 6 achieved a pregnancy. So admittedly, constantly heating the testicles is probably not a good idea, but there is very little evidence that heat exposure affects male fertility. Finally, a 1998 study looked at the influence of boxer shorts on male fertility and guess what? No effect! So, boxers or briefs or commando are okay.

Can the female join her mate now that he has been cleared for hot tub use — perhaps less frequently? The body has incredible temperature regulatory systems to prevent the core body temperature from rising. As a graduate student, Dr. R supplemented his income by being a subject for studies looking at the effect of heat and humidity on human physiology. The subjects walked on treadmills in an environmental chamber where the heat and humidity could be controlled. As the temperature and humidity were increased, the body's core temperature began to rise. A 1 degree Centigrade rise was enough to absolutely drive the subject to get out of the chamber and cool down, and no amount of threats or money could stop the subjects (meaning Dr. R). The ovaries reside well within the human body and thus are kept at core temperature. No amount of hot tub use can cause a significant rise in the woman's core temperature, and if for some reason it does start to rise, no amount of encouragement from her partner will keep her in that tub — sorry, guys.

Balancing the yin and yang of exercise

So your partner decided to work out stress by bicycling or playing rugby. This exercise should be a good thing, right? Wrong! Prolonged cycling can cause damage to the groin from constant pressure of the bike seat, and contact sports can lead to injury to the testicles and can damage sperm production. The emphasis here is on prolonged cycling, not recreational cycling. However, most studies evaluated the effect of cycling on semen parameters and not on reducing the fertility rate. For males with a normal semen analysis, exercise (especially recreational exercise) does not seem to alter the man's fertility potential. For males with mildly abnormal semen parameters, reducing exercising levels, especially cycling, may have a beneficial effect.

Women who exercise heavily may find that their periods have stopped. This condition is called *amenorrhea* (we get into this in Chapter 11) and is common among women who are very thin and exercise daily. Obviously, you can't get pregnant if you're not having periods; you're not developing eggs. Particularly concerning is the triad of no periods, heavy exercise, and bulimia. This triad requires treatment by a physician. So what can you both do to reduce stress that won't cause fertility problems? Exercise in moderation is fine — for both of you!

Dumping the douche

WARNING

Douching is a bad idea whether you're trying to get pregnant or not. Researchers found that women who douched regularly had an incidence of pelvic inflammatory disease (PID) of 13 percent compared to 6 percent for the women who did not douche. PID can cause damage to the fallopian tubes and uterus. The ectopic pregnancy rate is higher in women who douche regularly. One interesting study compared women who douched to those who did not, and after one year of observation, there was no increase in PID in the group who douched. There was, however, a 15 percent decrease in fertility, and for those who douched frequently, fertility decreased by 33 percent. Dump the douche!

Avoiding toxins at home and away

WARNING

Changing your job isn't always easy, but you do need to consider potential exposure to dangerous substances and take steps to protect yourself from them. Here are some examples:

» Think about substances that you're exposed to at work. For instance, if you're a home remodeler, bridge painter, welder, or solderer, you may be exposed to large amounts of lead. You run the same risk if you're remodeling an old house and scraping old paint off the walls. Lead exposure in men has been linked to low sperm count and decreased motility of sperm. In women, lead exposure may cause low birth weight in babies, high blood pressure during pregnancy, damage to the baby's nervous system, and developmental delays.

» Heavy, exertional work can lead to reduced sperm counts, but there is little evidence about the effect of this on actual fertility rates.

» The advent of OSHA (the federal Occupational Health and Safety Agency) has provided safe work environments for almost all occupations. Since this is true, it is hard to imagine that there are strong negative influences on fertility rates based upon occupations. In fact, even though OSHA lists a few known toxins that could affect fertility (nitrous oxide, lead, jet fuel, and a variety of pesticides), it clearly states that these substances may not affect all workers, or all workers in the same way.

» There are a few studies that identify some environmental toxins that *may* (emphasis on the possibility, not the probability) impact a person's infertility. These include hexachlorocyclohexane, polychlorinated biphenyls (PCBs), dichlorodiphenyltrichloroethane (DDT), some pesticides, and ingested heavy metals (mercury and lead).

REMEMBER

The impact of any potential toxin on a given individual's fertility potential depends upon the intensity of the exposure to the toxin. You cannot assume that casual exposure is at the root of your infertility problem. When in doubt, please check with your doctor about your specific concerns.

Making the connection between stress and fertility

Can stress keep you from getting pregnant? First of all, what is stress? One Google definition is "a state of mental or emotional strain or tension resulting from adverse or very demanding circumstances." However, a key factor resulting in elevated stress is the person's reaction to a situation. Some circumstances create more stress for some people than for other people.

STRESS AND ACTIVITY ARE NOT THE SAME

Dr. R: I remember one patient who had a very achievement-oriented, high-powered North Shore Chicago–type job. She found not being able to conceive at her command almost intolerable since for most everything else she had tried she was successful. Somehow, she was convinced by well-meaning friends and family that if she would only relax, she would become pregnant. So, she quit her job and stayed at home eating well and exercising. Since she was not working, she could devote every waking moment to her quest. After about two weeks of "rest" she was climbing the walls with boredom and her stress level was truly off the charts. She went back to work, adjusted her schedule to allow her to pursue treatment protocols, and fortunately, after considerable work and persistence, she had her first child. Child number two came as a complete surprise since not everything was perfect yet for that second child. The point: Many active people need to maintain a certain level of activity to control their stress. Don't confuse activity with stress.

Full disclosure: Dr. R is not a firm believer that stress is a significant cause of infertility. He is a strong believer that infertility causes stress. To that end, anything that will reduce your stress and allow you to pursue treatment is desirable.

REMEMBER

The literature about stress and infertility is not clear. A recent literature review concluded that there was no clear cause–effect relationship between infertility and stress. This was due to the conflicting results of the many studies and the lack of ways to objectively measure stress.

What can you do to reduce stress? We talk more about stress-reducing techniques in Chapter 9, but in general:

>> **Talk it out.** Stress increases when you hold everything in.

>> **Try to focus on the "big picture."** When you're trying to get pregnant, every failed month seems like a year — or the end of the world. When you finally do get pregnant, it won't matter whether you got pregnant in November or January. Remember that the odds are on your side, in most cases, and that you *will* get pregnant.

>> **Don't lose sight of the rest of your life.** While trying to have a baby may be a big part of your life at this moment, it's not the only thing you have going on in your life. Make time for your family, your partner, your friends, your hobbies — and anything else that helps you remember that you had a life before you started thinking about pregnancy, and you still do!

Getting Checked Out from Top to Bottom

Having a checkup even before you try to get pregnant is always a good idea, and it's essential if you've been trying for a few months and still getting "not pregnant" results on the home pregnancy tests. Sometimes simple imbalances in your thyroid levels, or other levels easily checked by a simple blood test, can be keeping you from getting pregnant.

Having a full physical

You can see either your primary care physician (PCP) or your gynecologist for a checkup — or both! Your PCP looks at the "big picture" while your GYN looks mainly at your reproductive issues. Either one can order blood work and do a physical exam. (See Chapter 8 for more on choosing a doctor to help you get pregnant.)

Do you need to book a full body MRI or CT scan to find out if you're in shape to get pregnant? No, a half hour with your doctor should do the trick. If you're putting off a visit because you're afraid of being "yelled at" because you're overweight, have bad habits you know you'll be lectured about, or are terrified of having blood drawn, now is the time to put those fears aside.

A routine checkup by your gynecologist or family doctor may be all you need to help you get pregnant; for example, your doctor can look at the following possible pregnancy stumbling blocks:

>> **Your weight:** Are you underweight or overweight? Being either over- or underweight may interfere with pregnancy.

>> **Your sexual practices:** Are you missing the big day each month because you've been misinformed about when you ovulate?

>> **Your sexual history:** Do you have a sexually transmitted infection (STI) that could be preventing pregnancy? (See the section, "Understanding Common Infections That Can Cause Uncommon Results" for more on STIs.)

>> **Your habits:** Do you douche right after sex? You may be washing some of the best swimmers away!

>> **Your blood pressure:** Women with high blood pressure may be prone to developing serious hypertensive disease during pregnancy.

The physical exam includes examination of the thyroid gland in the neck, breasts, heart, lungs, abdomen, and reflexes (for neurologic response). A pelvic exam includes a vaginal speculum exam to evaluate the cervix (this generally means a

PAP smear!), a bimanual exam to assess ovaries and uterus, and a rectal/vaginal exam. A transvaginal ultrasound frequently completes the initial pelvic exam so that your ovaries and uterus can be visualized.

Checking your blood levels

The good thing about having blood drawn is that a single specimen can be used to test for many different health conditions, including some that can interfere with getting pregnant; we look at a few in the next sections.

Looking at your thyroid function

Women who have an underactive or overactive thyroid may have trouble getting pregnant. Thyroid abnormalities can cause anovulation (no egg is released), irregular menstrual cycles, or short menstrual cycles. (See Chapter 2 for more about menstrual dysfunction.)

Hypothyroid, or low thyroid levels, can raise your prolactin level (*prolactin* is a hormone that helps control milk production in breastfeeding women). High prolactin levels can prevent ovulation; prolactin levels can be diagnosed with a blood test.

Running a chemistry panel

A chemistry panel tests your blood sugar to show if you have diabetes; it also tests your liver and kidney functions. Many health problems that can have impact on pregnancy can be found through a chemistry panel.

Checking your blood count

A complete blood count, or CBC, tests your hemoglobin, which shows if you're anemic. It also tests your white blood count, which can show chronic infection.

When you go for your routine checkup, your doctor will be doing the basic things to see if you are healthy overall. This is the starting point. Additional testing to assess why you are not getting pregnant is discussed in Chapter 11.

Checking your medications

Have you overlooked something that could be interfering with your getting pregnant? Think back a few months, especially when thinking about sperm production; the sperm being ejaculated today have been over two months in the making, so anything your partner was taking a few months ago could be affecting his sperm count today. Ask yourself the questions in the following sections about a few possible deterrents you may not have thought about.

Taking a closer look at prescription medications

What you put in your body may matter when you are trying to get pregnant. Taking a quick inventory of any ongoing or recent prescription drugs can identify if any of these are getting in your way:

>> Has your partner taken antibiotics, such as erythromycin or gentamycin, or antifungal medications, such as ketoconazole, or been treated for psoriasis with methotrexate? Has he been on anabolic steroids? These medicines can all affect sperm production.

>> Do you or your partner take medication for high blood pressure? Sometimes, when you've been taking a medication for a long time, you almost forget that it can have serious side effects. Men who take certain types of antihypertensives called calcium channel blockers may produce sperm that can't penetrate eggs well; other high blood pressure medications may cause *retrograde ejaculation,* a condition in which the semen is pushed backwards into the bladder instead of being ejaculated out; or they may cause an inability to get and sustain an erection. Some antihypertensives are dangerous in early pregnancy as they can cause birth defects. Other antihypertensive drugs are available that don't have these effects, so talk to your doctor about switching medications if possible.

TECHNICAL STUFF

By definition, medications are substances that are prescribed and regulated by the FDA. Many medications can have a negative effect upon fertility or on a pregnancy, but there is an easy way to check the potential for problems on FDA-regulated drugs. Medications are categorized as to their effect on a pregnancy with the majority being either category B (okay to use) or category C (use only if benefit outweighs risk). By using this categorization system, you can determine if the medications you are taking are worth it:

>> Category A is for drugs that have a proven safety record backed by research on women.

>> Category B drugs have shown safe use in animals, but there are no well-controlled studies in humans.

>> Category C includes drugs where animal studies have shown an adverse effect but there are no well-controlled human studies to tell us what happens in humans. This is where a risk-benefit evaluation helps to decide if the medication should be used.

>> Category D is where studies have shown an adverse effect for humans but where special circumstances may warrant the use of the medication.

>> Category X: Well, what do you think — does X sound good? You are right — the answer is "no." These medications have proven adverse effects on pregnancy and no amount of benefit outweighs the risk — just don't use them.

WARNING

Do not stop taking any prescription medication before discussing it with your doctor. You are on that medication for a reason!

TIP

Some of the commonly used medications for fertility treatment have very scary warnings on their labels. Do not freak out! These warnings don't apply to your situation (or else your physician would not be prescribing them) as long as the physician knows you are trying to get pregnant.

The good and bad of antidepressants

Considering how many people are using antidepressants, it is surprising how little research has been done on the influence of antidepressants on fertility. There are a number of categories of medications that are antidepressants. However, the largest group are the selective serotonin reuptake inhibitors (SSRIs). These work by increasing the levels of serotonin in the brain. Serotonin is a chemical in the brain that acts as a messenger between brain cells. Examples of SSRIs are Prozac, Lexapro, Zoloft, Paxil, and Celexa to mention a few.

A recent review identified 16 articles that studied the effect of SSRIs on fertility. Six of the studies demonstrated no effect on fertility, three suggested a negative effect, and one demonstrated an increase in pregnancy rate. Although the research methodology was considered poor, six of the studies demonstrated a negative effect on the semen parameters. So, what to do? First, ask yourself if you really need those little happy pills. If not, stop — under the direction of the prescribing physician since some cannot be stopped suddenly. If you truly need those pills, so be it. Just remember to notify your fertility doctor of the pills you are taking.

Reviewing nonprescription medications

It is amazing how often we grab an over-the-counter (OTC) medication to take care of a back sprain after playing pick-up basketball or a rash on the leg after hiking in the woods. Who checks with a doctor first? Well, things are different when you are trying to get pregnant and — as we warn you about vitamins and supplements in Chapter 9 — you need to pay a little bit more attention to what you are putting in or on your body. Your fertility clinic will no doubt give you a list of medications that are acceptable, but here a few general tips that you should think about before popping a pill or rubbing on salve:

>> Acetaminophen is generally considered safe to use as a painkiller for various aches and pains.

>> NSAIDS (non-steroidal anti-inflammatory drugs), including ibuprofen, may interfere with ovulation and can increase bleeding if taken prior to any procedures (like an egg retrieval). One study suggests that high doses impact sperm production. These should be used with clinic instruction only.

>> Aspirin can increase bleeding so use with direction only.

>> Milk of magnesia and antacids are usually fine to settle down that "icky" tummy.

>> Topical preparations for itches (like Cortaid) or minor skin infections (like Neosporin) can be used as long as you don't overdo it and ignore what is causing the problem.

REMEMBER

The best thing you can do is answer honestly when your doctor asks you "What medications do you take?"

Deciding if you need a mammogram

It's not essential to have a mammogram before getting pregnant, especially if you're over the age of 40 or if you have a family history of breast cancer. In fact, the American College of Obstetricians and Gynecologists (ACOG) recommends that discussions between physicians and patients of screening mammography to determine when to start them should take place around age 40, but definitely by age 50. Some fertility clinics are making mammograms "required" for all patients who will undergo IVF or are over a certain age, so don't be surprised if this test gets added to your list of things to do. You might think that having a mammogram "can't hurt." That actually is very incorrect. Every medical test has a certain "false positive" rate, meaning that the test says you have a problem when in fact you don't. So, every test has a trade-off between correctly identifying a disease when it is present and correctly telling you that you don't have a disease if you don't. Women who have a mammogram that gives them a false positive (the test says you have breast cancer, but in fact you don't), will undergo unnecessary further testing, interventions, and psychological trauma. The current recommendations for mammograms take into account the balance of false negatives and false positives.

During the time of your pregnancy (ten months), along with the time you plan to breastfeed, mammograms will not be a good option. This could be one to two years, depending on how long you choose to nurse. Talk to your OB/GYN about this before you get pregnant, as she may elect to do a baseline mammogram prior to conceiving.

Seeking other prepregnancy medical counseling: Do you need it?

If you have a chronic disease (diabetes or lupus, for example) or condition (such as heart problems), have had pregnancy or delivery problems in the past, or you are over a certain age, your doctor may want you to have further evaluation by another specialist before you begin treatment. Sometimes this is as simple as going to the doctor that handles your disease/condition to get what we call "medical clearance," or the go-ahead, to start fertility treatment. Medical clearance lets the clinic know that your condition is under control and that another specialist has looked at you and the proposed treatment so that all risks are identified and managed. Here are two other specialists that you may be asked to see.

Looking for input from maternal-fetal medicine (MFM)

MFM (maternal-fetal medicine) is a subspecialty of obstetrics. An MFM has done a four-year residency after medical school and then a fellowship of three to four years. All MFMs are board certified obstetricians. MFMs manage complicated maternal and fetal medical problems. Women with severe diabetes, heart disease, neurological disease, and so forth are managed for their medical condition. Frequently, MFMs work with the OBs to co-manage a person, with the OB actually doing the delivery. The most common path to an MFM is a referral from an OB or reproductive endocrinologist (RE) who has identified a problem that needs expert management. If a person knows that she is high risk for pregnancy, she may seek out an MFM without seeing a general OB first. IVF pregnancies may be considered high risk (especially multiples), but they can generally be comfortably managed by a general OB.

Pursuing genetic counseling

Genetics seems to be everywhere today, from prenatal carrier screening, a family history of a genetic disease, or a defined genetic disease with either parent, to a genetic disease of the developing fetus. Any one of these issues may be better served by genetic counseling. The field of genetics is moving so fast that the generalist or even the REI can't keep up with all the recent developments. Genetic counselors are extremely helpful in informing patients about the significance of genetic problems. Chapter 3 tells you more about genetics and your genes.

» **Weighing the decision to have another . . . and another!**

» **Climbing back on the infertility treadmill**

» **Understanding why having one child doesn't always reduce the emotional pain of infertility**

Chapter **5**

It Worked the First Time! Tackling Secondary Infertility

I n the immortal words of Baseball's Yogi Berra, "It's déjà vu all over again!" For many, Yogi's words perfectly describe the struggle with secondary infertility, or difficulty getting pregnant a second time . . . or a third.

Although exact numbers are difficult to pin down, according the most recent U.S. government statistics, (HHS.gov accessed November 2019) one in ten women ages 15–44 experience infertility. This means that 6.1 million women in the U.S. experience infertility, and 12–13 out of every 100 couples experience infertility.

In this chapter, we define secondary infertility and then take a closer look at its emotional impact, as well as what you can do to deal with the merry-go-round of infertility — take two.

Facing Secondary Infertility

Defining secondary infertility is not as straightforward as it may seem. Also, the term secondary infertility can be applied to a number of different situations. The Department of Health and Human Services (HHS) of the federal government defines secondary infertility as "infertility in a woman who has had one or more pregnancies, but cannot become pregnant again."

Secondary infertility can occur whether the first conception was difficult or easy. It can be due to female issues, male issues, or a combination of both. One problem with the definitions is just what is meant by pregnancy. Does pregnancy mean a rise in the HCG shortly after a missed period? Does pregnancy include first trimester losses? Does pregnancy mean having a normal, healthy child at term? Considering that the purpose of the exercise is to have a full-term, live birth, it would seem that the most appropriate definition of pregnancy would be just that — a pregnancy that ended in the delivery at term of a healthy child.

The situation is complicated by the history of the previous pregnancy. Was the pregnancy conceived within a normal time frame and thus the couple were considered to have normal fertility? Or was the pregnancy conceived only after a diagnosis of infertility was made and the pregnancy was a result of treatment? The history helps determine what course of action is most appropriate to try for the next pregnancy.

For people who conceived spontaneously within six months to a year of trying, the diagnosis of infertility is made if they have been trying for six months to a year for another pregnancy and they have not achieved a pregnancy. After all, infertility is infertility, whether you call it primary or secondary. The significance of this is that once the term infertility is applied, the course of action is the same whether it is primary or secondary: use diagnostic tools to make a diagnosis. However, if the couple had the diagnosis of infertility for the successful pregnancy, then the course of action is determined by that diagnosis. It is not always necessary to reinvent the wheel! Other problems may have arisen in the meantime, but many problems will persist. The approach is to make sure nothing *else* has changed and then apply the previous diagnosis to determine what the best course of action will be.

For example, if there is a severe male factor in a young couple and it took IVF with ICSI to achieve a pregnancy, it most likely will require the same process for another child. If the diagnosis was polycystic ovarian syndrome, then it may actually be more difficult to conceive again. Possible reasons for this are that age may play a role, but many women gain weight when pregnant and it is difficult to lose this weight. Increased weight may make the PCOS more difficult to treat.

Frequently, couples seek consultation because of secondary infertility, and they feel they are unique and alone . . . this only happens to them. They start to question themselves, and this can lead to a feeling of isolation and guilt or of not being as good as someone else. If you find yourself in this bad head space, take note: Secondary infertility is common! The actual number of people experiencing secondary infertility is hard to determine, but estimates indicate that at least 30 percent of couples seeking help for infertility have secondary infertility.

Whatever the exact nature of the definition, few disagree that secondary infertility, whether an adjunct to primary infertility or a new challenge all its own, can be a confounding and painful experience that can prevent many from creating the complete family of their dreams.

Wanting an Heir and a Spare?

PERSONAL STORY

After a hard-fought battle to conceive her first child, co-author Jackie smiled, nodded, and promptly began dreaming of more to come. She remembers her drive to "get started again" as follows:

"I want another child," Jackie cried out, only weeks after her long-awaited daughter was born (following a three-and-a-half-year battle with primary infertility). Those first few weeks of babydom were filled with all the promised dreams of baby food commercials everywhere. She and her husband often looked down upon their (then) sleeping baby and commented that if only they "could," they'd have many more. And then the long-awaited daughter "came to."

Jackie relates, "Seriously, the next few months were consumed with feeding issues, sleeping issues, adjustment issues, family issues, and so on. We could barely imagine how we could care for the child we had, let alone another.

"Four years later, our son was born. I was convinced that we were perched on the edge of Camelot. Yet, a mere three years later when trying to negotiate an all-out war between the siblings we had dreamed of, I told my then seven-year-old daughter, 'You're so lucky! I always wanted a sibling. I thought you would too.' In her inimitable manner, she stared at me before responding, 'But, Mommy, you thought wrong!' The best laid plans."

In case you're wondering about moving on down the road before you are even fully in the driver's seat, we give you some good reasons to not rush into trying for another child:

>> **Underestimating the responsibility and work of a new baby:** Perhaps this is one of the reasons why sex is forbidden in the six weeks following delivery. If it wasn't, maybe in that pink (or blue) cloud of new parenting, second babies would be sprouting up everywhere!

>> **Wanting to have a spare:** As a friend of multiples pointed out, doubling your child load doesn't halve your fears of bad things happening. It actually doubles your fears, since it doubles your love.

>> **Trying for that elusive son or daughter:** Trying again just for another gender is a sure way to set yourself up for disappointment. You need look only as far as Jackie's poor grandmother who birthed *seven* daughters prior to finally producing a male heir. Jackie's uncle didn't marry until much later in life and then decided to limit himself to one child whom he adores — who, by the way, is a daughter and will *not* continue the family name anyway!

>> **Giving your child a playmate:** As an only child myself, I (coauthor Jackie) always imagined the "luxury" of having a sibling to share my joys and the responsibilities of dealing with my parents as time went on. All I needed to clear up that misconception was time and eyesight. For as many inseparable siblings that exist, so do those who never speak at all. Biology is no guarantee of love or friendship. Nor is it a promise of commitment. Most families that I have encountered are made up of one child who bears many of the family burdens, including mending fences, dealing with aging relatives, and facilitating communication throughout the flock. Seldom are those responsibilities equally divided. The other lack of equality is in perception. I often wished for a sibling to share my views on my parents, our home, and life itself. Yet, it seems that there are as many different views of a family as there are members. Being raised together and/or in the exact same way does not guarantee a shared vision.

Ideally, the parents of multiple children truly enjoy the experience of raising each child as an individual as well as part of a family. Giving your child a playmate is an added bonus to having more than one child, but not a reason in and of itself. Wanting to share your love again and again is cause for trying again, whatever the process of again may entail.

OUT OF THE MOUTH OF AN ONLY CHILD

Co-author, John "Dr. R" says, "Having an only child has it ups and downs. During one of those father-daughter intense discussion sessions, I naively asked my daughter what I could have done better. As an aside, my suggestion is don't ask! But my daughter told me she often felt alone even though she never asked for a sibling and had lots of cousins nearby. We have a big house, and she had an entire side to herself. Somehow, I thought that was a good thing. Not so much! But her suggestion as to how I could have been a better parent was to have bought her a dog. How simple is that! So, my first tip to parenting may be as simple as the addition of a dog!"

So, if siblings and families bring no promise of inherited closeness through thick and thin, then what *are* the reasons to duplicate or triplicate your efforts in the area of reproduction? We give you some good reasons in the list that follows:

>> **There is a joy and warmth that *can* come in larger and extended families.** If having a houseful of people around all the time makes you happy, a houseful of kids will guarantee it — at least until they grow up and leave the nest.

>> **Siblings take off the pressure that only children are sometimes subject to** — the pressure to be all things to their parents, the total fulfillment of every pre-parent dream.

>> **Siblings can teach each other valuable life lessons** — as well as some not so valuable ones. Sibling influence isn't always beneficial!

>> **You just want another baby.** There's nothing wrong with that, as long as you remember that a new baby will, like the first, grow into an individual person with quirks and characteristics that may have you wondering why you thought this was a good idea in the first place.

Facing Secondary Infertility

Knowing *what* you're dealing with, particularly if it is secondary infertility, doesn't make it any easier. Often, if a woman had little to no problem conceiving a first or second child, the diagnosis of secondary infertility can be confusing. If there were problems the first time around, facing them again can be too much to bear. In the following sections, we discuss some of the different challenges that secondary infertility can present.

Wondering whether it will feel as bad as it did the first time?

Secondary infertility can be less stressful (you have a child), no different, or more stressful (you have a child who requires your time and efforts). Coping with secondary infertility after the stress of infertility sometimes seems unbearable. Perhaps you thought that despite the five years of trying to conceive baby number 1, baby number 2 would just miraculously appear one day. Sometimes that is the case, and conceiving and giving birth to number 1 seems to open the floodgates. More often than not, however, patterns tend to repeat themselves, including the pattern of primary infertility.

The obvious answer is to try the exact same plan that worked for you the first time after you have eliminated things which may have changed and introduced different barriers to pregnancy. If you want to try on your own, hoping for the possible reprieve from Infertility, Part 2, go ahead. But, for your peace of mind and for the sake of giving yourself the best opportunity within a reasonable amount of time, set some parameters. If you haven't conceived naturally within six months to a year (less time if you're over 40), consider going back to the drawing board and/or the original "architect," whether that be your primary physician, OB/GYN, or reproductive endocrinologist.

Until you've given the tried and tested method another go-round, this probably isn't the time to switch doctors, switch protocols, or go out on a brand-new limb. Give the old method at least a few tries before discussing moving to different options with your physician or before you discuss moving to a different physician with your partner.

TIP

If it took fertility treatments to conceive, that does not automatically mean you need to return to the same treatment. Maybe less aggressive methods are needed for the second pregnancy.

Dealing with disbelief: But it worked before . . .

Perhaps one of the most confusing physiological and psychological dilemmas occurs when something worked before and suddenly, apparently without reason, ceases to be effective.

Those struggling with secondary infertility commonly lament:

"We conceived the first month we tried."

"All my husband had to do was look at me and we got pregnant with our first two."

"Conceiving a child was never a problem with us."

Sometimes secondary infertility seems to defy proper or satisfying explanations; other than being a year or two older than you were the last time you had a baby, nothing seems to have changed. Other times, getting to baby number one may have been a challenge, and the fact that it's not going to be easier the second time around is disappointing, but not unexpected.

Begin with a careful review of your first successful go-round. Ask yourself the following:

>> Was it as easy as it seemed the first time or is that merely in comparison to the current struggle of secondary infertility?

>> Did you miscarry two or more times on the way to a healthy baby? Were these miscarriages investigated and found to be due to chromosomal abnormalities, which increase with age?

>> Was it ever suggested, prior to conception, that there might be issues that *could* cause a problem in conceiving or carrying a child (for example, abnormal hormonal levels; structural issues in the uterus, ovaries, or fallopian tubes; a family history of infertility; and so on)?

It's not uncommon to disregard a previous observation, even if it was made by a medical professional, particularly if their diagnosis proved to be wrong, and the proof — the child — is now pulling all the pots and pans out of your cabinet and trying to flush them down the toilet. It's even more common to ignore a family member's recollection of history (for example, every woman on your mother's side went into menopause at the age of 35) if you seem to be the exception.

Conduct your own investigation if you feel that you may have overlooked a comment or a speculation the first time around. Ask your partner if you can't remember correctly or check with the physician whose care you were under prior to the conception of your first child. You may also see this as an opportunity to open or reopen discussion with family members to get an accurate picture of your genetic history when it comes to reproduction. You may well end up finding out that you do indeed have a clean bill of health, but you may also uncover information that can help you get to the bottom of secondary infertility.

Looking for What's Different This Time Around

So, the reproductive system isn't working like it used to — what could be the problem? Similar to primary infertility, finding the answer to secondary infertility can take a while and fill up at least an entire book such as this one. But, for the sake of getting to the point, we list some quick and perhaps not-so-obvious possibilities.

Changes in age

Unless (or even if) your last child was born six weeks ago, time does march on! And from an infertility point of view, that's never a good thing. One of the primary reasons for secondary infertility is the age of the mother. But put this into perspective. If you had your first baby at 27 and now are trying for number 2 at 30, age is not the issue. However, if you had your previous child at age 38 and now you are 41, age becomes a major issue.

Age-related male infertility can also be a consideration, although Father Time does seem to be a bit more forgiving when it comes to the dads. Regardless of whose age we're discussing, by definition, both you and your partner (should both parties remain the same!) will be older when you try to conceive your next child. As we have seen in preceding chapters, fertility declines throughout the years, so the baby that popped up so easily in your 20s may not be as forthcoming in your 30s or 40s. The longer the interval between children, the more likely that time is not on your side. The fact that you have conceived, carried, and delivered a baby are certainly positive predictors of your ability to do so, but realize that many cite the age of the mother as the primary reason for reproductive success. Is this true? Only time will tell.

TECHNICAL STUFF

One interesting way to look at the effect on age is to look at the IVF data that the Society for Assisted Reproductive Technologies (SART) publishes. SART divides people using IVF into age-based categories. If you take the average delivery rates for each age category and graph them, they are almost a straight declining line. For the under-35 crowd, the average is about 45 percent per try. For the 45-and-over crowd, the average is 0. So for the ten years that this represents (35–45), there is a 45 percent drop, which because it is linear means that each year represents a 4.5 percent loss in fertility potential when using IVF. Based upon this logic, at age 38 your chance of a live birth using IVF is close to 20 percent per try, but by age 40 this has declined to 10 percent. So, in just two years your chance of success has been cut in half.

Remember, your age isn't an admonishment. Family planning is all about the spacing of children to fit with your lifestyle, finances, and capabilities. Having children back-to-back is not necessarily the best thing to do, for your health and well-being and that of your family. Most physicians recommend a minimum of one year in between pregnancies in order to allow your body to heal. Considering that sex is a no-no for the first six weeks after delivering, those who have a ten-month difference in the age of their children are ignoring *someone's* advice. While age is certainly a large factor in planning your family, it can't be the *only* thing.

So what now? You're older and having problems. As with primary infertility, if you are over the age of 35 and have not conceived after trying naturally for six months, it may be time to visit your primary care physician, OB/GYN, or reproductive endocrinologist. They will likely run the same battery of tests on you that they would on a patient who presented with primary infertility. Be patient. You want a thorough report, not a speedy one. Two weeks won't make a difference!

Changes in health

As with primary infertility, your overall health does make a difference. While you may still be living the clean life, it doesn't mean that your body hasn't undergone changes all its own. Have you had an increase or decrease in your weight? As we discuss in detail in Chapter 9, BMI (body mass index) can certainly play a part in your fertility or lack thereof. Have you suddenly become a marathon or long-distance runner? This too can affect your metabolism and your body's responses, including the reproductive ones. While these can be positive health changes, they can also upset the delicate balance to which your body may be clinging. Take a look at any lifestyle changes, good or bad, and discuss them with your physician to see if therein lies the culprit.

Occult, or not yet uncovered, chronic or acute illness can also play a role in reversing your fertility. Diabetes, autoimmune disease such as lupus, thyroid problems, and a host of other issues, large and small, can also affect your ability to conceive and may be brewing without your knowledge. If you haven't had a complete physical workup, as well as a gynecological one, now would be the time.

Are you fresh from your first, or last, pregnancy? Still breastfeeding? Or burning the midnight oil trying to rock Junior to sleep? Again, even subtle changes such as a shift in your sleep patterns can wreak havoc on your system, which can leave your fertility in less than fighting shape.

Another thing to consider and discuss with your OB/GYN is any lasting effects from your previous pregnancy(ies). Could you have developed adhesions as a result of a caesarian section? While it is possible to develop adhesions, this is relatively uncommon. One study reviewed the literature and reported a 10 percent increase in infertility after a C-section. However, if the delivery was complicated, then subsequent pregnancies may be difficult. For example, retained placenta requiring a D&C, especially if there was an infection, may cause uterine scarring. Did you have problems with excessive bleeding that may indicate unresolved issues? Make sure that you check out as normal from your last foray into baby making before jumping into the next.

The other large category of problems in secondary infertility is the status of the pelvic organs: Are you having abnormal bleeding (especially between periods) that may be indicative of a fibroid or a polyp in your uterus? Have you had any kind of abdominal surgery since your last delivery (appendectomy, gall bladder surgery, ovarian cyst removal)? All surgery is associated with a risk of scarring (adhesions), which may either block the fallopian tubes or pull them away from the ovaries so that they cannot pick up the ovulated eggs. The good news is that all of these conditions can be identified with the use of appropriate diagnostic tests that your doctor can order.

REMEMBER

Throughout the process of secondary infertility, make it a point to take optimal care of *yourself* through nutrition, rest, and exercise. You will need to be in tiptop shape to handle children in multiple forms; this would be a good time to start the process.

Changes in partners

No, we're not suggesting you go out and look for a new partner if you're not getting pregnant the second time. But you may be focusing on the wrong part of the equation, if you're only thinking about what's different with *you* this time around. Remember, primary infertility is split fairly evenly between women's issues, men's issues, and those issues that are shared by both. If you have changed partners since your last child, perhaps the problem lies with your other half. Has he recently taken up running marathons? Has he developed a passion for spending hours in the Jacuzzi? Has he built a Finnish spa in the backyard that he loves to sit in and binge-watch Netflix?

Just as with you, your partner's health status can change over time as well, having a less-than-desirable effect on his contribution to the baby mix. If you've been checked out in all areas, maybe it's time to check, or recheck, dear old dad.

Dealing with the Emotional Pain

"I'll be happy when . . ."

It's easy to place caveats on joy, particularly when it comes to getting what you want. Remember when you thought/said/prayed/swore that if you could only conceive this one child, you would never ask for anything again? Like many "foxhole prayers," it's easy to forget previous promises. It's human nature.

While some couples are more relaxed the second time around, others bring the same intensity to conceiving number 2 (or number 3!). As with everything in life, it's how you see the situation . . . is the cradle half empty or half full?

Longing for another child

"Another child is a bonus," a friend once said in describing her desire to have another child. She and her husband are forever grateful for their beautiful daughter, and their one and only has given them their dream and a wonderful life to go along with it. This friend has not conceived again since her four-year-old daughter was born, but she has stood by her promise. While she may occasionally dream of giving her child a sibling, she is ultimately happy and satisfied.

While this mindset may be an ideal, it is certainly not shared by most and more often forgotten by many. Secondary infertility can, and often is, every bit as painful as the first go-round. Some friends have said that it can be even more difficult. Suddenly, you are thrust into the world of children where everything seems to come in pairs, if not higher multiples. The "lonely only" child is regarded by many in the child-abundant world as somehow missing out, whether it be in social interaction or family dynamics.

REMEMBER

You can't miss out on what you don't have. Children without siblings tend to be higher achievers, quite social, and often leaders in society. And you can certainly have spoiled, lonely, or maladjusted children, even amongst large sibling groups. "I don't want my only child to grow up spoiled," whine many parents. Yet, upon having baby number 2, many of these families find that indeed they don't have one spoiled child anymore, they now have two! Remember, history repeats itself. Don't assume that another child will miraculously convert you . . . or your parenting skills. That's a job that *you* have to do, whether with 1 child or 20.

Losing support the second time

Another emotional dilemma of secondary infertility can be the lack of support from those who once mopped your tears. "Be thankful for the child you have," family and friends may snap at you impatiently. It's hard to explain that you're immensely grateful and through the joy of conceiving, delivering, and raising your first son or daughter, you have awakened your own inner parent, one that dreams of adding to the flock.

You can't quantify pain, particularly not that of another. Many women grieve as much for the inability to have child number 3 as others do for number 1. Dreams are highly personal and don't generally adjust themselves too easily to life's ups and downs. But, explaining that to family and friends who don't understand can be as challenging as any other aspect of secondary infertility. Even "classic" forms of support, including the internet, often disregard those suffering from secondary infertility, claiming that at "least" they have a child.

PERSONAL STORY

Dr. R says, "I once had a patient who consulted me at age 40. She had four children but wanted to have another. I was much younger then and far smarter than now, so I found this almost inconceivable — pun intended. As so often happens, she taught me invaluable information about the desire to have children. After much discussion and negative predictions, we attempted IVF. It did not work. Again, after considerable consultation and negative predictions on my part, we did IVF again and again and again. And guess what — on that fourth try she conceived and now has child number 5. This single case report is in no way endorsing endless IVF, but it does demonstrate the medical limitation to predicting the outcome. And it emphasizes that each individual has a different drive for children. As a follow-up, she knew when she started to try for number 5 that that would be the last. And true to her plans, five was enough — she did not return for number 6. She thanked me after the delivery because she acknowledged that she knew I did not think it would work. I tried to tell her how much her willingness to work with me helped so many patients who came after her."

You are not alone. Look for specific friends and organizations, whether online or in person, that address some of the issues of secondary infertility. You may be surprised, upon getting to know other parents in your child's playgroup, to find that others have or are dealing with the same issues.

After a particularly painful second-trimester loss of a second child, Jackie was swinging her daughter Ava in the park one day in between two pregnant mothers (just for the record, Jackie was there first!). As Jackie quietly bemoaned her fate, feeling sorry for herself and simultaneously jealous of these strangers, she found herself eavesdropping on their conversation. One of the mothers was sharing how she was just approaching the "critical" point of her pregnancy. As she appeared to be ready to pop, Jackie was a bit confused and continued her nosy vigil. Apparently, she had prematurely delivered her last child at seven months and the baby had not made it. This woman, who Jackie saw as filled with baby and with hope, had endured an even greater tragedy than Jackie had. This is a good reminder to not measure your insides against another's outsides.

Planning Treatment for the Second Time Around

Approaching secondary infertility is not that different from approaching primary infertility. First, what were the circumstances surrounding the previous pregnancy: Was it spontaneous or was it achieved through treatment for infertility? If there was an infertility diagnosis, is that a diagnosis that does not change as a result of a pregnancy? Have you tried long enough: six months if over the age of 35 and one year if younger? Has something changed in your life that would suggest a change in fertility?

Consult your doctor or, if you were working with an REI, consult with that REI.

At this point, diagnostic testing will usually be in order. Check all three areas associated with normal fertility: eggs, female anatomy, and — yes — the male.

Based upon the results of these tests, you can choose a path that gives you the best chance for another successful pregnancy.

Success rates for secondary infertility are the same as for primary infertility because they are based upon the diagnosis. If the diagnosis has changed — for example, age-related infertility — then the chance of success may be less than it was for the first pregnancy. Only your medical provider can determine this.

2
Taking the Initiative

Find out how to improve your efforts by looking at ovulation predictor kits and timing sex right.

Be aware of some special situations that may throw a wrench in your plans, including age and certain diseases.

Get modern medicine on your side.

Look at diets and supplements and what effect they may have.

Manage emotions and relationships while on the bumpy road of fertility issues.

Chapter **6**

DIY Methods to Increase Your Chances

After you start trying to get pregnant, you expect results — that's human nature. But Mother Nature isn't always on your timetable, and you may find yourself still trying after a few months and anxious to step up the pace a bit with some scientific aids. In this chapter, you can find out about some low-tech but helpful methods of trying to pin down an elusive positive pregnancy test.

Many women can read their bodies' signals well enough to pinpoint ovulation almost to the minute; others need scientific aids to help pin down exactly when they're ovulating. We discuss both the simple and the scientific in this chapter.

We also look at how all this planning may affect the romance in your relationship and give you some ideas for keeping the spark alive. In addition, we help you avoid sparks in your relationships with family and friends when you're under stress and give advice about living through major stressors like the holidays — or your friends' baby showers.

REMEMBER

Ovulation is the monthly release of an egg from your ovary. Ovulation is the one time during the month that you can actually get pregnant. Ovulation does not give you information about the quality of the egg that is released — only that it is released. Your window of opportunity is approximately two to three days.

Reading Your Body's Signals and Signs — An Incomplete Story

Do you cringe a little when you hear someone say, "I know exactly when I am ovulating"? How do they know? Is that why they can get pregnant and you can't? Well, it's not as simple as that. Knowing your body is helpful, but you also have to understand what to do with what you know.

Checking for signs that really matter: Your menses

One of the first signs fertility specialists look for on the road to conceiving is the average menstrual cycle length: the time from day one of one menses until day one of the next menses. If the cycle length varies, then help is probably needed, and it is time to consult a physician. But what if the cycle length is relatively regular? Somewhat surprisingly, the American College of Obstetricians and Gynecologists (ACOG) defines a normal cycle length as between 24 and 38 days. Most clinicians look at 28–32 days as a normal cycle length. What is important is not necessarily the actual length but the regularity. Longer cycles that are always the same length are probably better than longer cycles that vary by more than a few days or cycles that were previously 28 to 29 days and are shortened to less than 26 days. (We look at some menstrual irregularities in greater detail in Chapter 11.)

The International Federation of Gynecology and Obstetrics (FIGO) defines irregular cycles as disturbances in frequency, with too few (*oligomenorrhea*) being one or two menses within a 90-day period and too frequent being more than four menses within a 90-day period. So, the summation of all of this: If you have more than two menses but less than five within a 90-day window and your average cycle length is between 24 and 38 days, you have regular cycles. That was easy — *not!* Frankly, if you presented this definition to your gynecologist, that physician probably wouldn't agree with this cumbersome method of defining cycle regularity. A more common-sense approach is this: If you think your cycles are regular, then they are.

Did I ovulate or not? That is the question

So now that you have determined you have regular cycles, is there a way to improve pregnancy chances? Here comes that overly emphasized word: "ovulation." Technically, *ovulation* is the process of releasing an egg. With perhaps no (or at most very few) exceptions and contrary to what you may have been told, women with regular cycles ovulate. The real issues are when the egg is released and what its quality is. Releasing a structurally damaged egg each month on time will not result in a successful pregnancy. (This is dealt with in Chapter 16.)

So, what about timing? To begin, what are the absolute limits — the immovable force? Sperm last within the female for up to five days but reasonably at least two or three. The egg, on the other hand, lasts at best 18 to 24 hours after it is released. So, having intercourse less than every two or three days around the time of ovulation or not having intercourse until 24 hours after the egg is released will be unsuccessful — this is the basis for the "rhythm method" of birth control. So, if you have been using the rhythm method of birth control, just do the opposite and it should work — if only! Despite popular belief, not all women ovulate on day 14 of their cycles. And knowing when you ovulate is crucial to your success in getting pregnant because sperm and egg can only get together if they're both in the same place at the same time. Having sex too early — or as little as one day too late — can reduce your chance of success.

This doesn't mean you have to have sex at a precise instance, or even a precise day, to get pregnant. We hope this will take some performance anxiety off both of you!

Counting the days — correctly

Most women ovulate 14 days before the start of a new menstrual cycle. So, if your cycles are 28 days apart, you ovulate on or about day 14; if your cycles are 25 days long, you ovulate earlier, around day 11. If your cycles are long, like 33 days, you don't ovulate until day 19. This is why it's so easy to miss the right day for conception; most women don't have on-the-dot, regular-as-clockwork periods and may ovulate on a different day each month.

TIP

To figure out when you're most likely to be ovulating, you need to keep track of your menstrual cycles each month. Having an idea of when you're most likely to ovulate, combined with simple observation of your fertility signs, can result in success if you've just been missing the mark every month.

Some women can chart their periods back for years; they religiously mark an "X" on the calendar when their period starts, and they always know exactly when their next period is due. Others are always surprised when their periods start, either because their cycles are irregular or because they never mark anything down on the calendar.

There are also as many period tracking apps as you may have periods! They keep a detailed record of how long and how far apart your cycles are — based on the information *you* enter.

If you're the regular, record-keeping type, it will be easy for you to figure out when you're ovulating. If you're irregular and/or disorganized, it may take you a month or two to determine when you're ovulating. Never fear, though; your body has ways of telling you when ovulation is approaching, and we can help even the most irregular/disorganized women figure it out.

Determining the shelf life of eggs and sperm

Do you have to have sex at the exact moment of ovulation to get pregnant? No, thank goodness, or getting pregnant would be much harder than it already is! Fortunately, both sperm and egg have a lifespan that, although short, allows them to stick around long enough to meet even if your timing isn't perfect. But what if you were a rabbit? To release an egg you would need to have intercourse because they are what are called reflex ovulators — they must have coitus to ovulate. But having coitus for rabbits is not an all-the-time thing. No! The female undergoes hormonal changes that prepare the egg. When everything is set, the female is receptive to the male, which is termed "in heat," and will copulate. Female rabbits can come into heat at any time during the year as opposed to other animals that reproduce based upon the seasons. What if you were a roe deer? Deer are seasonal breeders so that they deliver when the fawn has the best chance of surviving. Here animals copulate in late fall then the males "rut." The egg is fertilized, an embryo is created, and then the embryo stops its development until the spring (*embryonic diapause*). Nature is truly amazing in the variety of ways to reproduce.

Sperm live longer than eggs; in the proper cervical mucus (we talk about cervical mucus more in the section "Observing cervical mucus"), sperm can live as long as five days, although two to three days is a more average lifespan for sperm. So, you can have sex up to a few days before ovulation and have sperm ready and waiting for an egg to appear.

Eggs, on the other hand, go bad fast; after ovulation, eggs live only 24 hours or so. That means that if you have sex more than a few hours after ovulation, there won't be time for sperm to reach the egg before it disintegrates.

Timing is everything — but don't make it too complicated!

The proper timing is necessary to get pregnant, but you don't have to have sex at the exact moment of ovulation to improve your chances. Pregnancy rates are the same whether couples have sex on the day of ovulation, the day before, or two days before. In contrast, having sex just one day too late (after ovulation) results in no pregnancies.

It's better (and probably less nerve-wracking) to have sperm waiting for the egg by having sex every other day around the time you're expecting to ovulate, or even all month, if you're feeling that energetic! Some people fear that having inter-course too frequently may decrease their chances for success. You may find it sur-prising, but some men actually increase their sperm counts by ejaculating more frequently. While frequent ejaculation more typically decreases the sperm count, it does not reduce the count to where it reduces the chance for pregnancy.

The point is that although timing is essential, you don't need to spend the whole month on pins and needles, wondering if now is the right time for conception. Predicting ovulation is a matter of watching the calendar and having a rough idea of when you may be ovulating and observing your body's natural signals that pre-cede ovulation.

Recording your basal body temperature (BBT)

Recording your basal body temperature (BBT) is one of the oldest methods of pre-dicting ovulation. A basal body temperature is just a long-winded way of saying your individual normal temperature. The theory of why recording your tempera-ture may help achieve a pregnancy is based upon the fact that progesterone causes an increase in temperature. Many other things throughout the day also raise the temperature. So, taking the temperature in the "basal" state (meaning an early morning period before any activity such as eating, moving, and so on) tries to remove all of the other influences on why the temperature changes and leave only a rise in progesterone.

The menstrual cycle has two phases separated by ovulation: In the first half, pro-gesterone is very low, whereas in the second half, after ovulation, the progester-one rises. Thus, measuring the temperature should identify when the cycle moves from pre-ovulation to post-ovulation. However, remember that intercourse needs to occur within 18–24 hours after the egg is released. So, the basal body tempera-ture (BBT) chart indicates ovulation after ovulation and not before.

A rather interesting study compared the day of temperature rise (in other words, the time to have intercourse) with ultrasound-documented actual ovulation. Ovulation occurred on the first day of the rise in temperature for 12 percent of the people and 69.5 percent ovulated more than 24 hours after the surge. In 17.5 percent, ovulation had occurred prior to the rise such that waiting for the rise to have intercourse would have made it too late. So, in roughly one out of five, the BBT would have reduced the chance of pregnancy.

TIP

Keeping a BBT is not harmful, but for women who have regular cycles, simply having frequent intercourse as described previously is all that is needed.

If you want to keep a BBT, then this method of predicting ovulation is simple but requires a certain amount of determination and a good memory. You need to remember to take your temperature every morning *before* you get up. Most doctors recommend that you not get up, eat, drink, or smoke before taking your temperature because any activity at all will raise your temperature, and eating or drinking will raise or lower it, depending on what you have.

TIP

Many charts are available to help you chart your temperature (you can just use the one we've provided in the front of this book!), but you can easily make one yourself, or, you can turn to your cell phone (again!) and seek out one of the *many* apps that can help you track BBT!

But, if you are feeling industrious, here's a DIY version:

1. **Draw a graph.**

   You can use graph paper or just draw the lines yourself; you're not going to be graded on neatness!

2. **Mark off spaces for 30 days.**

   Use more if your periods run longer. Mark these spaces on the bottom of the page (horizontally).

3. **Mark off spaces for temperature readings from between 97 degrees and 99.5 degrees in one-tenth increments down the side of the paper (vertically).**

4. **Take your temperature before getting out of bed in the morning or before performing any other activities.**

5. **Mark down your morning temperature to the exact one-tenth of a degree.**

6. **Connect the dots.**

   You'll notice that your temperature is lowest when your period first starts.

7. **Have sex every other day, to cover all the bases.**

8. **Look for a subtle drop in temperature, followed by a sustained rise in temperature, meaning a rise for more than three days.**

   Your temperature should rise at least 0.5 degrees and remain elevated. The drop occurs around ovulation, and the rise indicates an increase in your progesterone levels.

9. **If you're having sex every other day, you should be covered at the time of ovulation by having waiting sperm ready for the released egg.**

   If you've been a little lax in this, make sure you have sex the day of your temperature drop.

This method has a few drawbacks:

>> **You need to be scrupulous about taking your temperature and recording it so that you don't forget it.**

>> **You have to keep your chart for the whole month.** If you're the type who loses things easily, keep a few copies of the chart around in case you lose one.

>> **Your temperature can be influenced by factors other than hormones.** If you're sick, even small temperature fluctuations may make your chart inaccurate, and you'll think you've ovulated when you actually have the flu. Alcohol, too little or too much sleep, and subtle illnesses can all change your temperature.

Your BBT can also give you an idea of whether you're pregnant. If your temperature stays elevated more than 15 days, there's a good chance that you're pregnant — unless, of course, you have the flu.

TIP

If you're prone to losing paper charts, you may be interested in a digital thermometer that stores your previous temperature. This device is handy in case you forget to write your temperature down one morning. Digital thermometers are a little more expensive than glass ones, but not more than $10–20 for a reasonable one, although you can spend a few hundred dollars for a high-end model — not necessary! Or you can store your last temperature even with a glass thermometer by *not* shaking it down immediately after using it. This tip is especially convenient if you don't have time to record your temperature right away. The mercury will stay at your temperature point until it's shaken down.

Observing cervical mucus

Cervical mucus changes consistency around the time of ovulation. Right after your period stops, cervical mucus is very thick, which makes it difficult for sperm to penetrate. Cervical mucus is normally thick (viscous) because it protects the uterus from invading bacteria from the vagina.

Cervical mucus increases in amount and becomes thinner under the influence of estrogen. In the first half of the cycle, estrogen levels start low, and as the egg unit increases, the estrogen increases. After ovulation, the mucus becomes thick again under the influence of progesterone. Many women can assess the nature of their mucus and therefore can use changes in cervical mucus to determine when ovulation occurs and thus time their intercourse. One study found that 76 percent of the women monitoring their cervical mucus identified their ovulation within 24 hours of the actual ovulation. If the window was expanded by 24 hours, the accuracy increased to 97 percent — not bad for a simple examination of the cervix.

In addition to becoming thinner and stretchy, cervical mucus becomes more alkaline, because sperm live longer in an alkaline environment. You can check the acidity or alkalinity of cervical mucus with an over-the-counter product called TesTape, which comes in a long thin roll of yellow paper. You tear off a small piece of the yellow paper and wrap it around the end of your finger. Next, you reach into your vagina and touch the paper to the end of your cervix. Then you bring out the piece of paper to see whether it turns color. It will first turn an olive color a few days before ovulation and then turn dark green or blue when your cervical mucus is alkaline, as it is right before you ovulate.

After ovulation, cervical mucus again becomes thick, cloudy or white in color, and scant.

Feeling your cervix

If you have no idea how to find your cervix, it's pretty easy. You just carefully insert your clean finger into your vagina until you feel a firm bump that feels somewhat like the end of your nose. That's your cervix.

You'll notice that your cervix itself also changes at different times of the month; around ovulation, it becomes softer, feeling more like your lips in firmness, and feels slightly open in the center. You'll also feel an increase in moisture. All these changes, like the changes in cervical mucus, help the sperm get through the cervix.

The cervix also moves to a lower and more central position, so it's easier to find with your finger, which means it's also in a more direct line with ejaculated sperm.

OUCH! I THINK I OVULATED

About 20 percent of women have pain called *mittelschmerz* (German for "middle pain") when they ovulate. The pain seems to be caused by blood and fluid irritating the tissues around the ovary after it releases from the follicle. Sometimes a small amount of vaginal bleeding occurs with ovulation, too.

Mittelschmerz can be a very precise way of pinpointing exactly when you ovulate; the only downside of using mittelschmerz to help you conceive is that it usually occurs at the time of ovulation. In other words, once you've ovulated, the clock is ticking and your egg is on a countdown with destruction within 24 hours or so, so you've got to have sex quickly.

Keeping a Fertility Chart

Although a fertility chart sounds exotic and complicated, it's nothing more than a record of observation of your body's natural fertility signals: your temperature, your cervical mucus, and changes in your cervix itself. You can make a simple chart yourself, recording your daily temperature on a graph with cervical changes and mucus written in underneath, or you can download one of the many fertility charts found on the internet.

Maybe you write everything down on little pieces of paper and keep losing them and think you'd do better to keep track of your data on your computer. There are programs you can download to allow you to keep everything organized online — just don't let your boss see you poring over your "data" at work!

In today's digital world, keeping a chart is passé. There are numerous apps that people can use. For those who want to do charting, review a number of apps and choose the one that works well for you — there is no magic in data keeping. Whether or not you're using a good app in most cases won't change the etiology of your infertility and thus will not increase your chance for pregnancy. However, for couples just starting on their infertility journey, as many as 75 percent do not know when the fertile window actually occurs. Using an app may speed the process by targeting the fertile window, making it less likely to miss an opportunity. Interestingly, apps have proven effective for *contraception* — hardly what an infertility patient needs. Of course, you could use one of these apps and just do the opposite from what it says.

Predicting Ovulation: Kits, Sticks, and Software

Maybe a month of trying to get pregnant has gone by — or maybe two, three, or four months — and you're beginning to feel frustrated and even a little scared that you're never going to get pregnant. Go back and read the statistics in Chapter 1 to remind yourself that nature is inefficient and remember that everyone in your family took six months to get pregnant. You may be thinking, "That's all well and good to read about," but you want to do something *now.* There must be something more scientific and more successful that you can do. You thought that you hit all the right days to have sex for the last few months, but maybe you're still missing the right day or misinterpreting your body's ovulation signs. This section covers a few ways to monitor your ovulation cycle that are more scientific than stretching cervical mucus and counting calendar days. Hopefully, one will work for you!

Using an ovulation predictor kit

Ovulation predictor kits (OPKs) are a popular way to test if and when you ovulate. The tests measure the amount of LH (luteinizing hormone) found in your urine. LH generally rises 24 to 36 hours before ovulation; the rise of LH is called your *LH surge*. You should have sex the day or two before ovulation and the day of ovulation to improve your chances of getting pregnant.

OPKs are easy to find; every drugstore carries them. They use your urine, a cheap and abundant substance, to test for ovulation. The sticks are small enough to carry around with you.

The OPKs, or "pee sticks" as they're called, have some drawbacks. Certain women, such as women with polycystic ovaries (see Chapter 7), may have a high LH all the time, so the kits will always be positive. Women over 40 or those in premature ovarian failure (POF) may also have a higher than normal LH, because LH and FSH (follicle-stimulating hormone) both rise in POF. Some tests are also difficult to read, require several steps that need to be carefully done for good results, or start to show positive only when the LH reaches 40mIU/ml, the International Standard for an LH surge.

TIP

Most kits show a positive as a line as dark as or darker than the control line. Read the test at exactly the time indicated; sometimes the lines darken over a few hours, but that doesn't mean you're having a surge.

For many, reading an OPK can be a frustrating test of judgment and trial and error. Is the test line lighter than the control line? By how much? Is it darker today than it was yesterday? What about in bright light? All of these may seem like legit- imate questions when determining the right time of ovulation, but keep in mind that the best indication of a surge is a test line that is *as dark as or darker than* the control line.

The kits are harder to use if you don't have regular cycles; unless you know approximately when you ovulate each month, you may use up a lot of sticks trying to figure out when your surge starts. If you have regular cycles, you can start test- ing about 16 days before you expect your next period, but if your cycles are irreg- ular, you need to start testing earlier to make sure that you don't miss the big-O day. Table 6-1 can help you determine when to start testing. But once again, if you have regular cycles, do you really need to do testing?

OPKs aren't cheap; they cost about $4–5 per stick, and you have to buy them in multiples. Digital readers are about $40 for one reader and 20 test sticks. A stan- dard fertility monitor will cost $230 for one fertility predictor and $65 for 30 test strips. You'll use one stick each time you test, and you need to test every 12 to 24 hours around the time of ovulation to accurately catch your surge. Resist the urge to buy the cheaper kits. They may not register lower LH levels, and they may be much harder to read. As a result, you use up more sticks because you're showing all your friends and asking their opinion on which line is darker. In addition to using up a lot of sticks, you may use up a lot of friends, too!

TABLE 6-1

Counting Days, Saving Sticks

Length of Normal Cycle	Start Testing This Many Days After Your Last Period
40	23
39	22
38	21
37	20
36	19
35	18
34	17
33	16
32	15
31	14
30	13
29	12
28	11
27	10
26	9
25	8
24	7
23	6
22	5
21	4

So is it worth it? A recent study, called a systematic review, concluded from numerous articles that home urinary testing may improve the chances for achieving a pregnancy but couldn't give any further data as to how much it helped. Because this is a costly and time-consuming endeavor, you may want to think twice about using such an uncertain method to help you get pregnant.

OPKs register only when your surge has begun, so you won't be able to time sex as accurately for the two days immediately before ovulation. Also, the strips must be stored at temperatures between 59 and 86 degrees Fahrenheit to ensure their accuracy, so carrying them around in a purse can be problematic unless you live in a totally climate-controlled world.

Also remember that the test measures a concentration of LH in the urine. This means that if the urine is too concentrated (like first morning urine), the test may show a false positive even if you are not surging. Along the same line, if your urine is too diluted (like if you've just finished a 32-ounce soda), it won't show a positive test, even if you're ovulating. A good rule to follow is to do the test about two hours after eating, after you haven't had anything to drink for an hour or so, and the urine should look yellow, but not too dark.

Adding computer power with a fertility monitor

If you want to go a little higher tech than the OPKs, you may be interested in a fertility monitor. A fertility monitor works a little differently than the standard OPK. These devices are actually small computers that store data about your cycle to tell you when you're going to ovulate. They're more labor intensive; you need to start testing the first day of your period and test every day around the same time. Morning is recommended as the best time to test. Because they test both estrogen and LH levels, fertility monitors can better predict ovulation about five days before it occurs, giving you a better chance to have sex two days before ovulation.

The fertility monitor can be used if you're taking fertility medications, unlike some of the one-use OPK urine tests. It also "sets" itself to your cycle if you're somewhat irregular.

These monitors are expensive — about $300–400 for a good one — and you also need to buy the sticks. Like the less expensive kits, they may not be accurate if you are menopausal or breastfeeding, have polycystic ovaries (see Chapter 7) and a normally higher than normal LH level, or are taking tetracycline antibiotics, which means they won't be able to tell if you've released an egg.

Just spit here — the saliva test

This is one of the newest and most interesting ovulation prediction tests out there; it tests your saliva for a rise in salt content, which rises as your estrogen rises. This method has several advantages:

>> **Carrying this around isn't too conspicuous.** The tube that holds the lens you place saliva on and the tiny lighted microscope you look through are all contained in what looks like a tube of lipstick.

>> **Because the lens can be washed and reused, this is a one-time purchase.**

>> **According to the U.S. Food and Drug Administration, this method is about 98 percent accurate.**

>> **Unlike ovulation kits, which use urine, these can be used any old time, not just when your bladder is full.** Peeing on demand can be hard, but you always have saliva. Plus, you can use the saliva kit on the bus, which is out of the question with urine-based OPKs!

Disadvantages to this method include the following:

>> **It's fairly expensive, about $60.**

>> **It's slightly more complicated to use.** You have to take the lens out and put it back properly or you won't read it correctly. You also risk the possibility of breaking or scratching the lens.

>> **Also, as with OPKs and TesTape, this tells you only when you're about to ovulate.**

The saliva test can be done every day starting at day one of your cycle; at first, you'll see only little dots (of salt) when you look through the viewing piece. As ovulation gets closer, you'll see what look like ferns (see Figure 6-1); when the ferns cover the whole slide, you're about to ovulate. It takes about five minutes for the slide to dry so you can accurately read it.

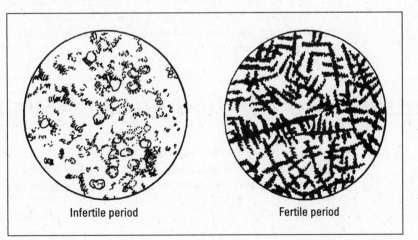

FIGURE 6-1:
Ferning appears on a saliva test when you're close to ovulation.

Infertile period   Fertile period

© John Wiley & Sons, Inc.

The saliva tests have an advantage over urine-based OPKs, which will only give you a yes or no answer as to whether you're ready to ovulate. The saliva test gives you more advance warning that ovulation is coming. With the saliva test, you can also avoid some of the false positives from LH kits and the fluctuations in temperature that can throw off results of the basal body temperature method (see "Recording your basal body temperature (BBT)," earlier in this chapter).

Even though the saliva test is initially expensive, it may be cheaper than buying ovulation predictor kits every month. And if you do get pregnant, you can use it after you deliver to *prevent* pregnancy until you want another baby! This method of birth control is approved by the Catholic Church and in some cases is thought to be more accurate than the rhythm method of counting days to avoid pregnancy.

Saliva monitors that store and analyze data, just like the urine monitors, are now available. These are quite expensive, however — $200 to $500.

TIP

If you already have a microscope and slides hanging around the house from a left-over science project or something, you can test saliva at home without any of the expensive packaged equipment. Put some saliva on a slide and take a look! You should also know that most doctors prefer the urine LH tests for accuracy.

Sperm testing at home

While you're doing all this home testing on yourself, it may seem like a good idea to get your partner in on the act with a little home testing of his own.

It's now possible to do a very rudimentary semen analysis at home; this method won't give you detailed information, but it will let you check out two semen samples to see whether the concentration of sperm meets the accepted fertility level of 20 million/ml. The simpler at-home tests cost about $50. Newer technology takes advantage of smartphone apps. A kit can be purchased, and the phone can be used for the analysis.

Getting through the Two-Week Wait

The *two-week wait* (2WW) is the time between ovulation and your next expected period, when you're on pins and needles waiting for enough time to pass to be able to look for pregnancy symptoms or to buy the ever-popular home pregnancy test.

You, like many women before you, may spend this time analyzing every possible pregnancy symptom ("Are my breasts tender?" "Am I peeing more?" "Was that a twinge of nausea?") looking for something — anything! — that indicates success in the pregnancy department.

The 2WW may seem like 1,000 years, and it's not likely that much will divert you from constantly thinking about pregnancy. If it's possible, putting pregnancy completely out of your mind may help you maintain your sanity; staying busy at work, going on vacation, taking up a new and incredibly complex hobby, or cleaning your house from top to bottom may help keep you occupied and away from the home pregnancy tests until two weeks have passed.

Looking for a Positive with Home Pregnancy Tests (HPTs)

If you think that you used a lot of ovulation predictor sticks, wait until you start using the home pregnancy tests (HPTs)! They're widely advertised on TV, depicting a couple excitedly waiting for the good news or a tense woman alone hoping for the happy news that she's *not* pregnant. The sections that follow give you all you need to know about HPTs.

Getting to know HPTs

The first home tests were available in the 1970s, and everyone probably would have been a little more squeamish about leaving them in the fridge next to the milk if they had known that they contained prepackaged red blood cells. These tests were very sensitive to movement, so you had to put them someplace quiet and leave them alone for a few hours. When you finally peeked into the fridge, you looked for the dark ring at the bottom of the tube — that's what appeared if you were pregnant. The clumping together of red blood cells if you were pregnant is what formed the ring.

TECHNICAL STUFF

All the tests, from the 1920s on, measured hCG (human chorionic gonadotropin), the hormone released by the implantation of the embryo and the growing placenta. The newest tests are very sensitive and are able to detect hCG concentrations of 10, 20, or 25mIU/ml (the smaller the number, the higher the sensitivity), which usually occur about ten days after ovulation or about four days prior to the time you would miss your first period. Even though most tests are accurate a few days *before* your period is due, a negative test at that time may not be accurate. You may have had a late implantation, or you may have ovulated a day or two after you thought you did. Another test should be done a few days later if your period still hasn't started.

TIP

The accuracy of any home pregnancy test depends on how closely you follow the directions, when you ovulated, and the sensitivity of the test. If you test too soon, you may get a false negative.

If you are pregnant, the average level of hCG 10 days post ovulation is 25mIU/ml; it is 50mIU/ml 12 days post ovulation, and 100mIU/ml 14 days after you ovulate. Keep in mind that these numbers are averages; your number may be higher or lower and still be perfectly normal. Also, as with LH kits, the concentration of the urine can play a large role in whether or not the test turns positive. Because any positive value is important, using first morning (most concentrated) urine is a good idea.

REMEMBER

Blood tests measure hCG with much more accuracy, detecting concentrations less than 5mIU/ml. (We talk about pregnancy blood tests more in Chapter 13.)

Using HPTs

Home pregnancy tests are available in every drugstore, so if you're buying in bulk because you're a compulsive tester, you can hit every grocery store and drugstore in town, and no one will know that you're compulsive — er, anxious to know! These tests give fast results, usually in two to five minutes. Most tell you to not urinate for four hours before you test so the concentration of the hormone will be high. Some kits suggest that you urinate in a cup and dip the wand into it, and other kits suggest peeing directly on the stick. Some show a positive as a little plus sign; others want you to drag all your friends back in to the bathroom (if you still have any friends left after ovulation) and have them compare the control line to the test line to see whether they match. Usually a positive is indicated by a test line that's as dark as or darker than the control, and many women drive themselves mad staring at the line trying to determine its exact shade of purple. Some tests now eliminate the "match game" by spelling out, "Yes, you're pregnant" or some variation if your test is positive.

Don't let the test sit around before looking at it, as some test results will change after an hour or two and will not be accurate. See Figure 6-2 for positive and negative results on a home pregnancy test.

Table 6-2 lists the common brands of home pregnancy tests and the lowest number they claim will register a positive result. Sensitivity is measured in units called *mIU*, which means milli-International Units per milliliter.

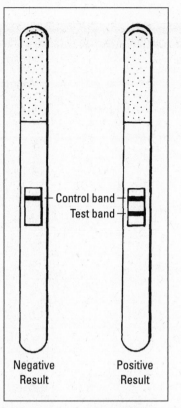

FIGURE 6-2:
Are you pregnant
or not?

Control band
Test band

Negative
Result

Positive
Result

© John Wiley & Sons, Inc.

TABLE 6-2

Home Pregnancy Test Sensitivity Levels

Home Pregnancy Test	Lowest Sensitivity Level
AimStick Pregnancy Test Strip	20 mIU
AccuHome Midstream Pregnancy Test	25 mIU
Answer Early Result Pregnancy Test	25 mIU
Answer Pregnancy Test (Cup)	25 mIU
Clearblue +/–	25 mIU
Confirm 1-Step Pregnancy Test	25 mIU
Equate Pregnancy Test	25 mIU
First Response Early Result Pregnancy Test	25 mIU

(continued)

TABLE 6-2 *(continued)*

Home Pregnancy Test	Lowest Sensitivity Level
One Step Be Sure Pregnancy Test	25 mIU
Walgreen Digital	25 mIU
e.p.t. Home Pregnancy Test (one line = not pregnant; two lines = pregnant)	40 mIU
e.p.t. Certainty Digital Test	40 mIU
Fact Plus Pregnancy Test	40 mIU
Clearblue Digital	50 mIU
CVS Cartridge Pregnancy Test	50 mIU
CVS Midstream Pregnancy Test	50 mIU
Drug Emporium Brand Pregnancy Test	50 mIU
e.p.t. +/− Test	50 mIU
early Pregnancy test	50 mIU
RiteAid Brand Pregnancy Test	50 mIU
Target Brand Pregnancy Test	50 mIU
Walmart Brand Pregnancy Test	50 mIU
Walgreens Pregnancy Test	100 mIU

Understanding false positives

False positive results are rare in home pregnancy tests. Today, HPTs have a greater than 90 percent accuracy. However, you may have a false positive if

>> You're taking injections of the hormone hCG to induce ovulation or for any other reason; it takes 14 days for 10,000U of hCG (a standard dose) to completely clear your system.

>> You recently had a miscarriage or ectopic pregnancy, and the hCG levels have not dropped to a negative range yet. (This can take up to four weeks.)

WARNING

>> You have an extremely rare form of cancer called a choriocarcinoma. Choriocarcinoma occurs in 2–7/100,000 pregnancies. The cancer is a cancer of the cells that would normally form the placenta. This cancer usually follows a full-term birth, miscarriage, or other pregnancy loss. This is a fast-growing cancer, so if you recently had a pregnancy loss of any kind and have a positive home pregnancy test and heavy bleeding, you *must* see a doctor immediately.

Understanding false negatives

The urinary test for pregnancy can show that you are not pregnant when in fact you are. These are called false negatives. The most common reason for this is that you test the urine too soon after ovulation. A second problem arises if you do not wait long enough to read the test. Finally, the urine may be too diluted. Using the first morning urine can decease the false-negative rate. The danger of a false negative is when there is an uncommon problem of an ectopic pregnancy, which is when a pregnancy implants outside the uterus — usually the fallopian tube.

WARNING

If you are undergoing fertility treatment, particularly IVF, you may be cautioned about using HPTs because of the false negative issue. If you use an HPT anyway (we know you might) it is best to check with your clinic before you stop any medication or start a new treatment cycle. Coauthor Lisa knows firsthand how "I got a negative" can turn into "Oh my, you're pregnant." She recalls one patient who had finished a Clomid/IUI cycle and reported a negative HPT and a menses. Later, when a baseline ultrasound was done to start the next treatment cycle (an IVF cycle), there was a gestational sac in the uterus! The patient had done the test too early and didn't explain that her "menses" was only spotting. This is why many clinics require a blood test to confirm whether you are pregnant or not. The real danger with a false negative is that the person assumes one negative test means there is no chance she could be pregnant and misses the presence of an ectopic pregnancy.

Chapter **7**

Considering Special Circumstances

Going through infertility treatments is generally about as "special" as one wants to be, but you may have other problems that make it harder than usual to get pregnant. Do you have issues? We have answers!

In this chapter, we talk about the effects of age on getting pregnant and look at some diseases that can make getting pregnant a challenge. We also help you decide what to do if you had a tubal ligation in the past and want to get pregnant now.

Calculating Your Fertility Odds as an "Older" Mom

More and more women and men are delaying childbirth until later years. In fact, over 20 percent of new mothers are now over the age of 35, and the average age for women to have their first baby is now over 25.

Checking out the statistics

But Mother Nature is apparently not one for statistics (see Table 7-1). For women, optimum fertility occurs when you're about 18 years old. It stays pretty constant in your 20s and then begins a gradual downward turn at about the age of 30. By the time you turn 35, the process has accelerated. When you hit 40, the slide becomes even more dramatic; 33 percent of women over 35 have some difficulty getting pregnant, and 66 percent of women over 40 have infertility issues.

TABLE 7-1 Statistics for Age versus Infertility, Miscarriage, and Chromosomal Abnormalities

Age	Under 30	30–35	36–40	41–45	Over 45
Percentage of women who have difficulty conceiving (trying to conceive naturally for one year without success)	20%	20%	33%	66%	95%
Miscarriage rate	15%	15%	17%	34%	53%
Rate of chromosomal abnormalities	1 in 526	1 in 385	1 in 192	1 in 66	1 in 21

TECHNICAL STUFF

Why the decrease in pregnancy and rise in miscarriage as you get older? It's because of the increase in chromosomal abnormalities in the embryos created by your eggs as they age. At age 20, your chance of having a baby with a chromosomal abnormality such as Down syndrome is 1 in 526. By age 30, the risk is 1 in 385; by age 35, 1 in 192; by age 40, 1 in 66; and by age 45, 1 in 21. And this is just the tip of the proverbial iceberg. Information from *pre-implantation genetic diagnosis* (PGD) strongly indicates that the majority of embryos in women over 40 are chromosomally abnormal. Of course, most of these don't implant, and those that do are usually miscarried. That's why the miscarriage rate increases with age.

Understanding how much age matters

We say this often throughout this book: Human reproduction is a very inefficient process *at any age*. When a woman is 35, one out of four embryos is abnormal; this number increases to one out of two at age 40, and five out of six at age 45. Although these statistics certainly show that age is a factor in conceiving, remember that you're an individual, not a statistic, and your odds may be better or worse than the statistics.

And remember, once you are pregnant, advanced maternal age (a lovely medical term!) contributes to an increased risk of chromosomal defects, of which Down syndrome is one.

PERSONAL STORY

BEING AN "OLDER" MOM — JACKIE'S PERSONAL OPINION!

Under the category of "things I didn't expect in life," having children in my 40s was certainly one of them! Infertility was another one. On the upside, I always hoped but never dreamed that I would find a partner as wonderful as my husband. And *he* was worth waiting for! That all said, I am the proud "older" mom of a beautiful daughter and son, and I wouldn't change a thing.

Being an older mom certainly has its downsides, primarily if you "aged" while waiting to conceive! But, for me, and many of my "older mom" friends, we see the glass as more than half full. As an older mom, we may lack a bit in energy (although truth be told, I'm in better cardiovascular shape than I was in my 20s), but I believe that many of us more than make up for this when it comes to maturity and stability in our finances, education, and careers.

I often said that I could barely figure out what I wanted to wear when I was in my peak reproductive years (generally classified as younger than 27 years old), let alone raise a child or two. While others in their 20s may certainly possess a more grown-up attitude than I did, we're not always ready for "things we don't expect, plan for, and can't control," like not meeting a partner on nature's timetable and ensuing age-related facing infertility. At the end of the day, we all do the best we can with what we have and what we "got," and being an older mom is a pretty amazing gift.

Consider Table 7-1 to give you a better picture of how age affects not only fertility but the risk of birth defects.

As with everything, there's good news and bad news to being an older mom . . . or dad. The best we can tell you is to use age as a suggested guideline. Fertility, most often, decreases *over time.* You will not become infertile overnight. Indeed, studies have shown that many women experience *perimenopause* (the stage prior to menopause, which can last up to ten years) and subfertility for as long as five to seven years before the onset of actual menopause (which *generally* signifies the end of your reproductive years).

The average age of menopause is 51. You can still become pregnant during perimenopause, although it may be more difficult and/or require medical intervention because you ovulate less frequently and the quality of your remaining eggs is not as good as it once was. That's not to say you should purposely delay childbirth until your "golden years." Common sense, and knowledge of the facts, can help you make the best decision for you and your family.

What's "older" these days?

We read a lot of ink on how 50 is the new 40 and 40 is the new 30. That's all well and good, but someone forgot to tell our ovaries, or for that matter, any other part of our body that is busy adjusting itself to our chronological age, regardless of what ages our faces, figures, or fantasies place us. The important point is that humans evolved hundreds of thousands of years ago. Evolution had to create a person who could reproduce enough children so that childhood death and maternal death would be compensated for, leaving enough humans to continue the species. In primitive societies, the average life expectancy for women was about 27 years old. So, evolution did not have to deal with women in their 30s or 40s.

In all fairness, however, we are seeing an extraordinary rise of pregnant women and mommies over 40, 50, and sometimes even 60. This isn't a reflection of the end of menopause as we know it, but rather the new technologies such as donor egg, sperm, and embryo, which allow women and men to bear children much later in life.

You can't pick up *People* magazine or turn on *Ellen* without hearing it: the great fertility debate over what age is appropriate when it comes to conception. Unfortunately, while there may be a modicum of truth, much of the *information* in magazines is inappropriate and just plain inaccurate. The chance to conceive in any given month depends upon both the age of the female and how long the couple has been trying to conceive. Evolution had to create the ability of a woman to conceive rapidly. So, the longer a woman has tried to conceive without success, the more likely there might be a problem such that she may never conceive.

REMEMBER

You wouldn't take medical advice from your car mechanic, so don't just assume that everyone who offers up an opinion, even a public one, knows anything more. Instead, ask your doctor, ask your nurse, or read a book (like this one) written by someone actually in the field.

But I don't look my age!

Whether you're dealing with fertility or fitness, age *does* play a role. Whether you *feel* like you're 15 or 50, whether you look your age or not, your body knows how old you are, and your ovaries do too.

In truth, there is only *one* answer to how old you are — and it can be found on your birth certificate.

REMEMBER

You can keep yourself in better baby-making shape (and better overall health) through good self-care, including nutrition and exercise. These measures will make a difference in your overall health and may actually improve your health during pregnancy and even decrease the risk of obstetrical complications (for example, losing weight may decrease the risk of gestational diabetes). We touch on these topics in Chapter 4. But ultimately, you can't fool Mother Nature. In other words, there is no known way to reverse the aging of the eggs.

Putting age in its (proper) place

Reversing the aging process is not an option, and if it you've found a way to do so, we recommend writing a book . . . and making a movie! But when it comes to conceiving at a later age, there are a few things that you can do to help the odds:

>> **Keep yourself in the best health and baby-making shape possible.** Get regular checkups, good nutrition, and plenty of sleep and exercise.

>> **Consult with a physician, be it an OB/GYN or a reproductive endocrinologist, who has experience in working with older wannabe moms.** Not all fertility doctors specialize in advanced maternal age or want to for that matter. Ask around and/or check with RESOLVE or online resources to find a doctor who has the latest and best information to help you address your individual issues. (If you're over 35, you should seriously start with a reproductive endocrinologist.)

>> **Don't compare yourself to younger women suffering from infertility, or any other woman for that matter.** Your issues may be entirely different and call for a completely different approach. Just because your friend's sister-in-law was successful with a high stimulation protocol at the age of 32, doesn't mean that this will work for you at the age of 39. It's important to work with a physician and a plan tailored to *your* needs.

>> **Coauthor Jackie was convinced that high-tech IVF with lots of drugs was the only thing that would work for her.** Luckily, Jackie's physician believed differently. Even so, it took Jackie quite a few months to believe him! After trying his lower-tech, low-dose medication protocol for a while, lo and behold, Jackie ended up with a bouncing baby girl. Being wrong was one of the few right things that she did in trying to conceive!

>> **Surround yourself with a good support team.** Whether it be friends, family, clergy, or professional help, this is not a battle that you want to fight alone. Your support team can help keep you sane and realistic.

>> **Consider your options.** Would you be willing to adopt? Use third-party reproduction (for example, donor eggs, sperm, or embryo)? A surrogate? Success can often be found in Plan B, C, and so on down the line.

>> **Set a timetable.** You don't want to make baby making a midlife project or crisis. Decide how long you want to spend trying and stick to it as best you can. Knowing that there's an end in sight can relieve a great deal of pressure.

>> **Investigate alternative treatment if you're interested.** Some women swear by acupuncture, naturopathy, or massage. Certainly, these are easier alternatives for your mind and body and just might deliver your baby to you as well. These measures are excellent for decreasing stress and helping you tune into your body's own signals. Just remember that alternative treatments can't reverse ovarian aging any more than traditional medications.

>> **Be patient.** Even at a young age, consider trying to conceive as a marathon, not a sprint. With each passing year, the time that this could take you is likely to be longer and the effort more intense. Don't set yourself up by expecting success the first month — or the second. If this does happen, you'll be pleasantly surprised, and extraordinarily lucky!

Modern ways to fight an "age"-old problem

There really are no ways to reverse aging. Science is working on this problem for several age-related problems. But aging continues. One recent development is the use of fertility preservation where eggs are retrieved and frozen when a woman is in her prime fertility years, which are under the age of 35. Most women won't need to use these eggs, but they serve as an insurance policy against age-related infertility. One hope was that the science of stem cells would solve the age issue if stem cells could be programmed to generate new eggs that could then be placed in a woman's ovaries and restore normal fertility. Each year it seems that science is a little closer to reaching this goal, but as of now, using some cells to reverse ovarian aging is a dream.

Calculating Your Fertility Odds as an "Older" Dad

Men do not have a similar loss of fertility as they age — unfair but true. Their peak fertility generally remains constant throughout their 40s. It does begin to decline over time, but at a slower pace than their female counterparts. Recent studies, however, do show a rise in chromosomal abnormalities in men over 35, and by age 50, most men show a 33 percent decrease in the number of sperm produced. So, although their problems may be less obvious when it comes to conceiving, the effects of the father's age may play a significant role down the road due to potential DNA damage in the sperm

Two recent studies address the impact of a father's age on his offspring. A study on *autism*, a spectrum communication disorder that can range from mild to severe, suggests that the age of the father plays a significant role1. In 2018, the CDC estimated the incidence of autism as 1 in 59 children. Fathers over 40 are six times more likely to produce a child with autism as those under 40. Autism spectrum disorder has been on the rise over the past few decades, with some experts pointing at environmental factors as well as possible links to preservatives used in vaccines. The "age" issue is an interesting correlation as the age of the average father, like that of the mother, has also risen over the years, which could be another explanation for the rise in the disorder. Another study looked at schizophrenia and reported a two to three-fold increase risk of schizophrenia in the offspring of men who have children when they are over the age of 50. The incidence of schizophrenia (number of times the disease occurred) was about 1 percent.

The problem with assessing the influence of male aging and adverse pregnancy outcomes relates to the fact that most older men are trying to conceive with women who are also older. One study tried to overcome this issue by measuring aneuploid rates (how often abnormal embryos occur) when the patient used donor eggs. They divided the males into three groups, <40, 40–49, and >49. They found that the over-50 group had a rise in the number of embryos that were trisomy 21, 18, and 13 (chromosomally abnormal). The authors concluded that the increased sperm damage due to aging increased the risk of having an embryo that had the wrong number of chromosomes. As with most studies, this study didn't really solve the issue. When the authors calculated the total aneuploid rate and compared the under-40 group to the over-50 group, the aneuploid rate went from 55 percent to 65 percent — an increase for sure, but one-third of the embryos had the correct number of chromosomes. One way to approach this therapeutically would be to do preimplantation genetic testing on the embryos. This might not correct all the subtle changes caused by male aging, but it would at least reduce the problem as much as possible.

Living with Diseases That Affect Fertility

Just a few generations ago, systemic diseases such as diabetes or lupus ruled out the possibility of having a baby. Now, pregnancies in patients with systemic disease are commonplace, and obstetricians or perinatologists who specialize in high-risk patients guide women with a history of cancer, kidney problems, heart problems, or just about any other health condition through successful pregnancies. Discuss the potential problems of pregnancy with your doctor beforehand so that you can be prepared for the problems you may face getting pregnant or carrying a pregnancy to term.

Polycystic ovaries

Polycystic ovary syndrome, sometimes called PCO or PCOS, although in "medicalese" it's known as Stein-Leventhal Syndrome, is the most common hormonal problem in women of childbearing age, affecting between 5 and 10 percent of women. PCOS is often associated with infertility but affects women in many other ways as well. PCOS is associated with weight, and since there is a rise in overweight/obese women, the incidence of PCOS is rising. This is especially important for young women who are overweight.

The diagnosis of PCOS has been standardized since 2003. Not all experts agree, but the general consensus is the application of what are called the *Rotterdam criteria* to make the diagnosis of PCOS. In the past, blood tests were used to make the diagnosis, but they are no longer part of the diagnostic criteria. They are, however, reassuring when present. The most common previously used test was the LH:FSH ratio. Normally, the ratio between these two hormone levels is 1:1, but in PCOS patients, the LH is frequently elevated, with a ratio of about 2:1 or higher. Additionally, insulin levels, free testosterone (a male hormone), and glucose may be high, and thyroid levels may be low.

The official definition of PCOS as determined by a workshop sponsored by ESHRE/ASRM (the European and American conferences on reproductive endocrinology) (Rotterdam criteria) in 2003 is that PCOS is present if two of the three following criteria are met:

>> Anovulation (no ovulation) or oligoovulation (ovulating only occasionally rather than every month, or fewer than 9 menses per year)

>> Excess androgen activity as seen by an elevated blood testosterone level or a history of acne or unwanted hair

>> Polycystic ovaries diagnosed by ultrasound where there are ≥12 follicles 3–9 mm in diameter in one or both ovaries in any pattern or an increase in ovarian volume

PCOS is a complicated metabolic disease. There is an as-yet-undefined genetic component and then some environmental or development trigger, which results in PCOS. Weight may play a role in some patients with PCOS. Not all PCOS patients are overweight, but estimates suggest 50 percent of PCOS patients have a BMI ≥30.

Up to 95 percent of PCOS patients who are overweight and 60–70 percent of PCOS patients have insulin resistance. Insulin is a hormone that regulates the body's use of starches and sugars. Women with insulin resistance, where the insulin is inefficient, produce an increased amount of insulin so that the blood sugar (glucose) remains constant. This is why one of the treatments for PCOS is metformin (Glucophage), a medication that is most commonly used for Type 2 (adult-onset, noninsulin-dependent) diabetes.

The unanswered question is, which came first, being overweight or the PCOS? The link between weight and PCOS is not defined, but because weight seems to be independently controlled, it may not be a cause of or a result of PCOS.

The overabundance of insulin production in women with PCOS causes the ovaries to make an overabundance of *androgens*, or male hormones. The excess of androgens leads to many of the symptoms associated with PCOS, which include the following:

>> Discoloration of the skin under the arms, breasts, and around the groin *(acanthosis nigricans)*

>> Excess facial hair

>> Acne

>> Thinning hair or male pattern baldness

PCOS can also affect women systemically, outside of the reproductive system, causing:

>> Type 2 (adult onset) diabetes

>> Heart disease

>> High blood pressure

>> High cholesterol levels

>> Sleep apnea

>> Depression

>> Gestational diabetes

>> Endometrial cancer

The increased androgens in the ovary slow or stop the normal development of eggs units, called *follicles.* Periods become irregular and, when they do occur, periods may be quite heavy because the uterine lining has become thickened as a result of not shedding on a regular basis. Normally a period of estrogen after menses causes the lining of the uterus to grow. Ovulation starts the production of progesterone, which opposes the estrogen and stops the increase in the lining of the uterus. If no pregnancy ensues, both the estrogen and the progesterone levels drop, and the uterus sheds the upper two-thirds of the lining of uterus. If the period of elevated estrogen production continues longer than it normally would and progesterone is either not produced because of no ovulation or infrequently produced due to longer periods, the uterus must shed an increased amount of lining resulting in heavy, painful periods.

This lack of regular shedding and thickening of the uterine lining can eventually lead to a risk of *hyperplasia* (a precancerous thickening of the uterine lining) which can, if left untreated, lead to uterine cancer. If you have PCOS and don't ovulate regularly, your doctor may recommend doing endometrial biopsies (a small piece of the uterine lining is scraped off and sent to pathology to be tested for abnormal cells) to check for cancer cells.

Women with PCOS may also have a higher rate of miscarriage and are more likely to develop gestational diabetes during pregnancy. Some women have an easier time conceiving if they take insulin-lowering medication; it's not yet clear if these same medications can also lower the risk of miscarriage in women with PCOS.

REMEMBER

If you have PCOS, you may need to see a fertility specialist to get pregnant. There are treatments that can help you get pregnant; the most common are

>> Medications like clomiphene citrate and gonadotropins to induce ovulation.

>> Medications to lower insulin resistance; these medications, Glucophage and Avandia, are also taken by people with diabetes.

>> Weight loss; the catch-22 is that women with PCOS have a harder time losing weight.

Endometriosis

Endometriosis is the growth of pieces of endometrial tissue (the inner lining of the uterus) outside the uterus. Endometriosis is commonly found in fallopian tubes, ovaries, the bladder, and sometimes even outside the pelvic cavity, in the abdomen. In rare cases, it has been found in the lungs, and even under the skin or in the brain! How does it manage to leave the uterus and travel to all these places?

There are many theories about how endometriosis travels; the most common are that endometriosis travels along with menstrual blood that flows "backwards" out of the uterus and into the fallopian tubes, ovary, pelvis, bladder, and abdomen. This theory doesn't explain how endometriosis ends up far from the pelvis; theories for how this happens range from travel through the lymph system to a theory that endometrial tissue doesn't travel to these places but is present in these locations from birth.

Endometriosis traditionally is a big player on the infertility field; around 30 percent of women suffering from infertility have endometriosis. Conversely, if you have endometriosis, you have around a 40 percent chance of having some degree of infertility. In addition, more than 30 percent of laparoscopic surgeries for unexplained infertility result in a diagnosis of endometriosis.

Endometriosis may affect fertility in a number of ways, including the following:

>> Blocking fallopian tubes so the ovulated egg can't reach the uterus

>> Destroying the *fimbriae,* the hair-like projections on the end of the fallopian tubes that guide the released egg into the fallopian tube

>> Causing cysts that may interfere with the release of eggs from the ovary

>> Creating an immune response in the pelvis that interferes with fertilization

>> Partially blocking fallopian tubes, so the embryo is more likely to implant in the tube (ectopic pregnancy)

Does all this mean you should throw in the towel on having a baby if you have endometriosis? Not at all! As many as 70 percent of women with minimal or mild endometriosis and infertility do conceive within three years of trying without any therapy.

However, you may not want to wait three years to get pregnant. And if you have moderate to severe endometriosis, your chances of pregnancy may be significantly lower without medical intervention. The good news is that there are treatments that can improve the chances for pregnancy. Treatment options remain controversial due to the predicted role surgery plays in the treatment of endometriosis. Treating severe endometriosis with surgery has become less common but remains a common form of treatment. Ultrasound can be used to diagnosis endometriosis in the ovaries causing a cystic structure termed an *endometrium.* The presence of an *endometrioma* (a tumor containing endometrial tissue) is staged a III (severe) on a scale of I to IV and can be surgically removed. This does improve pregnancy rates. An alternative is to use IVF instead of surgery, and some studies suggest the presence of the endometrioma does not reduce the chance of success. The only way to diagnoses a Stage I or II (mild, moderate) endometriosis is to directly visualize it through the use of the surgical procedure of laparoscopy. This form of treatment has been largely forgone and instead the use of oral fertility medications combined with intrauterine insemination or IVF has taken surgery's place.

In vitro fertilization (IVF) has helped many women with endometriosis conceive, even in previously "hopeless" cases. (Check out Chapters 15 and 16 for more info about IVF.) In spite of its other effects on natural conception, endometriosis does not diminish IVF success rates.

Diabetes: More than a "sugar" problem

Diabetes affects about 17 million Americans, or approximately 6 percent of the population. There are actually several different types of diabetes, including the following:

» **Type 1 diabetes,** which used to be called juvenile diabetes, usually develops before puberty, but can develop at any age. Five to ten percent of diabetics have Type 1 diabetes, which is an autoimmune disease. In Type 1 diabetes, the beta cells of the pancreas stop making insulin altogether, so people with this problem must take injections of insulin every day.

» **Type 2 diabetes** usually develops in people over 40, but it can develop earlier. It is often associated with being overweight; 80 percent of Type 2 diabetics are overweight. It develops more slowly than Type 1 and can possibly be controlled with diet and pills rather than injections.

Diabetes leads to problems with blood vessels, circulation, and nerve function. Therefore, men with diabetes often have problems with erection and ejaculation; some male diabetics have retrograde ejaculation, a condition in which sperm back up into the bladder.

Women with diabetes need to have well-controlled blood sugar levels during pregnancy. Even with good control, the rate of birth defects in women with diabetes is two to three times the normal rate. Women with PCOS may develop Type 2 diabetes later in life.

WARNING

Diabetics tend to have large babies, which can create problems at the time of delivery.

Lupus and other immune disorders

Systemic lupus erythematosus, commonly called lupus, is primarily a disease of women, although a small percentage of men also develop it. It is one of a group of systemic autoimmune diseases (SADs) that also includes multiple sclerosis, antiphospholipid antibody syndrome, rheumatoid arthritis, systemic sclerosis, Sjogren's syndrome, mixed connective tissue disease, idiopathic inflammatory myopathies, and vasculitis. These diseases can affect connective tissue, the tissue that binds together various tissues and organs. It can also affect the nerves, muscles, endocrine system, and gastrointestinal system. One of the outward symptoms of lupus is a facial rash, but lupus can affect every organ in your body. A few generations ago, women with lupus were advised not to have children because it was felt that pregnancy worsens the disease. More recent studies have shown this belief not to be true, although one-third of pregnant lupus patients have "flares," or increases in disease activity. About 10 percent of pregnant lupus patients find that their symptoms actually improve.

Fifty percent of women with lupus have normal pregnancies and normal deliveries; about 25 percent deliver prematurely, and another 25 percent experience miscarriage or stillbirth.

Miscarriage may be related to antibodies called antiphospholipid antibodies (discussed earlier in this chapter) found in some lupus patients. These antibodies cause clotting and interfere with the growth of the placenta. Baby aspirin and/or heparin may be given in pregnancy to help blood flow to the placenta.

WARNING

About 20 percent of lupus patients develop *toxemia*, a condition that results in high blood pressure, liver and kidney malfunctions, and premature delivery and can lead to eclampsia, which can cause maternal seizures and death.

REMEMBER

If you have lupus, you need to be followed carefully by an obstetrician who specializes in high-risk patients.

Dealing with autoimmune disorders can lead to lifestyle changes and higher vigilance to your overall health. While it is important to identify whether or not you or your partner have such a disease, a positive diagnosis does not necessarily mean that your fertility will be impacted. Here is a look at some of the other immune disorders that may or may not affect fertility:

>> **Ankylosing spondylitis (AS):** Ankylosing spondylitis is a type of chronic inflammation that affects the spine and sacroiliac joints causing back pain. It occurs two to three times more frequently in men than women. While its symptoms may affect a patient's mobility, the disease does not in and of itself impair fertility in females. Similarly, AS does not seem to impair male fertility; however, there may be a slight association with erectile dysfunction (ED) or reduced libido, which may impact the length of time to pregnancy.

>> **Rheumatoid arthritis (RA):** Male patients with RA tend to have lower testosterone and high FSH and LH levels. Like AS, RA males may have an increase in ED and decreased libido, but there is little impaired fertility related to RA itself. Some women with RA do have an increase in infertility with anovulation and unexplained infertility being the primary diagnoses related to this disease. Women with RA generally have fewer children than they had hoped for, and the time to conception is longer than in the general population.

>> **Multiple Sclerosis (MS):** Affecting women two to three more times than men, MS is a chronic, progressive disease that effects the lining of nerve cells in the brain and spinal cord. While it is extremely debilitating over time, MS alone has not been found to be a definitive cause of infertility. One study showed an increased incidence of childlessness in women with MS, but it was not determined whether this was by choice or due to an inability to conceive. There is some evidence, however, to suggest that undergoing fertility treatment may exacerbate MS relapses.

>> **Anti-phospholipid antibody syndrome (APS):** The finding of anti-phospholipid antibodies is usually seen and diagnosed after a pregnancy loss (which we talk about in Chapter 13). Some studies have suggested that APS may also play a role in embryo implantation, development of the placenta (called placentation), and early embryo development.

WARNING

Patients diagnosed with an autoimmune disease may be on medications that could interfere with fertility treatment or their ability to get pregnant. If you have one of these diseases you need to share this information, and information about any medications you are taking, with your fertility specialist.

Cancer and Fertility: The News Is Cautiously Optimistic

Just a few years ago, having cancer meant that you would probably not be able to conceive and carry a child. Surgery, radiation, and chemotherapy, the mainstay treatments of most cancers, could destroy ovaries and sperm cells as well as your hope of having a child.

Today, however, new advances have made it possible for cancer survivors to become parents, and the really good news is that more advances are being made all the time. The information of today may be obsolete soon, and the chances for parenthood will hopefully be better than ever. The good news even today is that there's no evidence that your baby will have a higher risk of birth defects or childhood cancer if you become pregnant after cancer treatment.

The cancer-fertility connections for women

Because women are involved not only in the production of gametes but also in carrying a baby to term, cancer in women who want to be parents can be more complicated than cancer in men. In the next sections, we look at different types of cancer that can impact future motherhood.

Beating breast cancer

Breast cancer survivors are now being told that pregnancy after treatment is possible, as long as their ovaries are intact and haven't been irradiated. Many doctors encourage patients to wait two years after treatment before trying to get pregnant. Pregnancy doesn't increase the chance of cancer recurrence, according to most recent studies, but doctors want to make sure that the cancer doesn't recur on its own.

WARNING

If you do have a recurrence of cancer while pregnant and require chemotherapy, you need to be aware that chemo in the first trimester may cause fetal malformation, while waiting till the second or third trimester may result in preterm labor or fetal loss.

TECHNICAL STUFF

Tamoxifen can be used during the stimulation form IVF to minimize the estrogen levels and perhaps reduce the risk of exacerbating the cancer.

Battling ovarian cancer

If you've been treated for ovarian cancer with radiation or ovarian ablation, your ovaries will not be functioning, and you'll need to use donor eggs to become pregnant. If you were treated with multiple-agent chemotherapy, there's a good chance you'll go into premature ovarian insufficiency (POI). One-third of women under age 30 and two-thirds of those over 30 go into POI. (We talk more about this in Chapter 11.)

It's sometimes possible to remove only one ovary or move the ovary not affected by cancer out of the way (surgically lift the ovary out of the pelvis), so it won't be affected by radiation treatment.

Fighting uterine cancer

The treatment for uterine cancer is usually removal of the uterus; this means you won't be able to carry a pregnancy, although if your ovaries are not removed, you can produce eggs that can be fertilized and implanted into a gestational carrier.

New therapy for very early endometrial (the lining of the uterus is called the endometrium) cancers involves treating patients with the hormone medroxyprogesterone and also performing repeated dilatation and curettage, scraping the uterine lining until it's free of cancerous cells. This method can be used only in cancer cases that are discovered very early and are confined to the endometrium. Because the cancer can return, very close follow-up is required.

Coping with cervical cancer

Early stage cervical cancer can be effectively treated by the removal of only part of the cervix; this process is called *cervical conization*. It may also be possible to remove the cervix while leaving the uterus intact when treating cervical cancer (this is called a *trachelectomy*).

The cancer-fertility connection for men

Although testicular cancer is rare, making up only 1 percent of all cancer, it's the most common cancer found in men between the ages of 20 and 34, with 7,000 new cases diagnosed each year. It is four times more common among Caucasian men than African–American men.

If only one testicle is removed surgically, the remaining testicle will produce enough sperm so that fertility won't be damaged. If both testicles need to be removed, several semen samples can be frozen before surgery and used for insemination later on. If only one testicle is affected, the man has a 2 to 5 percent chance of developing cancer in the other testicle.

REMEMBER

Some chemotherapy treatment causes temporary loss of fertility, but sperm counts may return to an acceptable level after two to three years. Radiation may also cause temporary infertility, but some men regain adequate sperm counts within a short time.

If certain lymph nodes are removed, the nerves that control ejaculation may be affected, although the sperm count may be normal. This condition may require sperm aspiration with ICSI and IVF to achieve a pregnancy.

Considering cryobiology

Recent advances in cryobiology have added a new dimension for cancer patients. Men who are to undergo chemotherapy and thus have their sperm destroyed can freeze sperm for use in IVF later. These specimens can last for an estimated hundreds of years.

Women who are being treated with chemotherapy or pelvic radiation can undergo IVF where the eggs that are removed are frozen for future use. For women, the use of chemotherapy that is toxic to the ovaries may not result immediately in menopause. However, some of the eggs will be destroyed, and thus the extent of the reproductive ability for the woman will be shortened.

Preservation of sperm or eggs must be done prior to the chemotherapy or pelvic radiation. The stimulation and retrieval of eggs can be initiated within days of the diagnosis so that treatment need not be delayed. Recent changes in the law require insurance coverage for fertility preservation for cancer patients who are to undergo treatments that would have a high chance of resulting in sterility. Fertility preservation is an insurance policy providing the possibility to have a child even if the person becomes sterile. The success rates depend upon how many samples are produced and stored for the male and how many eggs can be retrieved and frozen for the female. For women where 12–15 oocytes can be frozen, the overall success rates are estimated to be 75–85 percent for young women and less for women ≥40 years old.

Chapter 8

Harnessing the Power of Modern Medicine: Finding a Doctor and More

Two classic Norman Rockwell drawings show a family on vacation in the station wagon, pictures that may or may not remind you of childhood! In the first scene, the daughter's braids dance in the wind, and everyone is in clean new outfits and wearing big smiles. The second scene shows the return from vacation — everyone is dirty, bedraggled, and grumpy, and Dad looks like he's ready to drive the whole group over a cliff.

You may have started toward pregnancy in the vacation mode, thinking "Can't wait to do the nursery," "What kind of maternity clothes should I get?" and "I wonder who'll give me a baby shower?" After a few months with no pregnancy, you may resemble the return group, worn out and testy, wondering why you ever thought any of this was a good idea and how you went from being a regular person to being a potential fertility patient.

In this chapter, we look at the first tentative steps toward being a fertility patient and help you to cope with family, friends, and your partner at this difficult point.

REMEMBER

Achieving a pregnancy depends upon at least three things: the technology, the technologist, and the problem (diagnosis). In today's world, the technology is standardized. The technician can vary between the generalist and the reproductive endocrinologist (REI). However, the primary factor deciding whether you will achieve a pregnancy or not is the disease. So before you drive yourself nuts with choosing the best doctor or technology, look at your diagnosis.

Exploring Your "Doctor" Options

The American Society of Reproductive Medicine (ASRM) recommends that you should consult a physician if you haven't gotten pregnant in one year if you're under age 35, or six months if you're over 35. These guidelines must have been written for very patient people. If you're under 35 and patient enough to wait for a year — a *year* — before talking to a doctor about getting pregnant, we applaud you! The guidelines were established to help people seek assistance if assistance seems necessary.

The reason for the wait is that couples with normal fertility will achieve a pregnancy within the first six months of trying to conceive. The estimate is that for people who become pregnant and have a child, 85 percent conceive that pregnancy within the first six months of trying. This is true for all couples with normal fertility regardless of age. However, age plays a role because as women age, fewer and fewer have normal fertility. The danger of doing testing too early is that many of the tests will suggest that there is a problem when in fact no problem exists. This approach can cause a couple to use needless, extensive treatment, including IVF, when no treatment was needed.

Seeking professional help is a big step. You always thought you were an average sort of person, and now you find that you're part of the 20 percent of women who don't get pregnant in a year of trying. For the first few months, you could pretend it wasn't a big deal, but now, well, it's time to take the first step and call Dr. Basic or your ground floor fertility caregiver. (Which means that Dr. Basic could be your family physician or your gynecologist — you choose!)

When not to wait — even a few months

Sometimes even Conventional Wisdom, that conservative soul, says not to wait six months or a year before seeing a doctor about not getting pregnant. There are circumstances about your health that might suggest seeking physician assistance before waiting at all.

You might want to see a doctor from the beginning if you've had a previous ectopic pregnancy or have pelvic inflammatory disease. You may have damage to your fallopian tubes, which may make IVF necessary. If you're not getting your period, or getting it very irregularly, you may need help regulating your cycles so that you develop an egg every month. Lastly, if you have very painful periods, you may have endometriosis (see Chapter 7 for more discussion of all of these conditions) and may need treatment to get pregnant.

You may want to have your partner do a semen analysis early on if he has a history of trauma to the testicles, had undescended testicles, or knows that he had mumps as a child. Any of these conditions may have caused damage to his sperm.

Of course, if you've had your tubes tied or if your partner had a vasectomy, you need to see a specialist to discuss either reversal of the surgery (see Chapters 11 and 12) or in vitro fertilization (which we discuss in detail in Part 4). If you need to use donor sperm, you'll also probably want to see a specialist who can tell you how to order the sperm.

Same-sex couples or single parents have special needs, which usually mean they will need physician assistance sooner rather than later. The type of assistance will depend upon the circumstance of the couple or person seeking to have a child. We talk more about these circumstances in Chapter 20.

Choosing between a family doctor and an OB/GYN

So, who *is* Dr. Basic when you're trying to get pregnant? The average doctor has about nine initials after his name, so how are you supposed to know which one you should see when you're trying to get pregnant? Some of the more common abbreviations you may see include the following:

» **MD:** Medical doctor. Someone trained in traditional medicine with four years of medical school after college has earned there MD. However, in order to obtain a license to practice medicine, physicians must continue their education by completing, at a minimum, an internship (one-year postgraduate). In addition, most MDs pursue further education by completing a residency which allows the doc to specialize in a specific area of medicine. OB/GYN is one field of specialization.

>> **DO:** Doctor of osteopathy. These doctors used to be more trained in manipulation and homeopathic methods, but today's osteopaths train in programs virtually identical to traditional medical schools.

>> **OB/GYN:** This specialty combines obstetrics and gynecology into one residency training program. Obstetrics is the specialty that focuses on taking care of pregnant women and handling labor and delivery, and gynecology is the specialty focusing on the reproductive care of women's health. Obstetricians and gynecologists all start with the same four-year residency training after medical school, which incorporates the internship requirement. While some may choose to do one or the other, most practice both. Because OB/GYNs do surgery and deliver in a hospital setting, they are usually board certified in OB/GYN. Board certification requires extensive exams and review of their practice. Further, they must maintain their certification through reading and testing on a yearly basis.

>> **REI:** Reproductive endocrinologist and infertility specialist. This doctor is a graduate of an OB/GYN program who has chosen to specialize in reproductive medicine and infertility. Most fellowships are three-year training programs, so an REI has completed seven years of postgraduate training after medical school. Many REI physicians are not board certified in REI but must be board certified in OB/GYN. To be board certified requires taking the extensive exams required to achieve certification, and many who complete the fellowship feel that this extra step does not make them a better physician. So even though they have completed the 3-year fellowship, they simply defer the exam requirement for certification.

>> **FP:** Family practitioner. These doctors have chosen to specialize in the health of the entire family. In some parts of the country, they, rather than OBs, handle many women's health problems, including pregnancy and deliveries.

>> **FACOG:** Fellow of the American College of Obstetricians and Gynecologists. A doctor who has FACOG after his name is board certified and is a member of this national society.

You may also come across these terms when doctor–shopping:

>> **Board eligible:** These doctors have completed the required residency or fellowship in their specialty and can now take the tests to become board certified.

>> **Board certified:** These doctors have completed residencies and for REIs the additional fellowship, have practiced their specialty for at least two years and then taken the tests necessary to be certified, and have passed them.

TIP

If you live in a remote area, you may need to start with your family doctor because specialists may not have offices in your area. Also, you may feel more comfortable starting with a doctor who already knows you, such as your OB/GYN or family doctor. If your doctor believes that your case is more complex than he or she is qualified to treat they'll probably refer you to someone more experienced in your particular situation. When you're just beginning treatment, you can probably safely assume that your regular doctor or OB/GYN can handle your case, unless you already have reason to suspect that you have tubal issues or that your partner has sperm problems requiring higher-tech intervention.

REMEMBER

Most couples first look to their insurance plan to help in deciding on a doctor, as medical care is expensive. Infertility care is no different, and your choice of care-giver may be limited to which doctor is in your insurance network. We talk more about this in Chapter 15.

Bringing your partner along: Four ears are better than two

Back in the olden days of gynecology, say before the 1960s, you *never* saw a man in the OB/GYN waiting room. Today, however, the situation is different; some men accompany their partner to every OB/GYN visit. The magazine categories in the waiting room have been improved, and the decorating scheme doesn't scream "Rock-a-Bye Baby." Many doctors even specifically request that you bring your partner to a visit so that you can all get to know each other.

For male/female partnerships, if you decide to start diagnostic testing, he'll need to have his own testing done since male factors account for as much as 40 percent of all infertility, so he may as well get familiar with the doctor right from the start. Furthermore, how will you feel if you have been tested and taken a few months of Clomid "to help you get pregnant," only to find out he has very few or no sperm. For same-sex couples, you may want to consider turning the tables and using the other partner's eggs or uterus depending on what you find out. So, should you encourage your partner to attend your first why-aren't-we-pregnant visit? That depends on a few things:

> **»** **Will he feel horribly out of place, not pay attention, or say something you'd rather he didn't?**
>
> Some men don't like to go to the doctor, ever, for anything. Whether it's the loss of control, the digging into what they consider their personal business, or just discomfort in the face of an authority figure, many men are not assets at the doctor's office. You probably know by now whether your partner will do well at the doctor's office. If you're going to sit there (half naked, no less) worrying about what embarrassing thing he might say or do, go by yourself.
>
>
>
> **TIP**
>
> If you are part of a same-sex female couple, that's a bonus! Your partner already knows the way around an OB/GYN visit! Regardless of your partner's sex, if they are the person in your twosome who remembers detail, writes things down correctly, asks sensible questions, and provides moral support, by all means, take them to your first doctor visit.

>> **Are you going to have to impart information that you don't want your partner to know?**

For example, did you have an abortion, give a child up for adoption, have a sexually transmitted disease, or do any other thing you'd rather your partner didn't know about? Then go to the first visit by yourself, frankly explain the situation to your doctor, and take your partner to the *next* visit.

>> **Are you going to be embarrassed about undergoing an examination with your partner there?**

Even today, in this let-it-all-hang-out age, some of you aren't comfortable having other people, even your partner, present for a gynecological exam. If this situation is going to make you uneasy, maybe your partner can wait in the waiting room until the exam is over and then come in when you're dressed.

Making a list of questions for your first visit

Whether you go alone or as a team to your doctor's appointment, prepare a list of questions ahead of time so that you won't forget anything. Here's a starter list. You'll probably have other questions specific to your own situation.

>> **Do you treat many patients trying to get pregnant?**

Obviously, you don't want to have a doctor taking on your case whose practice mostly consists of gynecological surgery on women over age 50.

>> **Will you do any testing before we start treatment?**

Some doctors just start you on medication for a few months before putting you through more invasive testing. This is probably not the best approach because treatment should match the problem. As we mention earlier, treating a woman with clomid when the problem is male factor is frustrating and a colossal waste of time and energy. If you start down the infertility pathway, *make a diagnosis first.*

>> **What do you think my chance for success will be?**

Obviously, your doctor doesn't have a crystal ball but should have some general idea, based on your age and history, of what your chance of getting pregnant is.

>> **How long should we try this before we do further testing?**

If your doctor shrugs and gives you the impression that they would stick to simple methods forever, you may want to find another doctor.

Filling out forms and answering questions

Dr. Basic is going to have some questions for you, too. You may be asked to fill out a pretty extensive preprinted or online profile before you even get to the office. Either beforehand or at the time of the appointment, be aware that the doctor will want to know the following, so come prepared with the answers:

>> How long you've been trying to get pregnant.

>> Whether you have ever been pregnant

>> How often you have sex and whether you use any lubricants

>> Whether you engage in any unusual practices that could affect your fertility

>> How old you were when you first got a period

>> How long your periods last

>> How long your cycles are from day one of one cycle to day one of the next

>> The date of your last period

>> Whether your periods are painful

>> Whether your periods are heavy and how many pads or tampons you use a day

>> Whether sisters or other close relatives have children

>> Whether there are any known genetic factors in your family

>> Whether you have ever had a pelvic infection or any pelvic surgery

Dr. Basic may have a lot more questions aimed specifically at you. Don't be afraid to express your fears, concerns, and expectations. This is a good litmus test about the empathy of the physician. This is also a good time to get an idea about the philosophy of the practice.

TIP

If you have had any illnesses, surgeries, or started any testing for fertility, it is very helpful to your doctor to have a copy of your medical records. You can have your current doctor send these to your new doctor or you can bring a copy of your medical records to the first appointment.

Moving Up to Dr. Specialist

After doing some testing, you may have a better idea of what your fertility problems are, and you may decide that it's time to see a specialist. Or perhaps your testing hasn't shown any specific problems, and Dr. Basic has decided you should move on to a specialist in infertility (that's most likely the REI we describe earlier in this chapter).

Your family doctor or gynecologist may have already handed you a piece of paper with the name of an infertility specialist scribbled on it. "Go to this guy, he is the best," he may say, and you may do just that, without thinking a whole lot about alternative choices.

Before you set up your first appointment, you may want to ask your doctor *why* he thinks the person he has suggested is the best.

Although the name that Dr. Basic gives you is a starting point, you should check out other doctors, too, before making a final decision. At this point, you probably will be looking for a specialist in the field, such as a reproductive endocrinologist.

Yelp, Vitals, Healthgrades, *ad infinitum* are often a great spot to check out the "rep" of your referral. However, keep in mind that much of the "grading" is done on bedside manner and results. Put simply, your goal is to conceive a child, not a relationship with your provider. Know yourself and know just how important it is that you get warm fuzzies from your specialist. It would be nice if all physicians were equally capable *and* wildly personable, but medicine, just like any other field, has introverts and extroverts. Deciding how much handholding you need from your doctor will help you make your decision.

Likewise, oftentimes those who post to referral sites may be particularly unhappy with the outcome — that is, not getting pregnant. While some of this may be physician related, most of it is likely due to the patient's unique physiological makeup or timing — or both. Doctors can't always cure what ails you, no matter how much they may want to.

Getting Help from National Organizations

After you have a core list of infertility clinics near you, you need to check out each one. You can visit each one, hanging around the waiting room and questioning people as they come out the door. Or you can contact infertility support groups (just search the web and you'll be amazed at how many you find!) see whether there is information on any of the offices you're considering. For example, Resolve is one of the largest national organizations dedicated to the treatment of infertility, but also look at some of the "best lists" for fertility blogs and online support.

TIP

Finding your local Resolve organization is easy; the website is www.resolve.org. Just click on the local chapters hyperlink to find one near you, which can connect you with more inside scoop on nearby clinics – or at least tips on where you may not want to go.

The Resolve website and others contain clinic success rates published by the Centers for Disease Control (CDC). This information is compiled by the Society for Assisted Reproductive Technology (SART), which you can read more about in Chapter 15. These numbers give you some idea of your clinic's success rates, but keep in mind that these statistics are only for high-tech in vitro fertilization (IVF) treatment, not for medium-tech treatment such as IUI (intrauterine insemination).

Infertility support websites also contains a huge amount of information on insurance coverage for infertility, adoption options, and information on clinical trials and research studies being carried out around the country. Resolve is very vocal in lobbying for insurance coverage for infertility treatments.

Your area may have other groups that meet to help you deal with infertility. Some are informal groups that started out as a few friends meeting to commiserate and then grew into clubs with monthly meetings. You may also find local psychologists or therapists who have started groups for infertile patients.

All of these are good resources for information on who's good and who's not in your area. Always get more than one person's opinion on a clinic because each person may have a bias one way or the other, depending on her own outcome.

Going Online for More Resources and Information

Resolve isn't the only information source online. In fact, after you start surfing the net, your sources of information will be limited only by the amount of time you have to spend. Whether you're interested in reading scientific journals, chatting with new friends online, or checking out clinic websites, we guarantee that the internet has enough stuff to keep you occupied until your children leave for college!

Chat rooms and bulletin boards

Perhaps one of the greatest sources of information and strength on the road to baby that I (coauthor Jackie) found came from the countless women I encountered in cyberspace, some of whom became friends in real time as well. I happened upon this wealth of relating and resources right after a failed in vitro fertilization attempt and a subsequent high FSH (follicle-stimulating hormone) reading, which, at the time, seemed a death knell to any future attempts.

PERSONAL STORY

After a good cry, I logged on to Google to see what I could find in reference to my new diagnosis of high FSH. Convinced that I was the only one to suffer from this odd disorder (actually a measure of diminished ovarian egg reserve), I was surprised at how quickly Google returned a result listing over 38,000 web pages on the topic. Okay, so maybe a few others out there had the same problem after all. The first listing, High FSH E-mail Group, connected to me a very lively, upbeat chat room. Through teary eyes, I asked one and all if I was doomed. I logged off in despair and went to work my way through the other 37,999 sites. After visiting two more sites, I went back to the chat room and was amazed to find at least ten responses to my wail. I read each and every one, printed them all (and have saved them to this day), and spent until the wee hours of the morning reading every message of encouragement and every link to more information on high FSH, low FSH, infertility, and the best medical and nonmedical sources for help, including doctors, clinics, acupuncturists, and herbs.

I never left that site through the remaining years of my fertility battle. From it, I garnered hope that I could conceive despite what my doctor had told me. I also found a new (and improved) doctor who (eventually) successfully treated me. I also discovered insights on new treatments and medications and located a 24/7 support network that accompanied me through fertility, pregnancy, and all the stressors in between. I developed a core group of friends from all over the country who were the first ones I called when the pregnancy test came back negative and when it finally came back positive. I can honestly say that my high FSH diagnosis was a blessing, one that led me to a much greater place.

The beauty of the internet is the availability of libraries full of information right at our fingertips. Bulletin boards help provide links to this information, along with the kinship so helpful in thriving through infertility. Man or woman, whatever the problem that ails you, you can be almost certain that the internet offers a chat room/bulletin board filled with others facing the same struggles.

Doctors' websites: Separating the glitter from the goods

Now it seems as if every infertility clinic has a website. Some are pretty basic, giving not much more than name, rank, and serial number, and others run a 24-hour-a-day media show, complete with question-and-answer sessions with the doctors, links to published articles, and testimonials from happy clients.

Some clinics list their website right next to their phone number in the phone book; others direct you to their website when you call the office. Some websites give detailed and frequently updated pregnancy rates. Other sites either don't supply or don't update statistics.

WARNING

Here's what *not* to be impressed by when looking at clinic websites:

>> **The way the doctor looks:** That picture may have been taken decades before. And really, you are looking for a doctor, not a dating service.

>> **Testimonials from patients:** Unless you know the patients personally and can verify what they say, you have no way of knowing who wrote these glowing reports.

>> **Great graphics:** Splashy visuals may indicate that the doctor has a son or daughter who knows a lot about websites, but those graphics don't reveal anything about a doctor's medical ability.

You can be impressed by the following website information:

>> Clearly written, frequently updated success rates

>> A list of clinic services, plus how many procedures are performed in a year

>> The doctors' degrees and the schools they were obtained from

>> Research and peer-reviewed articles by the doctors or staff

>> Lab certifications

>> Ancillary services like genetic counselors and psychological services

>> Insurance plans accepted

WARNING

Understanding success rates can be very confusing and misleading if you do not know what you are looking at. Also, and unfortunately, some websites are unclear or like to boast — to put it mildly. We talk more about how to understand success rates in Chapter 15.

Discussing Dollars with the Doctor

PERSONAL STORY

When I (coauthor Jackie) visited Dr. Badadventure for the first time, I was quickly whisked away to meet with Mr. Dollars and Sense, the finance guy. It should have been a warning. Needless to say, my fertility experience with Dr. Badadventure cost considerable dollars and yielded pennies in results.

We're not saying that you should turn tail and flee when the mention of payment comes up. Fertility doctors and clinics are for-profit institutions, so they're permitted and expected to make money from their patients. Most clinics ask for payment up-front for certain procedures, including extensive testing, surgery, and in vitro fertilization. Don't be offended. Because many insurers don't cover fertility, doctors do need to guarantee payment for their time, services, and staff and you need to know the costs upfront to make good decisions about your care. If your doctor determines, after careful review of you and your records, that high tech is the way to go, expect the issue of cost and payment to come up. You don't want to be surprised by a bill in the tens of thousands of dollars.

Understanding What Your Doctor Says

Doctors and nurses aren't *really* trying to confuse you when they spew forth a list of initials or shortcut terms. But when your doctor says something like "Get an HSG and a sono, and then if your APA and FSH come back okay, we'll start the stims," your immediate reaction may be "Huh?"

TIP

Whenever you don't understand what the doctor or nurse just said, ask the person to stop and explain. Don't write it down, thinking that you'll look it up later, or nod just to look like you know what they're talking about. Please ask! You may find it helpful to take some notes when your doctor is speaking, or to record conversations with your doctor. This can be a helpful tool in relaying this information to your partner or to your cousin who is a doctor. Always ask your doctor if doing so is okay, particularly when it comes to taping your discussions. Most doctors are glad to accommodate your notetaking; however, most *people* (including doctors) become a bit unhinged if they find out that they were being taped secretly.

You may find it helpful to enlist a second set of ears as well. This can be a perfect spot for your partner to participate! Fertility is an emotional subject. Especially if the doctor is addressing problems that *you* have, you may be too close to the situation to hear and understand all the options that are available. Your partner or a friend may be a bit more detached and better able to comprehend and communicate the information to you.

Knowing When to Switch Doctors

So, you've tried and tried and tried some more with your initial doctor of choice. Despite your efforts, she isn't sensitive to your needs, whether they're physical, emotional, or financial. Perhaps your doctor is stuck in a time warp of sorts, insisting that *eventually* you'll conceive naturally, or with minimal intervention, despite the fact that you've been trying for months or years with no success and a loudly ticking biological clock. Or else your doctor is pushing for expensive, invasive treatment that you don't feel prepared for.

Either of these reasons, or no particular reason at all, is perfectly understandable in your decision to switch doctors. The personalities of some patients and doctors just clash. For many, this alone can be a reason to run.

Keeping Your Own (Hit) Records

Fertility is certainly a project that can generate a lot of paperwork. Old records, profiles, test results, instructions, consent forms — "aye yai yai"! The good news is that so much of this is digital now that lugging that binder around may not be necessary anymore. But keeping track of your own info is still important.

PERSONAL STORY

After initially relying on only my doctor's records, I (coauthor Jackie) eventually discovered the need to keep my own records as well. The process was simple, but the organization was not. After every doctor's appointment, monitoring visit, or blood test, I asked for a copy of my records from that day. My records often consisted of nothing more than my notations from the day's blood work results, which I would date and keep in a separate folder. My records proved invaluable during the course of my treatment. Seldom did I have a question that couldn't be answered by reviewing my own information. And, when the time came to switch doctors, I had my own history to present to my new doctor at our first visit.

In today's world of electronic medical records and patient portals, your information is obtainable with a click and a smile. Regardless, consider copying records and storing them in your own files. Doing so also allows you to double-check doctor's instructions and test results if the communication with your clinic is less than perfect.

As a cautionary note (from one who knows!), try to avoid making your records nighttime reading. If you bring this information to bed with you, you may be becoming a wee bit obsessive about the process. This type of behavior will not help your cause or your sleeping patterns. A lighthearted magazine or book that has nothing to do with fertility is a better sleep aid.

REMEMBER

Reviewing your information periodically and having an extra set of records for your files are very helpful to your treatment. Trying to diagnose yourself based on your past performance is a job better left to the pros. Your records are your backup. Your doctors are still the front line.

Facing the Stranger in Your Sex Life — Treatment and Your Loss of Privacy

When going through fertility treatment, you open the door to your private life — yes, including your sex life — for all the medical world to see. This loss of privacy is bound to happen and takes some getting used to.

Talking sex with clinic staff

The frequency of intercourse, the quality of your menstrual cycles, and your past history of pregnancies, whether by hit or miss, are crucial bits of information in piecing together your reproductive profile. Offer information gladly because doing so only helps to educate your medical team. Feel free, however, to leave out the details that truly define intimacy. Remember that sexual intercourse is a biological process. Intimacy may occur in or out of the bedroom, and the specifics of that are all your own.

REMEMBER

Your doctor (and his staff!) would rather discuss things other than your sex life. They will not discuss your private life in their private lives. That's part of that little thing called HIPPA (the patient privacy act), which makes sharing your information not just an ethical breach but a legal one as well. Their job, however, is to help you conceive a baby, and their inquiries are part of the process.

Figuring out who gets to know what

One of the hardest things to come to grips with is who to talk to and how much to tell. You know you have to come clean with your doctor and the clinic staff in order to optimize your treatment. Family and friends are another story and, frankly, this is where "need-to-know" tactics come into play. You get to decide what you want to share and with whom. If you are working on a second baby and you'll need Grandma to watch Baby #1 while you go through treatment, or you always talk about what's going on in your life, you'll probably share more. If you are a "keeps herself to herself" kind of personality, then follow your head and heart with what feels right.

REMEMBER

While everything else about being in the infertility club feels out of your control, you still get to manage most of who knows what. Talk to your partner, the clinic staff, and other people on your support team to find your comfort zone. Take a look at Chapter 10 for more specific ideas on how to handle this in your life.

Chapter **9**

Improving Your Odds with Diet, Supplements, and Exercise

Nothing has worked so far, and your doctor (or your partner!) may be suggesting stepping up the pace — but you're not quite there yet. Isn't there anything else you can add? Well, maybe. Alternative therapies, which can include everything from acupuncture to traditional Chinese medicine, from massage to meditation, have become a popular means of either supplementing or substituting for the standard "Western" approach to infertility (doctors, tests, and blood work). *Complementary and alternative medicine* (CAM) includes a diverse group of medical treatments, which include acupuncture, massage, herbal medicine, mind–body techniques, and Chinese medicine. CAM is used not just to enhance fertility but also to treat the stress that fertility treatment often causes. Various studies from around the world show that roughly 50 percent of fertility patients use some form of CAM. The most commonly used CAM treatments are herbal medicine, acupuncture, and nutritional supplements.

WARNING

Not all research has the same quality, and research is categorized into four groups, with Level I having the highest level of reliability. While there are numerous research articles evaluating CAM, the majority are Level III or IV, with relatively few Level I articles. Conclusions based upon the less reliably performed research should raise questions about how useful the findings of those studies are in treating infertility.

Some clinics are offering alternative services to their patients through liaisons with providers. Others, while not adding to their staff, are allowing outside providers to come into their clinics and service patients upon request, such as acupuncture treatments before and after IVF embryo transfers.

In this chapter, we talk about those "other" ways to consider, alternative measures from basic to beyond, and help you decide which ones are worth trying and which ones may just result in expensive urination.

Eating for Fertility

Common folklore ascribes considerable emphasis to diet and infertility. "You're too thin, you're too fat, you don't eat frequently enough, you eat too frequently." So, which is it? One thing to keep in mind is that evolution crafted the modern human under deplorable conditions. And yet here we are. So, what does science have to say about diet and infertility?

Considering BMI

Common sense would say that extremes of weight could reduce a woman's chance of achieving a pregnancy. So, what about too thin? If a woman's body fat is reduced enough and her BMI (body mass index — an indicator of total body fat calculated by height and weight) is too low, she may stop having periods. The loss of periods means that for this woman, the brain has stopped telling the ovary to mature an egg and therefore she will not get pregnant. One form of this is the athlete's tirade, which is no periods (*amenorrhea*), eating disorder, and loss of bone (*osteoporosis*).

The original definition of eating disorder was modified to say "low energy availability." Low energy availability can be due to low food intake, such as extreme dieting or bulimia/anorexia, or increased energy expenditure such as extreme exercise (think marathoners or professional ballerinas). One study of professional dancers in the United States demonstrated that 55 percent had delayed onset of menses and 20 percent had amenorrhea.

TIP

Most fertility clinics today calculate a woman's BMI to help determine diagnosis, the appropriate treatment, and medication dosages. This is easily done by using an online BMI calculator, app or graph. These tools look at your height and weight (in kilograms and meters — so make sure to do the conversion) and, using the formula $BMI = kg/m^2$, come up with a final number. Table 9-1 explains what that number means.

TABLE 9-1 ## BMI Table

Underweight	Normal	Overweight	Obese	Extreme Obesity
Under 18.5	18.5–24.9	25–29.9	30–39.9	40 and higher

If you're underweight

The good news for women who are too thin and not menstruating is that the problem is with the control of the reproductive system. The eggs are perfectly okay. So, overcoming infertility can be accomplished by using FSH/LH, which is what the brain should be doing. This approach may help a person achieve a pregnancy, but it doesn't correct any underlying problem that could put the woman at serious risk such as anorexia nervosa. (The mortality has been estimated to be around 10 percent, with suicide being the leading cause of death.) Women who are diagnosed with being too thin should ask their physician to evaluate them for risk factors. After all, no mother wants to leave her child with one less parent if the problem is diagnosable and treatable.

What about obesity?

Obesity is on the rise and has a number of health-related issues. Obesity has a negative impact on people with polycystic ovary syndrome (PCOS; further discussed in Chapter 7). Early studies demonstrated that a PCOS patient with irregular periods and obesity can increase her chance of conception considerably with a 10 percent body weight loss. The pregnancy rate for this group of people who do lose 10 percent of their weight is the same as the pregnancy rate using clomid. Not too shabby!

But what about the person who is overweight (BMI 25–30) or obese (BMI > 30; BMI > 40 is severe obesity) and does not have PCOS? One interesting study tried to answer some of the questions about obesity by studying the use of donor eggs. Using donor eggs removes the eggs as part of the problem of reduced pregnancy in obese patients. The study found that when using donor eggs, weight did not correlate with pregnancy. In other words, it was not the uterus that could be the problem — the chance of getting pregnant was the same no matter what the weight.

Obesity is associated with a reduced pregnancy potential. The extensive Nurses' Health Study found that being obese at age 18 had a negative impact on future fertility. The study suggested that the composition of the diet was significant with a low glycemic diet and nutrient content diet being positive for achieving a pregnancy.

Obesity is associated with adverse pregnancy outcomes such as subfertility, recurrent pregnancy loss, gestational diabetes, preeclampsia, and stillbirth. Thus, regardless of whether it is the egg or the uterus, obesity is detrimental to motherhood and the composition of the diet is important for maximal fertility.

So, what should I put on my plate?

Eat meat if you want to get pregnant with a boy, and eat sugar if you want a girl, an old wives' tale states. But what if you just want to have a baby — of *any* kind?

When coauthor Jackie first ventured online to find out more about this road that had become a little longer than she had first anticipated, she found an entire civilization of people trying to conceive by using a variety of dietary means, claiming that diet changes put them in tiptop reproductive shape. These women (and men) had purged their diets of red meat, dairy products, white flour, sugar, and a host of other staples that she viewed as necessary. She was terrified. Their list of don'ts was Jackie's diet in a nutshell.

Some people swore by omega-3 fatty acids, found most commonly in salmon and other fish, as the magic potion for improving and/or restoring fertility. The only fish Jackie consumed were Goldfish (those popular snack crackers, that is). She thought she was in big trouble. The prospect of shots, whatever they were made of, seemed more attractive to her than a complete overhaul of her diet, but she didn't want to skip what could be a crucial step.

But is your diet a factor when trying to get pregnant? A good rule of thumb is to treat your body as though you were already pregnant. That's food for thought! If you wouldn't put it in your body while pregnant, why do so before (or after for that matter)? By acting proactively when it comes to "cleansing" your diet, when you actually get pregnant, you'll already be in tune with your new state!

There is no one definition of a healthy diet, but most studies defining a healthy diet suggest diets that have whole grains, fruits, vegetables, fish, and olive oil (the Mediterranean diet comes to mind). A recent study evaluated the impact of various dietary components on blastocyst formation. The following had a positive impact on blastocyst formation: cereal, vegetables, fruits, and fish. The following had a negative impact on blastocyst formation: smoking, alcohol, weight-loss diets, red meat, and higher BMI. Here's a brief look at some foods and our recommendations (our recommendations may not help, but they certainly won't hurt, and they do represent a "common sense" way of eating):

WARNING

>> **Red meat:** Studies show that red meat neither helps nor hurts your chances of getting pregnant. But you must be cautious about how it is prepared.

Do not eat raw or undercooked fish, meat, or poultry when trying to get pregnant or during pregnancy. These products have a higher-than-normal chance of carrying listeria, bacteria that may make a mom somewhat ill but wreak havoc on an unborn child's nervous system. Listeria has also been linked to an increased rate of spontaneous abortion.

Many pregnant women are also advised to heat up luncheon meats (sliced turkey, bologna, and so on), which can also carry listeria. If you choose to do so, heat the meat in a microwave and eat it while it's still hot. Once it cools, the bacteria can reform.

>> **Dairy:** Many women trying to conceive cut dairy products from their diet, but there's no conclusive medical or scientific data that supports the notion that dairy foods compromise fertility. Use organic products if possible. If you're lactose intolerant, dairy products can create havoc on your system, so be aware of your personal dietary needs.

>> **White flour and processed sugar:** No studies have proven that refined sugar or processed flour decreases fertility. We recommend limiting their intake. However, for women with an increased BMI and PCOS, reducing the amount of carbohydrate may help improve insulin resistance. Following a lower glycemic index diet is the optimal choice. Flour and sugar raise the glycemic index, so any reduction in these food substances will improve the chance for pregnancy. An easy way to determine what to eat is to limit anything made from something white. Brightly colored vegetables and fruits are better than lighter colored vegetables and fruits.

>> **Artificial additives:** Despite hot debate, no definitive studies prove that additives such as aspartame and MSG are harmful. Limit or eliminate these additives from your diet if the controversy worries you. Fewer additives in any area of your life is a good thing.

>> **Omega-3 fatty oils:** Studies are underway to evaluate the use of omega-3 oils in male infertility and in women with endometriosis. Omega-3 oils, present in fish, soybeans, flaxseed oil, canola oil, wheat germ, and walnuts, have been shown to reduce heart disease. We recommend (and the FDA/EPA guidelines also suggest) that you eat no more than 12 ounces of fish each week and limit canned tuna to an occasional serving. Avoid shark, swordfish, king mackerel, and tilefish (also called golden or white snapper), tuna steak (fresh or frozen), orange roughy, Spanish mackerel, marlin, and grouper because these fish are at the top of the food chain and contain the highest levels of mercury.

>> **Soy:** Some older studies showed that a very high soy intake may decrease fertility. However, more recent evidence suggests just the opposite, and soy may actually improve the chance of conception. As with most dietary matters, keep the intake in moderation.

REMEMBER

Good nutrition is something that you should *not* ignore. Consider it common sense, as well as medical sense, that the healthier your body is, the healthier all its systems, including the reproductive system, are. Nutrition is part of the bigger picture that also includes such basics as getting enough sleep, exercising, and nourishing your body as well as your mind. Although good nutrition is rarely the sole factor that brings about a baby, it does help to better preserve your overall health so that you may enjoy your future child as well, and as long, as possible.

If you choose to opt for a complete nutritional overhaul, realize that this is a long-term commitment and is unlikely to produce a quick fix for your fertility issues. If you want to try a complete dietary overhaul, you should consult your doctor or a nutritionist first to make sure that you get the proper balance of vitamins and minerals. For most people, this is a major lifestyle change and may lead to better overall health.

On the fertility front, however, keep your expectations in check; diet changes alone are unlikely to get you pregnant. And conversely, it is unlikely that your dietary habits, whatever they are, are playing a large role in your infertility. However, a good diet is a good idea whether you're trying to conceive or not.

The Controversy over Estrogen

The debate over possible side effects from the use of estrogen supplementation in menopause and in birth control pills (estrogen is the main hormone responsible for female sex characteristics) has been raging since time began. But, really, it only *seems* that way. Estrogen comes in several different forms; the form most familiar to women is the synthetic estrogen called ethinyl estradiol, which is found in birth control pills and some forms of hormone replacement therapy.

WARNING

In 2005, the National Institutes of Health released the results of a long-term study of more than 11,000 women on the effects of estrogen on post-menopausal women undergoing hormone replacement therapy to relieve common menopausal symptoms such as hot flashes, depression, and low libido. The study has since been severely criticized for a number of reasons. Unfortunately, the damage done remains, and patients entering menopause need to discuss the pros and cons of hormone replacement therapy with their physicians.

However, menopausal estrogen therapy has very little to do with fertility therapy. After all, your ovaries make estrogen (in the form of estradiol), and this is a very important function. You look like a woman because of estradiol! And estradiol is necessary to develop a healthy egg, to thicken the endometrium to get it ready for embryo implantation, to change the cervical mucus to the thin stretchy kind, and so on, and so on!

So, when your doctor prescribes estrogen to help the uterine lining or to "support the luteal phase," this is the same estradiol that your ovaries would be making if everything were going well. The brand name that is often prescribed is Estrace.

So why is there a warning on the estrogen-containing oral contraceptives used frequently for IVF or to help manage irregular cycles saying you should not take them during pregnancy? Unfortunately, if women accidentally take birth control pills during early pregnancy, the hormones may have a negative effect on the fetus (girl fetuses can have changes in their genitals that make them look more "masculinized"). Birth control pills contain not only synthetic estrogen in the form of ethinyl estradiol, but also a synthetic progestin (usually a derivative of testosterone), which could cross the placenta and have effects on the developing fetus. Even though this has nothing to do with natural estradiol, the drug companies are obliged to put a warning on all forms of estrogen.

REMEMBER

Hormones are not necessarily bad; in fact, they are needed to make pregnancy happen. If in doubt, ask your doctor, and make sure that all the hormones you take are natural and not synthetic.

Considering Supplements — Vitamins, Minerals, Herbs, and More

The old adage is "you are what you eat." Really? However, there is a strong belief that what a person eats or does not eat can significantly influence their health. Two points about that: First, humans evolved in an environment where they were constantly hungry, so the human body was not designed to deal with upper limits on calorie intake. Secondly, lack of essential nutrients can cause severe disease. The disease scurvy is caused by a lack of vitamin C and results in swollen gums and open wounds. This was particularly a problem for sailors of the 18th century, when they were on ships without fresh fruit for months. Simply by providing the sailors with citrus fruit, scurvy was avoided.

In today's advanced societies, there are seldom circumstances where conditions are so severe that essential nutrients are unavailable. If anything, the dietary concern today is one of excess. However, special circumstances may arise where deficiencies of nutrients may occur, and thus it pays to study the influence of nutrients on fertility.

Dietary supplements are very popular; one survey shows that over 75 percent of all Americans use some form of supplement. Dietary supplements include herbs, vitamins, minerals, amino acids, enzymes, and extracts. Because they're considered a dietary product rather than a medicinal product, they aren't regulated by the U.S. Food and Drug Administration the way prescription medications are. This lack of regulation means that the ingredient amount may vary from one pill to the next. Supplements have also been found to be contaminated with animal parts and toxic molds in some cases. It is difficult to do sound scientific research on dietary supplements and how they influence infertility. Because of the limitations, there is considerable controversy about the value of dietary supplements.

WARNING

Because they're sold over the counter, without a prescription, supplements are often viewed as harmless. Studies have shown that many supplements are far from harmless. Some supplements, such as ephedra, have been implicated in causing death, and others, such as comfrey, can cause severe liver damage.

Taking vitamins

What are vitamins and why are they important? Vitamins are substances that the body cannot make but are required for proper body functioning. The body uses proteins to do work. These proteins are called enzymes, and they take one substance (like cholesterol) and change it into something the body needs (like estrogen). In order for these enzymes to work, they need help, and that is what many vitamins provide.

TECHNICAL STUFF

So, consider you have a cholesterol molecule and it attaches to an enzyme. The enzyme needs one molecule of a vitamin to convert the cholesterol to estrogen (this is a hypothetical case . . . biochemists relax!). What happens if you don't have that one molecule or vitamin? No conversion occurs. You can correct this by making sure your diet has enough of that vitamin or by taking vitamin supplements.

What if you add ten molecules? Those extra nine molecules are of no use. Supplemental vitamins don't increase how the enzyme works. But lipid soluble vitamins are not simply urinated away. They can collect in cells and actually damage them. Vitamins A and E have been associated with toxicity to both mothers and fetuses. For example, polar bears have very high levels of vitamin A in their liver. Eating polar bear liver is a no-no and can cause hair loss, blurred vision, skin peeling, birth defects, vomiting, and in rare cases, death. Seal and walrus livers are a no-no as well — in case you were thinking of substituting!

Multivitamins are a good way to supplement your diet, but they're not a substitute for good nutrition. While you're trying to conceive and when you get pregnant, you need both. Much has been written about the importance of folic acid in early pregnancy. It has been shown to diminish certain birth defects, such as spina bifida.

REMEMBER

Overdosing on vitamins *through foods alone* is highly unlikely. Because most foods contain small amounts of any individual vitamin or nutrient, you would have to eat bushels of bananas, oranges, or spinach to get too much. Overdosage of any particular vitamin, mineral, or nutrient is generally only a danger if you consume it in a concentrated form, such as vitamin pills or powders.

TIP

Is taking a prenatal vitamin when trying to conceive premature? Not really. The primary difference between multivitamins and prenatal vitamins is the greater concentration of folic acid and iron in a prenatal vitamin. Folic acid is crucial in pregnancy to help prevent spinal and neural tube defects, while iron is often needed as a supplement for the loss of iron due to pregnancy.

An excess of iron *can* result in constipation, which can be remedied through the introduction of additional fibers, fruits, and vegetables in your diet, a good thing no matter where you are on the baby-making quest.

Over the counter (OTC) prenatal vitamins may boast that they contain even higher levels of the necessary vitamins and nutrients. In order to achieve this, however, the OTC brand may require dosages up to three times a day while prescription prenatal vitamins pack their punch in one dose per day. If you're feeling childlike, even though you're not with child yet, you can also get the same ingredients of a prenatal vitamin by taking three Flintstones Complete vitamins per day.

WARNING

If you're taking a standard multivitamin rather than prenatal vitamins while pregnant, make sure that it doesn't contain extra ingredients such as herbs. Many health food stores sell blends that contain herbs. Don't take these types of vitamins during fertility treatment or pregnancy.

Are certain vitamins, taken in greater (or lesser) quantities, more likely to result in increased fertility? At the time of this writing, no direct evidence supports this. We advise you to stick with a standard multivitamin or prenatal vitamin. Your local pharmacist can recommend a good OTC brand, and your doctor can steer you toward a good prescription choice.

Some studies have shown that liquid prenatal vitamins are better absorbed than pills. They may also be less likely to make you nauseated after you become pregnant.

REMEMBER

All the vitamins in the world can't get you pregnant, but they can help you keep your body in the best nutritional shape possible, along with proper diet, exercise, and the right fertility treatment.

Herbs

Although herbs have been used for centuries, studies on their safety and benefits have been few. That's beginning to change, with the National Institutes of Health (NIH) now studying many herbs and other alternative medications. Herbs aren't always benign, and someone with some knowledge of their interactions should oversee their use. Practitioners in this area may include chiropractors, osteopaths, nutritionists, and naturopaths (those who employ a drugless approach to keep the body in balance). Keep in mind, however, that herbs are, in essence, drugs in and of themselves. The big difference? They aren't regulated by the FDA!

A large review article published in 2013 found that Chinese herbal medicine did improve the pregnancy rate. However, the authors found that the research was so biased that the results were questionable, which is less than helpful. Unfortunately, much of the research in this area concludes with statements that large, better controlled studies need to be done. Until such time as these studies are actually done, the best approach is to be cautious when using herbal preparations.

Plants have hundreds of hormones, just like people, and not all of them are useful for treating infertility. It is illuminating to remember that progesterone, a key component of the birth control pill, was originally isolated from a tuber of the same family as yams.

Here's a look at some of the more popular herbs used in the treatment of infertility. This list represents a small sample of herbs that can be used and represents herbs that are both Western in origin as well as Chinese.

>> **Black cohosh:** An herb with estrogenic qualities, black cohosh is often used to relieve the discomfort associated with menopause (hot flashes, for example). Studies have been mixed on whether black cohosh is effective. Black cohosh is also recommended to boost estrogen production, although there's no proof that this works. Side effects of black cohosh are dizziness, nausea, low pulse rate, and increased perspiration.

WARNING

>> **Dong quai:** Dubbed the "ultimate herb" for women, dong quai is used for everything from restoring menstrual regularity to treating menopausal symptoms. Dong quai is a blood thinner and should not be taken during an IVF cycle or by women who have very heavy periods.

>> **False unicorn root:** Native Americans used this herb to improve menstrual irregularities and to alleviate problems associated with menopause and problems with infertility due to irregular follicular formation.

>> **Nettle leaves:** This herb is considered to be an overall uterine tonic that better prepares the uterus for implantation of the embryo. (There is no scientific evidence for this.)

>> **Primrose oil:** A fatty acid, primrose oil may increase cervical mucus to make it easier for sperm to get to the egg. An unwanted side effect of primrose oil may be thinning of the uterine lining, making implantation more difficult.

>> **Red clover:** This herb is often used to boost estrogen in a women's body. This exogenous, or outside the body, form of estrogen may raise your estrogen levels artificially, which is meaningless if the rise isn't caused by the production of a mature egg.

WARNING

>> **Red raspberry leaves:** Another uterine toner, this herb reportedly increases the uterine lining thickness (in order to make the uterus more receptive to the embryo). Red raspberry causes uterine contractions and absolutely should not be used in early pregnancy.

>> **Vitex:** Also known as chaste tree berry, this herb has been used by herbalists for many years to help regulate women's hormones. Some use Vitex to increase luteinizing hormone levels and help an egg release. According to others, Vitex can also increase progesterone levels and should be used only after you ovulate — not before. If taken earlier, it may keep you from releasing an egg. If taken in the luteal phase, after you ovulate, it may regulate and lengthen your cycle to give the embryo a chance to implant. Vitex is slow acting, so it may take several months for any effect to occur.

>> **Wild yam:** In large doses, wild yam is used as a contraceptive; in smaller doses, it may promote progesterone production. Don't take wild yam until after ovulation occurs.

WARNING

The following herbs stimulate the uterus, so you absolutely should not take them after you get pregnant:

>> Black cohosh

>> Dong quai

>> False unicorn root

>> Feverfew

>> Goldenseal

>> Pennyroyal

In addition, avoid these drugs if you get pregnant:

>> **Blue cohosh:** May cause fetal heart defects

>> **Mugwort:** May cause fetal abnormalities

WARNING

Herbal treatment of infertility is not a do-it-yourself approach! Let all your doctors know if you're taking any kinds of herbs, whether they're the over-the-counter variety or prescribed to you by another source. Undesirable reactions may occur between one herb preparation and another. In addition, they may all cross-react with the drugs your reproductive endocrinologist is giving you. Deciding what to take on your own is complicated, because the same herb may be described as useful for two entirely opposing actions. Telling your doctor that you are taking supplements is the very least that you should do!

Folic acid

Folic acid, a B vitamin, is essential when trying to get pregnant. Many studies have shown that 0.4 mg of folic acid a day cuts the chance of having a baby with neural tube defects by 50 percent. Neural tube defects occur in 6 of 10,000 births in the United States and include problems with the spine and brain. Neural tube defects develop very early in pregnancy, in the first four weeks, so taking a good multivitamin containing this amount while trying to get pregnant is essential. Many foods, including leafy green vegetables, fortified cereals, orange juice, and lean beef, contain folic acid, but overcooking can destroy folic acid, so take a vitamin even if you eat well.

The folic acid story provides a great example of the frustration in trying to decide whether supplements are useful in infertility. Folic acid is used in processes that alter DNA. Some people have a gene that causes lower activity in the use of folic acid, and this was originally found to influence the quality and number of oocytes in IVF. Based upon this, it was hoped that supplementation with folic acid would improve the pregnancy rate and reduce the miscarriage rate. Shortly after these original articles, the following studies suggested that folic acid actually increased the risk of fetal death. Of course, there then followed a number of articles refuting the negative effect of folic acid. So today we are on neutral ground. Maybe yes, maybe no. Overall, supplemental folic acid is important for the normal development of the baby.

Wheatgrass

For coauthor Jackie, it was a litmus test. When she dropped a wheatgrass pill on the floor, her basset hound (also known as the canine garbage disposal) raced toward it. Before she could grab it, he had it in his mouth. Then, to her disbelief, the dog, who has been known to view dead squirrel as a delicacy, dropped the wheatgrass pill and scurried away. It was not a testament to taste.

What is wheatgrass anyway? Wheatgrass is a dark, leafy green vegetable (think kale, also categorized as a "super food," but in and of itself, does not a healthy diet make) that can be harvested, dried, and bottled in pill form. Some people attest that the homegrown or fresh-grown variety is better and raise their own wheatgrass from seed, later shaving off the grass and blending it into a questionable-looking "mix."

REMEMBER

Regarding the claims that wheatgrass lowers FSH levels and thus improves the number and/or quality of eggs, remember that you're born with a limited number of eggs that only decreases over time. There is virtually no way to increase that number or to change a bad egg into a good one. FSH is merely a measurement of ovarian reserve and is generally checked to determine the probable response to stimulation via fertility medicines.

WARNING

Just because something is touted as "natural" does not mean that it has no harmful effects. Many "natural" products are advertised for very narrow purposes with exaggerated results and do not have any scientific basis for how they work. So, often, they just don't work. Always ask your doctor before you embark on any "natural" treatment program.

L-arginine

L-arginine is another example of a product that has received cult status over the past few years for treating everything from immune disorders to sexual problems. L-arginine is a nonessential amino acid found in whole wheat, rice, nuts, seeds, corn, soy, grapes, carob, and other foods. Nonmedical individuals in the fertility community have used L-arginine (also known as arginine) in concentrated pill form during fertility cycles in efforts to improve egg quality. Some studies also show increased blood flow to the uterus. In males, some studies (but not all) have shown increased sperm motility and production when taking L-arginine.

A study published by the professional journal *Human Reproduction* pointed out a negative effect of L-arginine if you're taking fertility medications. The study showed that in a small test group, the use of L-arginine supplementation was detrimental to embryo quality and pregnancy rate during a sample cycle when the test also used fertility medicines.

WARNING

If you're prone to cold sores, L-arginine may exacerbate them. Use with caution.

Like many supplements, L-arginine can cause adverse reactions at higher doses when taken in pill form as a supplement. It is virtually impossible to overdose on the amount of L-arginine found in foods, as even foods that contain it have it only in trace amounts. However, L-arginine can reach less-than-desirable levels when taken in more concentrated forms, such as pills. Pregnant women are advised not to use L-arginine.

WARNING

A walk down the aisle at a local "health food supplement" store to peruse the ingredients in all the bottles may shock you! There are "natural" remedies that were made from animal thyroid glands, adrenal glands, and other parts of animals. Yet nowhere on the label does it warn the consumer that products made from animal thyroid glands contain thyroid hormone, which is identical to the one made by humans! This thyroid hormone is available without a prescription, in purity that could not be assessed and in doses that could not be determined! And products made from adrenal glands of course contain adrenal hormones, which include steroids (such as cortisol), adrenalin, and so on. All of these can and do have real physiologic effects on humans, and those trying to conceive are especially vulnerable.

Vitamin D: Is all the hype justified?

Who hasn't had their vitamin D level checked recently? There has been a significant increase in healthcare concerns about vitamin D in a lot of different areas of medicine. Research suggests that these concerns may be justified. So, what is vitamin D and should a person care?

TECHNICAL STUFF

Vitamin D is not really a vitamin based upon the definition of vitamin. A vitamin is a substance that the body needs in very small amounts but cannot produce. Vitamins are therefore essential micronutrients that must be derived from the diet. Vitamin D can be synthesized in the body and thus is more properly viewed as a hormone. Classically, vitamin D has been associated with the intestinal absorption of calcium, magnesium, and phosphate. But it has been implicated in a number of biological processes, including some related to reproduction.

Vitamin D deficiency has been implicated in a number of reproductive processes, and there is a large number of publications concerning Vitamin D. Relying upon systematic review and meta-analysis, two recent studies agreed that vitamin D does play a role in the success of IVF. It will take a while before a definitive answer can be found, so the decision about the measurement of vitamin D levels in women undergoing IVF and the subsequent choice to treat low levels becomes a question about the danger of the treatment. Vitamin D treatment for women with low vitamin D levels seems to be safe. Therefore, currently, measuring vitamin D levels and treating seems to be the most prudent way to go.

As with so many questionable treatments in medicine, the use of vitamin D has come under attack. A recent editorial in the *Journal of the American Medical Association* demonstrates how early correlations many times are found not to be causes when more rigorous scientific testing is done. The authors (Lucas & Wolf [2019] JAMA 322:1866) note that publication of randomized controlled trials (RCTs) failed to substantiate some of the suggested beneficial health claims for vitamin D. These studies have not addressed infertility, but hopefully in the near future RCTs will be performed to assess the importance of vitamin D in the treatment of infertility.

Myoinositol and PCOS

Recently there has been considerable interest in the use of myoinositol (M-inositol, M-IN) in the treatment of infertility for polycystic ovary syndrome (PCOS) and IVF.

M-inositol is actually a sugar that is found in a number of human organs. The body can make as much as 2 grams of M-IN a day from glucose with the kidney. Other tissue can make M-IN, but the highest amount is found in the brain. M-IN was formerly thought to be vitamin B8, but since it is made in the body and is not an essential nutrient, it cannot be a vitamin. M-IN is involved in several molecular functions in the body. It is involved with neurotransmitters, as second messengers in various cells, and in the synthesis of some hormones. Inositol functions as a second messenger in several cells. One type of second messenger is involved with insulin, and since insulin plays a central role in the pathology of PCOS, it seems reasonable that M-IN might help in the treatment of PCOS. The results from a couple of meta-analyses agree that M-IN helps in the treatment of PCOS.

M-IN is a safe, over-the-counter substance that may help in the treatment of PCOS or in certain circumstances when patients are undergoing IVF. One treatment suggestion was to use 2 grams of M-IN twice a day. Metformin can be added to this regimen if deemed necessary. This, combined with lifestyle changes such as a 10 percent loss of weight, a reduction in carbohydrate consumption, and an increase in daily mild exercise, can improve the chance of obtaining a successful pregnancy. When successful, the pregnancy usually occurs within the first six months of consciously trying to conceive. If after six months there is no pregnancy, then other treatments are available such as letrozole and IVF. Overall, cumulative success rates of pregnancy for women with PCOS are extremely high given today's knowledge about PCOS and the technology available.

Coenzyme Q10 (CoQ10)

Coenzyme Q10 is a molecule that is required in order for some proteins to do their work. The body has many of these substances, and they are called cofactors. CoQ10 is involved with the molecular system that cells use to generate energy, which occurs primarily in structures within cells called *mitochondria*.

The process of embryo formation requires considerable energy. Some young women undergoing IVF respond poorly to the stimulation protocols used in IVF. One suggestion is that these women have poor energy generation, and thus it may be possible that the addition of CoQ10 could improve the responsiveness to the protocols. Decreased levels of CoQ10 occur as women age, and the addition of CoQ10 has been suggested to improve male fertility. Based upon an understanding of the physiology in the egg, a study was done to determine if the addition of CoQ10 could improve the response for a group of young patients who had experienced a poor response in their IVF cycle. The study was a randomized control trial and did show that the addition of CoQ10 results in the reduction in the amount of FSH required, more eggs retrieved, and more high-quality embryos. However, while there was a trend for higher live birth rates, this trend did not reach clinical significance. CoQ10 is relatively inexpensive, readily available over the counter, and safe. The study involved a particular group of patients and may not be applicable to other patients undergoing IVF. Until more is known, the use of CoQ10 seems reasonable.

Supplements for better sperm production

Fertility is not just a female issue. In fact, 40 percent of the time, male factor is responsible for a couple's failure to conceive.

So, women aren't the only ones who may venture onto an alternative path for treating medical problems related to infertility. Keep in mind that studies have been mixed (at best) as to the efficacy of taking supplements. Also remember that in male problems where surgery is deemed necessary (to fix a varicocele or any other structural issue), diet and/or supplements won't do the trick. These tips, however, can benefit overall health, which can contribute to better reproductive health. A man produces new sperm every three months, so what you do today can theoretically affect conception down the line. The following supplements have been suggested to benefit sperm count and motility in some studies (but note that as with women, no conclusive evidence exists, and, just as with women, too much of a good thing can be quite toxic, never mind counterproductive):

>> **Zinc:** Suggested to increase sperm motility and sperm count

>> **Vitamin B12:** Suggested to increase sperm count

>> **Vitamin C:** Suggested to increase sperm count

>> **Vitamin E:** Suggested to increase sperm motility

>> **Selenium:** Suggested to increase sperm motility

>> **L-Carnitine:** Suggested to increase sperm motility and sperm count

>> **L-arginine:** Suggested to increase sperm motility and sperm count

>> **Folic acid:** Suggested to increase sperm motility and sperm count

>> **CoQ10:** Suggested to increase sperm motility and sperm count

A good multivitamin generally contains an adequate amount of all of the preceding.

REMEMBER

When supplements are labeled as "natural," they should be used with caution as they have limited FDA regulation, which means you may not know what's really in the "compound" you buy; they may interact with the medications prescribed by your fertility doctor and, most important, some have serious side effects.

Exploring Alternative Medicine from China and Beyond

Complementary and alternative medicine (CAM) is widely used. Much of the current CAM is based upon Chinese medicine that has been practiced for over 5,000 years. Some of the forms of this are acupuncture, herbal medicine, and massage. Many practitioners of CAM believe that the body will heal itself if kept in proper balance, and herbalists tout supplements as a way to achieve the proper balance and thus help to get (and stay) pregnant. Internet sites abound with happy moms claiming that supplements were responsible for their pregnancies. So, who do you believe, and are there any supplements that you absolutely should not take? The most important consideration for the use of CAM is that it must not reduce the chance for a successful pregnancy. Beyond that, there is considerable debate about the use of CAM, but one way to view it is as a complement to the more traditional Western medical approach.

Traditional Chinese medicine

Traditional Chinese medicine (TCM), often referred to as Eastern medicine, works on a different set of principles and beliefs than Western medicine (that which is practiced in the United States and many other parts of the world). Traditional

Chinese medicine views the individual as an integral mind/body organism and, in essence, believes that a delicate balance, the yin and yang, is necessary for optimal health and well-being. TCM divides the body into various *meridians,* or pathways, along which *qi,* or energy, flows. For example, fertility problems may be explained by liver qi stagnation, that is, congestion in the liver meridian. Primary treatment in TCM includes the administration of herbal formulas and acupuncture to clear the body passageways and restore normal function.

Although traditional Chinese medicine has been practiced since 204 B.C., only during the past two decades has it been recognized in the United States and other parts of the world. According to Western medicine, anecdotal evidence, as demonstrated in TCM, awaits confirmation in randomized clinical trials.

Despite this lack of scientific evidence, many patients, suffering from diseases ranging from cancer to chronic fatigue to infertility, have found a haven in the TCM community, which many times is warmer and fuzzier than the classic Western doctor/hospital setting. Some who have given up on Western medicine (or on whom Western medicine has given up) have found palliative relief, remission, and results under the guidance of a traditional Chinese medicine doctor.

WARNING

Before you jump on the TCM bandwagon, check the credentials of the practitioner you select. TCM doctors must complete training, just as they do in Western medicine, and should be licensed or certified (if your state offers this). In addition, they should be nationally certified through the National Certification Commission for Acupuncture and Oriental Medicine. To confirm certification, visit the commission's website at www.nccaom.org.

Help from herbal formulas

Your TCM practitioner may prescribe an herbal formula containing up to ten different herbs. The combination of herbs to create a formula is one of the main differences between the Western and Eastern views. TCM relies on this ability to modify formulas in order to customize an individual approach based on a patient's needs. TCM herbal formulas are also available in pills that can be purchased from your TCM practitioner; however, they're considered to be less effective due to the extraction process necessary to convert them into this form.

Because there are over 6,000 herbs from which to choose, this formulation is a science in and of itself and, unlike the single-ingredient, Western herb approach, can't be self-administered.

Most TCM practitioners also use *moxibustion,* in which small mounds of herbs are burned over certain areas of the body, in the treatment of infertility. TCM practitioners also treat male infertility issues, so feel free to go as a couple.

REMEMBER

WARNING

Don't view traditional Chinese medicine as a shortcut. Nothing in medicine ever is.

We also recommend that you "pick your poison," for lack of a better term. Whether your treatment is traditional Chinese medicine or Western medicine, don't try to combine the two. Many herbs, when taken with fertility medicines, can cause adverse reactions. Particularly when combined with treatments that involve surgical procedures, such as in vitro fertilization, the ingestion of herbs or other tonics can cause more severe problems, such as bleeding, or simply complicate matters. As a result, both your TCM doctor and your Western doctor may find it impossible to accurately define and treat your condition.

If you choose to try both TCM and Western medicine simultaneously (despite our suggestions to the contrary), make sure that all of your practitioners, doctors, and nurses are aware of your protocol. Not revealing this information is an ideal way to confuse the people whose goals are to help you conceive.

On pins and needles — acupuncture for infertility

Perhaps one area of traditional Chinese medicine that has benefited the most from the recent interest on behalf of Western medicines is acupuncture. The use of acupuncture has certainly created considerable controversy almost creating a divided nation of believers and doubters.

The rule of thumb is that the more controversy a topic creates the less likely that it will be possible to answer any question with a yes or no response. The answers will be in the gray zone and of the order of "maybe, but we need more information," or "not necessarily." Acupuncture is based on the belief that a person's health is determined by a balanced flow of energy (qi) in the body. This 5,000-year-old practice is most often used to relieve chronic pain by inserting needles into a variety of pressure points on the head and body. Acupuncture is also used for treatments for everything from the common cold to drug addiction.

Acupuncture has long been a popular alternative form of treatment for infertility. Women have found that acupuncture has been crucial in helping them relax through the trials and tribulations of fertility treatment. There are numerous studies about the usefulness of acupuncture on the treatment for infertility (for example, some say it increases blood flow to the uterus), *but* there is no consensus amongst this vast amount of research.

An example of some of the research is a recent randomized control trial (RCT) where acupuncture was compared to sham acupuncture. The study failed to show an improvement in pregnancy rates when using acupuncture. However, other RCTs did show an improvement.

When such a situation occurs in medicine, scientists have developed ways of statistically evaluating all studies and combining their results to give a more accurate answer about the usefulness of a treatment. These studies are called systematic reviews and meta-analyses. Three such studies (2008, 2013, 2013) all reported similar results concluding there was no evidence that acupuncture improved pregnancy rates. A more recent meta-analysis (2018) evaluated 20 trials and included 5,130 women. The study found that acupuncture did improve outcomes for embryo transfer in IVF when the control group had no sham control. Applying a sham acupuncture as a control group removed this positive effect.

REMEMBER

Whether its effects are actually physiological or not, acupuncture can be an adjunct to a fertility regimen as a means of relaxation (if you are someone who relaxes by becoming a human pincushion, that is!) However, be sure that those performing the treatment are certified. Many fertility clinics work in conjunction with an acupuncturist and/or can recommend someone who specializes in fertility-based treatment.

Many states have their own acupuncture society, and some states have specific requirements that must be met. For example, in Indiana, people need a prescription from a physician in order to be treated by a certified acupuncturist. You can check online for your state's rules and regulations, as well as for acupuncture societies, which may also provide you with specific recommendations.

If you're scared of being stuck with acupuncture needles, take heart! The average acupuncture needle has the thickness of a human hair. You may feel a small stick, but it's far less discomfort than a blood test. But if you're still a bit apprehensive and too needle-phobic about the procedure, you may be better off skipping this particular form of treatment. Remember that the goal is to relax.

TIP

Bring along a favorite tape or CD to listen to during acupuncture treatment. Most acupuncture treatments require you to lie still with the needles in place for a short period of time, usually 20 minutes or less. This may also be a great time to use your visualization techniques.

Chanting Your Way to Conception: Meditation and Yoga

For those who need a little more help than self-help, consider the structure of a class such as meditation or yoga. Although they're not cure-alls, these ancient arts can go a long way in easing your mind, body, and spirit.

Staying sane through the process is a goal that can carry you through your fertility rites. This goal is something you *can* control, and meditation or yoga can help. Check with your local gyms or wellness centers to see whether they have classes. Or ask your family or fertility doctor to recommend a particular class or instructor. You may be surprised at how many medical folks use the same techniques to bring peace to their own lives.

In today's world, you can practice meditation or yoga by simply summoning the correct app! Our entire book could be dedicated to listing all those that exist. Utilize your googling and search skills and you can be on your way — without leaving your house!

HOW DO YOU SPELL RELIEF? R-E-L-A-X

Medical researchers have known for some time about what's called *relaxation response or mindfulness,* which is defined as a series of physiological changes that occur when a person blocks out intrusive thoughts by repeating a word, a sound, a phrase, or a prayer. Relaxation response can cause a decrease in metabolism, heart rate, rate of breathing, and brain wave activity.

When used in conjunction with nutrition and exercise, relaxation response has been proven to be effective therapy in treating the stress brought on by a number of conditions, including infertility and its treatments.

Some research says that infertile women are twice as likely to experience depressive symptoms as fertile women.

Coauthor Jackie participated in a six-week program that applied the techniques of relaxation response conducted by a nurse who worked for a local fertility clinic. Although she (Jackie) was initially skeptical about the benefits, she did find the relaxation techniques, nutritional information, open dialogue, and camaraderie to be helpful. Partners were invited to participate in the last class of the session, where everyone focused on communication skills to better express their individual problems and fears related to their infertility and treatment. She enjoyed this opportunity immensely, and her husband appreciated the refreshments.

To find out more about workshops in relaxation response in your area, ask your doctor (ideally your OB/GYN or a fertility specialist) or contact your local chapter of Resolve at www.resolve.org.

Both meditation and yoga can carry you through your pregnancy as well. Meditation can help relieve the discomfort and pain of everything from morning sickness to labor, and yoga can keep your gestating (or pregnant!) body fit and focused all the way through.

Seeking Help from On High

When you're caught up in the minutiae of fertility management (and there's plenty of minutiae!), you may have trouble seeing your daily struggles as part of a larger plan designed by a power greater than yourself. Whatever your faith, solace and relief are available to you.

Coauthor Jackie has witnessed many women online and in person walking through the fertility process with confidence as they placed their fears and worries in the hands of their God, a special saint, or an icon. Many chat rooms started their own prayer group. And although many people claim to be disbelievers, the old adage "there are no atheists in foxholes" seems to be true. Online prayer groups grew at a lightning pace, bearing the names of those who were pious by nature, as well as those who just figured prayer couldn't hurt. And it can't.

Through the ages, certain groups have turned to the power of prayer for healing the sick and giving sight to the blind. A study was released in the United States in early 2002 that claimed that patients in a test group who were prayed for by outside individuals made a quicker and better recovery than those who weren't. Some physicians scoff at this notion. However, many people find credence in the idea that prayer helps patients relax and, in doing so, helps them to release whatever stranglehold they may have on their condition and to stop trying to force results. This type of help may make whatever road you travel a little less bumpy.

Individuals and couples may also benefit from the moderation of a third party, such as a priest, rabbi, or other religious figure. These professionals often act as counselors to help an individual or couple work through problems resulting from outside stressors, such as fertility. Religious leaders also respect your privacy and maintain confidences just as a therapist or doctor does. Their consideration of all things spiritual may also help to reveal another point of view or option. If nothing else, your local clergy can provide additional support, something that you can never get enough of, regardless of your situation.

Putting Your Body in Motion:
The Benefits of Exercise

PERSONAL STORY

Jackie found that one of the most difficult parts of infertility and its treatments was the loss of certain aspects of her life. As an avid runner, coauthor Jackie questioned her exercise routine and wondered whether the constant jarring might be preventing her from getting pregnant. She asked her doctor, who recommended moderate exercise. Jackie's not the type of person who understands the word *moderate*, regardless of its context. She decided not to take any chances and replaced running with a workout on a stair-climbing machine. After a few more months of failed attempts at pregnancy, she reevaluated the stair-climbing workout as well. And so it went until she was reduced to walking, which also became a personal no-no during the two-week wait after the time of ovulation. As the fertility bar seemed to get higher and higher, her stress management tools, such as exercise, had diminished to almost nothing. It was not a pretty sight.

Regular exercise is a good thing when trying to conceive, just as it is at almost any time in your life (except maybe when you're in traction). The key is to participate in moderate (there's that word again) activity that's consistent with your past routines. For example, if your previous exercise plan consisted of wind sprints to the refrigerator and back, training for your first marathon while trying to conceive isn't a wise idea. Some doctors recommend keeping your heart rate under a maximum of 140 beats per minute. You can use this as a guide to help build your exercise plan. When it comes to nonaerobic activity, the sky is (virtually) the limit. Again, use common sense when making your choices. Full-contact boxing may be a bit more precarious during this time (actually during any time!), but kickboxing for fitness could be a good compromise.

WARNING

If you're someone who over-exercises as a means to lose weight, your behavior could affect your fertility. Check with your doctor to make sure that you're within the proper weight limits. Carrying too little weight can affect your menstrual cycle as well as your hormones, therefore compromising your ability to conceive.

TIP

Above all, no matter what exercise you engage in, stay well hydrated at all times. Doing so is especially important when trying to conceive and even more so while pregnant. Wear comfortable clothing and be aware of how you feel at all times. Exercise shouldn't be painful — ever! If it is, stop, rest, and consult a trainer or exercise physiologist before resuming your routine.

Ironically, after tiring of her lack of exercise and treating her body as though it was spun glass, Jackie began running again during her third year of trying to conceive. After one month of resuming her former exercise routine, she found out she was pregnant. Go figure.

Chapter **10**

Are We Having Fun Yet? Managing Your Emotions and Relationships

While making a baby certainly has all the right ingredients for a good time, once infertility is stirred into the pot, fun becomes a concept reserved for those for whom sex has remained — well, just sex.

In this chapter, we discuss how to traverse the lost and found sections of the couple's fun department. While infertility certainly has its share of growth opportunities, which are anything but a good time, your relationship can actually grow in a positive manner, helping you and your partner find ways to support and love one another through the rough spots. Consider all these learning experiences good practice for the many challenges that child rearing will offer you!

Holding Your Relationship Together during Treatment

Experiencing infertility can take your relationship to a whole new level — one you could probably live without. Human relationships are rarely improved by the addition of stress, frustration, anger, and recriminations, at least not until the crisis is over and some perspective on the situation can be gained. In hindsight, we realize that our relationships aren't really strengthened by the good times, but instead the bad ones, or in the words of an old adage, "What doesn't kill you makes you stronger." So, buckle up, buttercup!

The potential loss of a dream as big as a family of your own can be devastating in a number of ways. The pitfalls you fall into while trying to navigate the uncharted waters of infertility depend on your personalities, the way you relate to each other normally, and sometimes just on the time of day or the weather! In the next sections, we look at some of the common relationship challenges couples dealing with infertility may face.

Easy does it when conceiving gets harder

Most couples start trying to get pregnant with barely a thought that success may not be immediate. Most couples are more afraid to start trying too soon, worrying more that they'll get pregnant the first month of trying. It usually comes as a complete shock to discover that pregnancy can, even under normal conditions, take up to six months or more to achieve.

A few months of negative pregnancy tests can be hard to process, intellectually and emotionally, when everyone else seems to be able to get pregnant so easily. "I never thought I'd be at this point," coauthor Jackie remembers lamenting to herself and anyone else who would listen. Married at 34, she had been trying to conceive for two years to no avail. Her local doctor had been convinced, and convincing, that she would get her baby through the low-tech intrauterine insemination (IUI) procedures. "You have stingy ovaries," he would say with a wink. "We'll just push you a little harder and hope you don't end up with more than one."

After three failed attempts and increasingly higher doses of medication, that dialogue began to wear thin. Her faith in him and in herself had waned, and she was off to find a new doctor and a more direct line to a baby. Now, here she stood contemplating in vitro fertilization (IVF), a $15,000-plus, two-month procedure for what she thought would have been accomplished in one night after a bottle of cheap wine. The mountain was indeed much higher than she thought.

REMEMBER

Failing to get pregnant month after month can be especially difficult if one of you is still in the "No problem, we'll just keep trying, it'll happen eventually" mode while the other partner is ready to move on — to a new doctor, medical intervention, or a high-tech procedure like IVF. If you're a couple with one laid-back partner and one gung-ho partner, you probably know this already. How to cope with mismatched ideas of how to proceed when what seemed easy turns out to be really hard? Talk to each other! One of you may need to lighten up a little and the other may need to "get off the pot" so to speak, so you can proceed at a pace with which you're both comfortable.

Avoiding the blame game, round one: It's not my fault

Perhaps the most destructive force in any relationship is blame, whether it is deserved or not. All of us can take responsibility for our actions, but for the most part, our reproductive system is what it is, regardless of anything we did or didn't do. Remember, infertility is not punishment; it's biology.

There's almost a perfect balance between male factors and female factors as causes for infertility; 40 percent of the time the problem is due to male issues, 40 percent of infertility is due to female issues, and 20 percent is unexplained — or a combination of the two. With the scales so evenly balanced, there is no rational reason to play the blame game, but inevitably, many couples end up in this no-win scenario.

Avoiding the blame game, round two: We should have started sooner

Ah! Another one of those useless diversions . . . we should have known we would have problems and started earlier! With such perfect 20/20 hindsight, none of us would need gainful employment.

Waiting until age 50 to conceive may not be the brightest of ideas, unless, of course, you are completely willing to use donor eggs, sperm, or both. But, other than an extreme case such as this, second guessing your decision to (pick one) wait for the right person with whom to build your life, put off having a baby to finish school, become financially stable, or improve a tumultuous relationship before bringing a child into it is futile. These are probably all excellent reasons for putting the brakes on baby making.

Revisiting these choices when you encounter problems is similar to replaying an accident over in your mind, trying to imagine what might have happened had you taken another route. It's over — move on and make the next right decision. Don't waste your time and energy rethinking your motives. Resist the temptation to reinvent history. It doesn't work.

Same game, more blame: Why one of you just isn't into it

You probably won't be surprised to learn that people react to things differently. While one partner's emotions may often rise and fall with each test result, the other person's feelings may not.

One common view of some partners is that the proof is in the baby, not in the myriad details. Your partner may not want to hear daily about your cervical mucus, your possible nausea, your maybe-slightly-a-little-bit-sore breasts, or your latest discussion with your mom about how long it took your cousin Susie to get pregnant. It's not that your partner doesn't want a baby, it's just that they don't want to hear about it ad infinitum.

If you're a micromanager (and many are, especially when it comes to something as big as getting pregnant), this seeming nonchalance, if not outright indifference, to the process of baby getting may infuriate you. You may goad your partner with "You just don't care" accusations, which probably aren't true and will probably provoke retaliation in kind, which isn't going to help either of you.

Some individuals want to talk about something once and then let it go until something actually happens. Others may want and need to talk things out not just once, but daily, hourly, or sometimes even every few minutes. Many people seem better able to compartmentalize the things that are going on in their lives than others. Like being able to put aside baby concerns when watching the Super Bowl, for example. You, on the other hand, may find the Super Bowl a perfect time to talk about baby.

Once you've been assured — or reassured — once or twice by your partner that yes, they really want a baby, and yes, they really do care about you and your future offspring, more than life itself, how about watching the Super Bowl now without thinking about how hard it must be for the players' wives to get pregnant when they're on the road all the time? Really, your partner's extreme desire to talk about the game rather than your ultrasound results when the game is in overtime is in no way a reflection of what kind of a parent they'll be.

WARNING

If, on the other hand, you notice real foot dragging on your partner's part when it comes to matters of infertility, you may need to have a serious discussion. Maybe they have concerns that haven't been brought up; maybe they aren't really as committed to having a baby as you are. If that's the case, it's time to put on the brakes until you can talk things out and find out what each of you is really thinking. Having a baby when one partner isn't sure about the idea is rarely a good idea.

Healing Your Relationship: Band-Aids and Longer-Term Solutions

So, sex isn't fun anymore. Dreaming about your family-to-be causes your eyes to mist up. So how do you bring the fun back into your relationship and your life?

It may be hard to believe, but it's the partner of the fertility patient who primarily faces the problem of loneliness resulting from the pursuit of a baby. While one partner is trying to cope with the possible loss of fertility, the other partner is dealing with: the loss of a partner who is immersed in the facts, figures, and minutiae that can become all-encompassing when trying to conceive. Many partners experience their own immeasurable pain watching the one they love struggle with infertility and feeling unable to fix it.

For the fertility patient, the struggle with fertility may bring a great deal of fear and pain, but it can also deliver new friends (real and cyber), enough reading and research to fill a lifetime, and a litany of emotions to sort through. A woman may find herself so busy with these activities that she doesn't even have time for a quiet night with her partner in front of the television.

TIP

To help solve this problem, we recommend "fertility-free zones," times and places where the subject is off-limits. Although detaching from what appears to be such a looming issue may be hard, the space created by these mini vacations allows you to recharge yourselves as a couple and remember what brought you together in the first place.

Remembering the joy

Fighting with your fertility is a battle best won with kindness, toward yourself and your partner. Here are our suggestions for marking time:

>> Take the time to appreciate good health; it's not a guarantee, whether you conceive or not.

>> If you don't have a baby to love yet, direct that energy toward the children and adults who are in your life today. Doing so involves no risks, and the rewards will carry you through this difficult time.

>> Are you angry? Makes sense to us. Perhaps you can channel that anger into a letter to your congressman lobbying for better healthcare coverage for fertility patients. Or, physical activity — paint a room, join a gym!

>> Do you feel it's unfair that people you consider undeserving parents get to have the children that you dream of? Consider underserved kids! Volunteer to be a Big Sister or Big Brother for a child who will truly benefit from your good parenting skills. Or, offer to babysit for your neighbor or sister!

>> Pamper yourself and your body. Get a massage, enjoy fine (and healthy) dining, read a good book, go for a walk, or play with a puppy.

>> Create a support network. While your old friends are like gold in getting you through this, no one can truly comfort and sustain you quite like another person experiencing the same thing.

Coming together as a team

REMEMBER

To get pregnant is not a job, a cause, or a *raison d'etre* (okay, Jackie, you need to explain the French: It means the most important reason for your existence!).

It's a means to an end with the idea of creating a family as the goal. When your mind is too caught up with too many details concerning the problem, you have lost sight of your objective. Step back and let go. It's a great way to get some perspective and some space, for you and your partner. If you need further advice on exactly what you can do to support your partner, here are a few tips from coauthor Lisa for those of you who are type A to the max:

>> **Plan for the downtime (like when you are waiting for test results).** The worst thing in the world is to be waiting with nothing to do. Now is the time to see that movie or try out that new restaurant together.

>> **Do something small for your partner that lets him or her know they are important to you.** In my house that means I empty the dishwasher or bring the garbage cans in! It's not the act but the thought that counts.

>> **Cuddle.** Don't underestimate the power of touch to reinforce positive emotions.

Dealing with Buttinskies (a.k.a. Friends and Relatives)

There's no question that dealing with infertility is a strain, and it's a strain that can turn into a major emotional drain when friends and relatives decide to involve themselves in your situation. In the sections that follow, we give you some tips on how to cope with these situations and people that try your patience.

TIP

You can try, nicely but firmly and, one hopes, unemotionally, to let relatives know that their concern is welcome, but their advice and opinions are not. Most often, you'll find they don't really want to know all the details. They just want to feel like they're an important part of your life and that you care enough about them to include them in what's going on.

Bringing friends and family onboard

You may be faring pretty well and your partner may be a rock, but your mother, sister, or best friend may be a royal pain in the proverbial you-know-what, wanting to know all the details of how things are going, how you're feeling, how your partner is reacting, and so on.

The obvious way to handle this situation is to just tell everyone to stay out of your business, but as you well know, this is much easier said than done. Some families consider this sort of interference as sort of a family right. Inquiring into your reproductive plans may have started the minute your relationship with your partner began. A polite "I'd rather not discuss it" isn't going to work in this kind of family. Before you know it, the whispering has begun, and the word is out in the family that something is wrong with you.

How much you tell is up to you and your partner. Usually your partner isn't as eager to blab the details to one and all as you may be, but you may want to consider that even the most prying parents and friends may turn out to be a real source of support after they know what you're going through.

PERSONAL STORY

You may be surprised to discover someone else in your circle of family and friends has been in your position or is going through fertility issues now. Coauthor Lisa has been working with fertility patients for almost 30 years and has often commented on how "things have changed" when it comes to sharing medical information. Early in her career, Lisa had a patient — a nurse who worked in the hospital where the clinic was located — who made her promise never to tell anyone why she was coming to the clinic. "Lie if you have to" was the watchword. Today, Lisa has patients who openly catalogue the details of their fertility journey on social media, and there can even be a gathering of friends in the doctor's waiting room. Talking about fertility is easier than it has ever been — but it has to be easy for you! Share what you can handle!

Surviving the holidays

Holidays bring their own special challenges to almost everyone, but those trying to conceive may be particularly affected. The summer holidays always seem to be the perfect setting for family picnics, reunions, and other get-togethers where carefree children frolic and nosy relatives coyly ask when you will be eating for two. Winter provides little relief as Thanksgiving, Hanukkah, Christmas, and Kwanzaa all seem to focus on extended family, the latest children's toys, and holiday newsletters that share every painstaking family detail, from birth to potty training to Junior's first car accident.

REMEMBER

Some of this family updating is normal, but you may be especially sensitive to the topic while you're trying to conceive yourself. Try as best you can to determine whether the conversation is the speaker's way of trying to connect or reconnect with family and friends or whether you're face-to-face with an insufferable boor. If you discover it's the latter, realize that you can't do much to guard against people like this, whether they're related to you or not. In such situations, the art of the smile, the nod, and the hasty exit will serve you well.

TIP

If you plan on spending extended time with your extended family, consider cluing in a few folks about your situation. They can be helpful in deflecting family or friends who are notorious for ill-timed comments. Arriving late and/or leaving early is another way to minimize your contact with difficult people and situations. You may want to plan something special for you and your partner or a friend after your family affair. This activity will give you something to look forward to throughout the family function.

COMPARING AND CONTRASTING

When coauthor Jackie's college friend, Leslie, got married at 39 and began planning her family, Jackie was still on the infertility treadmill that had taken up three years of her life. They were the same age, and Jackie anticipated that her friend would also be faced with the same uphill battle. Two months later, Jackie asked her friend Leslie how her low-tech attempts were faring. "Jackie," she said, her voice breaking, "I'm pregnant. It happened the second month."

Jackie loves her friends and wishes them the best. And despite this, Leslie's success seemed to be Jackie's failure, even more so than the unsuccessful years of trying. Luckily, Jackie had her network in place. A call to her friend Susan, who was also experiencing infertility, quickly salved Jackie's wounds, at least temporarily. "Susan had spent the last five years in low-, medium-, and high-tech fertility treatments with no baby to show for it (although she has since given birth to a healthy baby girl, who came about in a completely unplanned, nontechnological way!). Susan's ability to immediately understand helped Jackie to begin to put the situation in perspective. Sharing with the newly pregnant Leslie that she (Jackie) felt happy for her *and* jealous also eased the pain. When all else fails, try to see another's pregnancy as a chance to observe just what you're getting yourself into! Perhaps you can put this more intimate knowledge of the pros and cons of being pregnant to good use in the future.

Coauthor Jackie was certain that, after attending family functions solo for years, her discomfort would end if and when she was married. How was she supposed to know that there was still another hoop to jump through? What she did discover was that there will *always* be another obstacle, if she allows it. Even if Jackie were to arrive with her perfect family in tow, some new challenge would always await. Holidays can become a time for comparison rather than a time for joy if you choose to compete. Instead, consider meeting those ill-timed comments and people with a hug and an expression of good wishes. Your grace may just stop the others in their tracks.

Rather than ignore the children playing with their new toys, get in there and play with them. You may just discover some of the fun of being with children and sharing their joy before giving them back to their rightful owner after the excitement wears off! Consider this your gift of the holiday season.

Declining invitations

If a family member or friend is expecting, you may find it difficult to attend any gathering that this pregnant woman attends. Don't chide yourself for your absence. A little denial can go a long way toward helping you gracefully deal with a painful situation. You may decide to bow out of a family dinner or two and count on the understanding of those who love you. Either way, you'll preserve your integrity and that of your family relationships by not forcing yourself to handle even one bit more than you think you can. This too shall pass.

Forecast: Baby showers likely

TIP

Definition of a baby shower: A seemingly benign tradition that can wreak havoc in the hearts of infertile women everywhere (many men claim this as well, no matter what the circumstances). Here's some advice on the topic:

>> **If you choose to attend (and remember you don't *have* to), don't go it alone.** Sometimes that may mean sharing your situation with the pregnant guest of honor. Although it is *her* day, a little bit of knowledge goes a long way toward sensitivity.

>> **If you don't choose to confide in the lady of the hour, hang with a friend.** Face it: Baby showers can be very emotional, but they can also be very, very humorous, particularly when shared with someone who understands your situation and can help you see the (inevitable) comedy of errors that often surrounds the pregnant population. This tactic can help you to laugh your way through situations that you may have spent months dreading. Remember though, be nice — isn't that how you want to be treated when you're pregnant?

>> **If no allies are in attendance, your phone can be a wonderful thing.** Try to make a difficult situation tolerable by calling a trusted friend before, after, and sometimes during (that's what bathrooms are for!) the event. Cell phones are wonderful for this purpose and have helped many a pregnant woman through a tough spot. Texting is another brilliant way to garner the support you need and not disrupt the party.

>> **If you're going solo to the shower, you can always use the bathroom, the porch, or your car for temporary refuge.** Or for a good cry if you need it.

>> **You don't have to stay until the last present is unwrapped either.** Making an appearance is sufficient, particularly when you're under pressure. You can be the life of the party another time. Your friends will understand.

Getting Professional Help for Very Personal Hurts

Everybody needs a shoulder to cry on from time to time. It really is okay. Those of you going through fertility treatments may need more than one person's shoulders.

Continued communication between you and your partner, devoid of blame and misdirected anger, is key to working through the infertility battle as a team. But sometimes, the hole feels a little too deep, and you may need further professional intervention.

Being in the club you didn't ask to join

Don't minimize the stress you're under. By acknowledging how difficult this may be for you, realizing that it may not be that difficult for your partner, and recognizing all points in between, you can define your starting point, a necessary step in determining your direction.

Although many of the more complex decisions in fertility treatment require medical guidance, you may find yourself getting stuck in areas that seem far simpler. Perhaps you're overwhelmed, a natural response when the path in front of you seems confusing. Talking about your options with your doctor is certainly one way to get clarity. A therapist, however, can help prevent you from getting bogged down with the small stuff and often help you to realize what's behind it all.

Consulting a professional therapist

Couples counseling is a great place to have your thoughts and feelings translated into a language that your partner may better understand. Do you find yourself snapping at every mail carrier and store clerk in town? Therapy may be a good place to unburden your frustrations before people scatter at the sight of you. Are you resentful of your or your partner's fertility problems? Telling one another over dinner may exacerbate the problem, but the helpful mediation of a therapist can allow you to acknowledge your feelings and your partner's and move on.

Many fertility specialists advise the couples they treat to consult a counselor or psychologist, especially one who specializes in fertility. These counselors are particularly adept at dealing with differences in the way men and women deal with the stress of infertility. And because a counselor is not the physician treating you, that person is often in a better position to offer objective advice about types of treatments, adoption, and so on.

TIP

When looking for a counselor to help with your fertility issues, it is helpful to find someone who is licensed (that shows they have had the proper education) and who has experience in infertility (that shows they've probably seen at least one other person with your concerns). You can find great referrals in your area from your fertility clinic or from the professional organization that provides guidance to fertility clinics and patients, American Society of Reproductive Medicine (ASRM). You can read more about ASRM at www.asrm.org. More importantly you can reach ASRM's Mental Health Professional Group at https://connect.asrm.org/mhpg/home?ssopc=1.

PERSONAL STORY

Throughout their many years of struggling to conceive their first and then second child, coauthor Jackie and her husband actually *did* gain a deeper and more loving understanding with one another. As their marriage continued, they discovered that life had even more ups and downs than trying to conceive. What they learned through the process of creating a child, however, made them better suited to face other challenges as well.

Seeking social support from your world and the rest of the universe

Ah! Social media and the 21st century: a gamechanger — or is it? Despite going through infertility "only" 13 years ago, social media has completely changed the landscape for finding information, support, and comparisons!

While some use these "tools" such as Facebook, Instagram, Twitter, and more to keep up with family and friends, others misuse them as methods to "keep up with the Joneses"! Funny that a picture of an old friend living a perfect "Facebook Life" with a partner, 2.5 kids and the requisite adorable dog, does little to boost any-one's mood, unless they too are similarly posting. It's important to remember that most people *aspire* to live lives as charmed as they appear on social media. As a good friend once said, "I don't post the bad stuff . . . no one wants to read about that!" Another friend who works as a psychotherapist shared that most of his patients are living perfect lives on social media — just not IRL (in real life . . . or his office for that matter!).

When trying to conceive, social media *can* provide information and *tons* of support with pages dedicated to almost every circumstance. That's the good news. Proper use (which would not be considered hourly checks on the progress of others) can yield a community of individuals experiencing the same trials, tribulations, and joys. The bad news is that it can trigger a sense of competition in an area where nothing can be truly validated as real. Lean on it for what it's worth; an extra option for support, not your only lifeline.

Taking a Break from Your Fertility "Job" — You Deserve It

When all else fails to help you relax, consider taking time off, whether that's a break from your efforts or a real vacation!

REMEMBER

Fertility often becomes a job with uncertain outcomes and at times difficult work-ing conditions. Just like any job, time off is necessary in order to clean your mind, refresh your spirit, and come back to greet another day with your best efforts.

Getting away from the daily grind helps you to gain a better perspective and make decisions that best suit you, your partner, and your living style. Some people can do this by taking a fertility-free weekend that includes no discussion of anything to do with physicians, fertility, treatments, or future plans. You'll be amazed by the perspective and peace that you can gain from a much-needed vacation. And although we don't advise planning a vacation with the hidden agenda of making this getaway the one that does the trick, perhaps it will.

TIP

If you have frozen eggs or embryos, you actually have even more time to "escape."

3

Seeking Answers, Identifying Causes, and Dealing with Disappointments

Understand what tests a woman may need to undergo to determine infertility causes and treatments.

Focus on fertility tests for males.

Look at what all those test results mean for your fertility potential.

Figure out how to manage the highs and lows of a pregnancy that doesn't get you a baby.

» Taking a look inside

» Diagnosing problems with ovulation

Chapter **11**

Ladies First: Female Testing Basics

If you haven't gotten pregnant after several months to a year, it may be time to start doing some tests. Your doctor may suggest these tests to you, or you may suggest them to your physician if you feel that time is slipping away and you want to find out why you haven't gotten pregnant yet or why you can't stay pregnant.

In this chapter, we give you a rundown of the tests that fertility doctors do on women most frequently, why they do them, and what you can expect to find out from the tests. If you're wondering why all the emphasis on you when there are two of you involved in the baby-making process, never fear — we address male issues in Chapter 12.

REMEMBER

For about 30 percent of couples trying to get pregnant, several problems contribute to infertility. This fact is especially important to remember if one of you has a known factor, such as previous tubal surgery or a known sperm problem. Many couples come to a clinic and tell the staff, "I don't need to do any testing — we already know the problem is him (or her)." You may think that you already know the problem, but keep in mind that for 30 percent of you, tests will reveal another problem, and pregnancy won't occur until both problems are addressed.

Understanding the Limits of Testing

The tests used to find a problem causing infertility are not what you might expect. For example, they rarely tell you exactly what is wrong. Many times, they are designed to identify a general area that may have an undefinable problem. This information can then be used to help make predictions about what may or may not work. Treatment for infertility is successful if its applied to the correct problem. But first you have to identify the problem.

Making a diagnosis becomes a critical first step on the road to resolving fertility issues, but not all tests are equally reliable. Medicine uses statistics to determine just how accurate test results are. Suppose an excellent treatment is discovered for a very lethal disease (for example, AIDS), but the treatment has a number of risks and side effects. There is a simple blood test for the disease. Suppose 1,000 patients are tested for the disease and the test identifies 100 people as having it. After following the entire group for a number of years, it is determined that the test missed three people. So, the chance of the test missing people with the disease is 3/1,000 or 0.3 percent — not bad!

This type of test is termed a *screening test,* and the 0.3 percent is the sensitivity of the test. But what about the 100 people who tested positive and were told they had this very dangerous disease and would need to go on dangerous and extensive treatment? By following these 100 people, it was determined that only ten actually had the disease. In other words, the test correctly identified people with the disease 10/100 times or was only correct 10 percent of the time. Not good considering what those 90 people went through. This statistic is called the *specificity.*

Ideally, a test would have a very high ability to correctly identify people with the disease, or in statistical terms, a high sensitivity and specificity. That rarely happens. More commonly, the initial screening uses a test with a high sensitivity so that only a limited number of people with the disease are missed. A test that has a very high specificity (called a *diagnostic test*) usually follows so that false positives can be correctly identified. This type of result can be quite annoying and worrisome as a person waits for the results from the second test, which usually takes more time than the initial screening test.

REMEMBER

Commonly then, in trying to determine a cause for infertility, a screening test is done first and if that test is positive, a diagnostic test is performed.

Testing Your Blood for Clues

It's never fun to have blood drawn, but there's a wealth of information in those little tubes. Blood tests are one of the most noninvasive ways to see how you're doing, reproductively speaking, by testing your hormone levels at different times of your menstrual cycle to see whether you're measuring up to fertility standards.

There are some subtleties when trying to determine what the results of hormone testing mean. For example, a normal test value does not always mean that everything is normal. A 40-year-old female may have a normal Day 3 FSH and yet have very few, if any, normal eggs. However, if that same person had an FSH that was elevated, it would confirm the concern about the eggs' quality.

Baseline blood tests

"Let's get some baseline bloods," your doctor may say when you first start looking for an answer to the "why am I not pregnant" question. This test is one of the simplest tests you can have done. You simply wait until your period starts, go to the lab on Day 2 or Day 3 of your period, and have blood drawn. Within a day or two, you usually receive the results, which give you quite a bit of information about your fertility.

The first tests you'll probably hear about are testing for egg quality. But beware: There are no accurate tests to determine whether a woman has eggs that can produce a child. There are tests that indicate there may be a problem with egg quality or the number of eggs remaining in the ovary. These include Day 3 (of menses) LH, FSH, and estradiol (E2); antimullerian hormone (AMH); and an ultrasound to count early eggs units called *antral follicles* (antral follicle count [AFC]). The major purpose of obtaining Day 3 labs is to assess ovarian reserve, the supply of eggs in the ovary that could be used to achieve a pregnancy. As women age, the reserve diminishes, and the assessment of the ovarian reserve may help a couple decide to move quickly to treatment or to choose another option.

To understand what the tests mean, reviewing the basic physiology of the egg unit (*follicle*) is helpful. The follicle has four main components: the egg, a fluid-filled space called a *cyst*, an inner layer of cells called *granulosa cells*, and an outer layer of cells called *theca cells*. The follicle starts as a very simple structure, which enlarges as the egg matures. Measuring the cystic part of the follicle can give an indication of how mature the egg is, and this is what an ultrasound of the ovaries determines.

The egg rules, in that it is responsible for the development of a normal follicle. If the egg is damaged, then the follicle won't develop normally, which forms the basis for testing the products from the follicle. The egg unit produces steroid hormones. The egg uses cholesterol, which the outer cell layer converts under the influence of the hormone LH (luteinizing hormone) to make hormones (androgens). The androgens are then converted by the inner cells to estrogen (specifically estradiol). The more mature the egg, the more cells, and thus the estrogen levels increase, giving an indication of how mature the egg is and also how well the egg formed the follicle.

Estradiol

The estradiol the follicle produces is actually used for three diagnostic purposes but on Day 3 it is used to try to determine how healthy the egg is. A structurally damaged egg will make an abnormal follicle and the estrogen level will not be where it should be. Early in the cycle, during menses, there should only be very small follicles and thus the estrogen should be low. Estradiol on Day 3 of your period is normally less than 30 pg/ml. An estradiol level that is very high (>75–100 pg/ml) may indicate a poor ovarian reserve.

Follicle stimulating hormone (FSH)

FSH is released by the pituitary gland at the base of the brain and is necessary for a follicle to continue to develop. FSH causes the granulosa cells to convert the androgens from the theca cells to estradiol. The normal fate of most follicles is death. But at the start of a woman's period, approximately 20–30 follicles are still developing. At this point the brain releases a surge of FSH, which allows one of the developing follicles to take the lead, become the dominant follicle, and continue to develop. The other follicles die. The brain monitors estradiol to know how much FSH to release, so a normal egg developing a normal follicle will have a level of estradiol that determines the FSH on Day 3 of a menses. Experts vary about what is considered a normal value, but most accept ≤10 mIU/ml as normal. A damaged egg creates a damaged follicle, and the brain perceives this as not working hard enough so it releases more FSH. Therefore, a high Day 3 FSH indicates poor egg quality and a reduced ovarian reserve. When there are no more eggs, menopause ensues and FSH levels rise about 20–40 mIU/ml.

Luteinizing hormone (LH)

Luteinizing hormone (LH) is also produced by the pituitary. LH has two major functions: The first is to help the theca cells convert cholesterol to androgens, and the second is to cause the follicle to release the egg (ovulate). Day 3 LH levels usually are 1–2 units less than FSH, although these levels may be higher in women with PCOS which we talk about in Chapter 7. LH levels rise near midcycle, usually going over 40 when you're almost ready to ovulate. LH causes the follicle to make proteins that dissolve the wall of the follicle, and the egg escapes. LH also causes the egg to complete the final stages of its development. The surge in the release of LH at midcycle has been used to predict ovulation. This is the basis of many home urinary LH tests which are reviewed in detail in Chapter 6.

AMH

The most recent hormone tested to evaluate the ovarian reserve is AMH. AMH is a protein made by the small egg units. The more eggs units, the higher the AMH — so a high result is actually a good thing. The advantage of AMH is that, while it is usually a part of the initial work-up on Day 3, it can be measured at any point in the cycle: however, if you are taking oral contraceptives they will negatively affect the AMH level. The ability of AMH to predict a clinically significant decline in ovarian reserve is age-dependent with better accuracy as women age. Low values in younger women do not always mean a problem of ovarian reserve. The utility of AMH testing has seen a decline because while AMH correlates very well with the response to stimulation in IVF, it does not correlate with pregnancy. Thus, age remains the best predictor of ovarian reserve.

Progesterone

Progesterone traditionally was measured in the second half of the cycle, after ovulation, to determine whether ovulation had occurred, and the ovary seemed to be producing enough progesterone to maintain a pregnancy. This was called a *luteal phase progesterone level* and is seldom used today. Progesterone is a result of the development of a normal follicle in the first half of the cycle called the *follicular phase.* The development of a normal follicle is dependent upon a normal egg. So, measuring progesterone is an indirect way to assess normal egg function.

Today, luteal phase progesterone has given way to follicular phase testing of other hormones. However, if a luteal phase progesterone is used, it is critical to time the measurement correctly. One way to do this is to monitor ovulation and then measure the progesterone 6–7 days after an LH surge. At this time a sign of ovulation is a progesterone that is >3 ng/ml, but normally if the egg and follicle are normal, the progesterone will be >8 ng/ml.

Prolactin

Prolactin is a hormone produced by the pituitary gland that is released when women are breastfeeding. However, some women have elevated levels of prolactin even if they have never been pregnant. When the prolactin levels become significantly elevated, the woman may experience irregular cycles, anovulatory cycles (no follicle develops), and breast discharge.

The increased release of prolactin (called *hyperprolactinemia*) may be due to a growth in the pituitary called a *prolactinoma.* These are almost always benign but occasionally can become enlarged. Because of where they are located in the brain, the enlargement may press upon the optic nerve, causing a unique type of peripheral (side) blindness, which the physician can assess easily in the office.

There are other reasons for an elevated prolactin, including rare growths in the brain (therefore women with elevated prolactin levels need to have an MRI of the pituitary to determine whether there is a prolactinoma and, if so, how large it is); or, using drugs such as antidepressants and antihypertensives.

REMEMBER

Two medications are routinely used to lower prolactin levels as patients move through their fertility treatment: bromocriptine (Parlodel) and cabergoline (Dostinex).

Thyroid tests

The best state to be in with your thyroid is *euthyroid,* which means that your thyroid is in balance. Thyroid problems are very common, with one out of eight women diagnosed with a thyroid problem at some point in their lives. Your thyroid can be either overactive (hyper) or underactive (hypo). Both hyper- and hypothyroid conditions can cause infertility problems.

A thyroid that is hypoactive usually causes fatigue, dry skin, and weight gain. A hyperactive thyroid causes a rapid heart rate, anxiousness, sweating, and weight loss.

Women with thyroid problems may experience an increased rate of miscarriage, lack of ovulation, or irregular periods. Hypothyroidism can cause an increase in prolactin, the hormone responsible for maintaining breast milk production in pregnancy. High prolactin can cause a decrease in fertility.

REMEMBER

Thyroid imbalances can be treated by daily medication, radiation, or, in severe cases, surgery. Your thyroid medication may need to be adjusted if you become pregnant.

Testosterone (Yes! For women, too.)

Testosterone is usually associated with males. And rightly so because it is the hormone that makes men develop as men. Women make a form of testosterone and then change it into estrogen. The general category of hormones that testosterone belongs to is called androgens, and there are many kinds of androgens. If the ovary fails to convert the androgens to estrogen, then the cycles can become irregular and a woman may show the effects of testosterone such as unwanted facial hair and acne. Increased ovarian androgens are the core issue for women with PCOS. Women who have PCOS and an elevated testosterone level can be placed on oral contraceptives and the testosterone level will decrease. There are very rare ovarian tumors that produce testosterone, but these tumors produce a lot of it. Frequently, women with one of these tumors will experience rapid changes such as loss of hair, increased body hair, and deepening of the voice.

DHEA-S

Androgens are produced by the *adrenal glands* (small glands sitting on top of the kidneys responsible for stress hormones and electrolyte regulation). The androgens produced by the adrenals is changed by the liver into a hormone called dehydroepiandrosterone sulfate (don't even try to remember how to say or spell this – it's DHEA-S). This hormone can be measured when a woman has elevated androgens and distinguishes the person with an ovarian problem, where the DHEA-S is normal, from a person who has an adrenal problem, where the DHEA-S is elevated. Once determined, the underlying problem needs to be treated.

Fasting insulin

So, what does insulin have to do with getting pregnant? Insulin is used to regulate blood sugar (glucose) levels. In all fairness, many physicians do not use fasting insulin in the management of their patients. However, some physicians find measuring fasting insulin levels useful for the management of women with PCOS. Over 95 percent of obese PCOS patients and 60–97 percent of nonobese PCOS patients have insulin resistance. If insulin levels are up, the levels of androgens increase in the ovary causing irregular cycles, anovulation, and reduced fertility. There's more info on this in Chapter 7.

Testing for immune disorders

Immune testing in infertility is considered controversial because rigorous studies have not definitively proven a role in infertility. However, some doctors feel that it can be valuable.

In most cases, only a blood sample is required. However, interpretation of the results isn't always simple. Some tests are widely done, and the results almost universally accepted. Other tests are done only by doctors specializing in immune disorders, and not all doctors believe the results are important. Here are some of the most common immune tests, with information on what the tests mean and how you're treated if the tests are abnormal.

Antiphospholipid antibodies (APA)

You'll most likely be tested for antiphospholipid antibodies (APA) if you've had multiple miscarriages or repeated failure with IVF. The test for APA actually tests for a number of different antibodies; a moderate or high reaction to two or more antibodies is considered a positive reaction. Antiphospholipid antibodies can interfere with the embryo implanting or can cause miscarriage; they disrupt the normal clotting of blood and the adhesion of the embryo to the uterus. Treatment is either baby aspirin, heparin (an anticoagulant, or blood thinner), or a combination of the two.

Antinuclear antibodies (ANA)

A high positive antinuclear antibodies (ANA) test can mean that you may have a disease called systemic lupus erythematosus (SLE). At lower positive levels, especially if the pattern is speckled, ANA can increase your risk of miscarriage. A positive ANA level may be treated with low-dose steroids, but this therapy is not proven to decrease miscarriage rates.

Antithyroid antibodies (ATA)

Antithyroglobulin antibodies (ATA) can cause problems with your thyroid function. Because the thyroid is so important in maintaining your hormone levels, antibodies that interfere with the thyroid's functioning may reduce the chance for conception. Antithyroglobulin causes continuous stimulation of the thyroid independent from the normal control mechanism for normal thyroid functioning. This results in hyperthyroidism (Grave's disease). Antimicrosomal antibodies can destroy the thyroid and result in hypothyroidism (Hashimoto thyroiditis).

Antiovarian antibodies (AOA)

If your doctor suspects that you're in premature ovarian failure or early menopause, you may be tested for antiovarian antibodies (AOA).

Vitamin D

A newcomer to the infertility scene is vitamin D. As we discuss more in Chapter 9, Vitamin D is not really a vitamin, but it has been implicated in a number of biological processes, including some related to reproduction. It may play a role in the success of IVF.

Infectious diseases

Your doctor will often want to make sure that there are no infections that may be complicating your chances of getting pregnant and so may order a battery of infectious disease testing. If you are a known IVF candidate, this type of testing will be required by the FDA oversight of the embryology laboratory. More information on all of these tests is found in Chapter 4.

Addressing Female Structural Problems

Women's infertility issues can be very complex because so many different systems can be at fault. Is the problem uterine, tubal, hormonal, age-related, or ovarian? Any one of these problems can cause enough trouble to prevent you from becoming and staying pregnant.

Picturing a healthy uterus

Maybe you had an HSG to evaluate your fallopian tubes and uterus, which we discuss in the later section "HSG (Don't even try to spell out the word)," or maybe you had a hysteroscopic surgery for an even closer look into the uterus. Looking at the uterus is an integral part of any fertility workup because the uterus nourishes and holds a baby for nine months.

Finding fibroids in the uterus

Fibroids, or benign tumors, are commonly found inside or on the outside of the uterus. They're extremely common, with 40 percent of women between the ages of 35 and 55 having at least one. Fibroids are even more common in African-American women, with 50 percent having at least one.

Fibroids can cause bowel or bladder problems, very heavy bleeding, or pain. Fibroids can be either inside or outside the uterine cavity; their location determines whether they cause a problem with your ability to get or stay pregnant. Fibroids completely outside the uterus, such as *pedunculated fibroids,* which are attached to the uterus by a stem, don't usually cause a problem with fertility. Submucosal fibroids grow through the lining of uterine wall and can cause a miscarriage.

Fibroids can be surgically removed, a process called a *myomectomy.* A small fibroid inside the uterus can usually be removed by hysteroscopy, a procedure in which a thin telescope is inserted into the uterus through the vagina. This is outpatient surgery and is relatively atraumatic. In contrast, large intramural fibroids require an abdominal incision and a hospital stay. You generally need to deliver by cesarean section after an abdominal myomectomy.

Removing polyps

Polyps are small fleshy benign growths found on the surface of the endometrium. Very small polyps usually cause no problem with getting pregnant, but larger polyps or multiple polyps can interfere with conception.

Polyps can cause irregular bleeding; they can be diagnosed via sonohysterogram or hysteroscopy and can be scraped off the endometrium. Polyp removal is called polypectomy.

Clearing out the fallopian tubes

Most women have two fallopian tubes, one on each side of the uterus, next to the ovaries. Because these tubes are the transport path from the ovary to the uterus, a problem with one or both tubes can have a big impact on your baby-making ability.

Understanding how fallopian tubes should work and what can go wrong

Fallopian tubes are not just tubes. If they were, then repair would be much simpler and far more successful. Tubes actually have jobs to do: specifically, to transport and culture. The tube is where the sperm and eggs meet, and fertilization takes place. So, the tube must allow sperm to migrate through the uterus and into the tube. The tube also must pick the oocyte from the surface of the ovary when it is ovulated and move it nearer the uterus. Finally, once the fertilized egg, now called an embryo, has developed for two to three days, the tube must move the embryo into the uterus.

The inside of the tube is lined with cells that have hair-like projections that move in a wave-like fashion to transport the embryo. (Think beach ball at a football game moving around the crowd.) Infections can damage these hair-like projections and decrease or destroy the tube's ability to perform the transport function. This is a microscopic function and therefore cannot be diagnosed.

Also, the tube acts as an incubator for the early development of the embryo. The environment in the tube, designed specifically for the embryo, is unlike anywhere else in the body. This function also cannot be seen or diagnosed.

WARNING

Sometimes a tube is surgically removed after an ectopic pregnancy, a pregnancy that starts to grow in the tube rather than in the uterus. If this pregnancy is found early enough, it may be possible to dissolve the pregnancy with a chemotherapy agent called methotrexate. However, if the fetus grows large enough undetected in the tube, the tube can burst, causing life-threatening bleeding (we discuss this in Chapter 13). The only way to stop the bleeding is to remove the tube.

You can get pregnant with only one tube but having one ectopic pregnancy leaves you at a higher risk to have another. Frequently, when a tube is removed, the surgeon will look at the other tube and find that it looks okay. For a person with an ectopic and one remaining tube, the pregnancy rate is estimated to be about 70 percent, of which 10 percent are another ectopic. So why don't the other 30 percent conceive? Probably because the tube may appear normal and be open, but damage on the interior of the tube has caused it to malfunction and not be able to perform the job it needs to do. When women become pregnant after an ectopic has been removed, they usually do so within the first year. Beyond that pregnancies can occur but they are rare, and the couple may want to pursue IVF.

Investigating damaged tubes

Women who have only the left ovary and the right fallopian tube can get pregnant because the egg can "float" to the remaining tube. Of course, this also applies to women who have the left tube and the right ovary. (One study estimated that the egg gets picked up by the opposite tube about 30 percent of the time.) Sometimes fallopian tubes are seen to be enlarged on ultrasound or during an HSG. If the tubes are very swollen and dye doesn't flow through them, you may have a *hydrosalpinx*, the medical term for a tube filled with fluid (see Figure 11-1). If both tubes are dilated, the condition is known as *hydrosalpinges*.

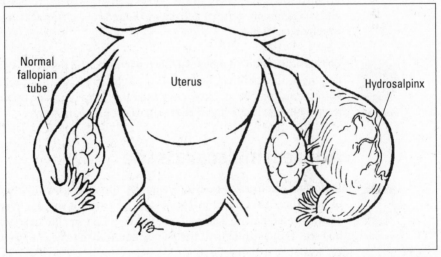

FIGURE 11-1: A hydrosalpinx can affect your ability to get pregnant.

Illustration by Kathryn Born

A hydrosalpinx interferes with pregnancy in two ways:

>> The egg cannot be picked up by the dilated tube, whose *fimbriae* (the end) is blocked by scarring.

>> The tube has an environment that damages the development of the embryo.

The treatment for a hydrosalpinx is surgical. In mild cases, the end of the tube can be opened and the ends peeled back like a flower. Surgical repair of damaged tubes has a low chance of success primarily because surgical repair does not address the damage on the interior of the tube. However, in severe cases, the tube will not work even if it is opened. In these cases, the tube or tubes must be removed, and you need to have IVF. This diagnosis is a hard thing for many women to accept because it definitely ends any chance that they'll be able to get pregnant on their own. However, well-done studies have demonstrated that pregnancy rates are lower for women with bilateral hydrosalpinges. Having one hydrosalpinx and one open tube still reduces the chance for a successful IVF cycle. The reason why the hydrosalpinx reduces the pregnancy rate is unknown, but theories propose that the fluid in the tube can leak into the uterus prevent implantation.

In very rare cases, women can be born without any fallopian tubes; often the tubes are missing as part of a syndrome in which the external sex organs look normal, but the vagina, uterus, and fallopian tubes are missing. Of course, if you've had two ectopic pregnancies, you may have had both tubes surgically removed also.

Sometimes fallopian tubes look fine on an X-ray but may be surrounded by adhesions (scarring) that prevent them from picking up the egg. *Endometriosis*, tissue growths found anywhere in the pelvis, can grow in or around the fallopian tubes and is a common cause of adhesions around tubes. Normal tubes can't be visualized by ultrasound.

REMEMBER

Because the fallopian tubes play such a large role in getting pregnant, you'll probably need intervention, such as IVF, to get pregnant if a problem is discovered with them. Removal or absence of the tubes, or a blockage that can't be removed, makes IVF inevitable if you're trying to get pregnant.

Addressing scar tissue

PERSONAL STORY

In dozens of surgeries over the years, Dr. Rinehart saw firsthand how scar tissue, or adhesions (as shown in Figure 11-2), can form in your reproductive system. Many women having a second or third cesarean section delivery or other surgery had scar tissue throughout the pelvis that needed to be cut away before the delivery team could get to the uterus.

Adhesions form when blood and plasma from trauma, such as surgery (like an appendectomy, tubal removal of an ectopic pregnancy or fibroid), form fibrin deposits, which are threadlike strands that can bind one organ to another. They can be removed, but surgery to correct adhesions may result in — you guessed it — more adhesions.

The amount of scarring depends upon the surgical procedure done but can occasionally be extensive. Adhesions can cause pelvic pain; cesarean sections can cause adhesions, but they tend to be anterior (or in front of) the uterus, and thus may cause difficulty during a subsequent C-section. However, C-sections don't usually cause problems with tubes (which tend to be behind the uterus), and thus don't usually cause infertility.

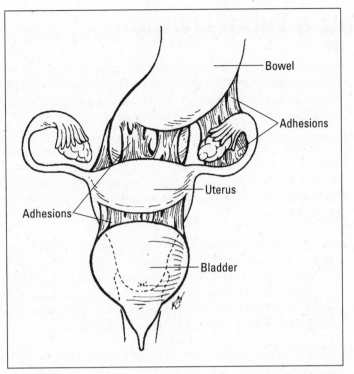

FIGURE 11-2:
Adhesions in the female reproductive system.

Illustration by Kathryn Born

REMEMBER

Your chances of getting pregnant after adhesion removal are highest in the first six months after surgery, before extensive adhesions form again. Some adhesions can't be removed without damaging the tubes or ovaries, and you may need IVF to get pregnant. Since the advent of IVF, surgical repair for pelvic adhesions is uncommon.

If you have adhesions in the uterus itself, you may be diagnosed with Asherman's syndrome, also called uterine synechiae. Asherman's can follow a dilation and curettage (D&C), an abortion, or a uterine infection. It can be diagnosed during an HSG but is best diagnosed with a hysteroscopy, where the inside of the uterus can be visualized. Asherman's is also suspected if you have scant or no menstrual flow or recurrent miscarriages following uterine trauma. There are varying amounts of scarring in Asherman's syndrome. Some people have very few adhesions, and these are filmy and easy to remove. That person has a very good chance to conceive. If the mild to moderate adhesions are removed surgically, you have a good chance, probably 75 percent or better, of becoming pregnant and carrying to term. Severe adhesions may destroy nearly all the normal uterine lining, and pregnancy may not be possible. Less frequently, a person will have extensive intrauterine scarring, and that person will have a very poor chance for achieving a pregnancy. A gestational surrogate (discussed in Chapter 20) may be needed in these cases.

Reversing a Tubal Ligation

Nearly 40 percent of American women of childbearing age have been surgically sterilized. Unfortunately, at least 10 percent regret their decision down the road. Can tubal ligation be reversed? The answer is yes, no, and maybe, depending on when the surgery was done and what kind of surgery it was.

REMEMBER

If you want a tubal reversal, look for a surgeon skilled in microsurgery (find them through the Society for Reproductive Surgeons website at www.reprodsurg.org). Depending on the surgeon and type of surgery done, your surgery can take several hours to perform and may require several weeks of recovery. However, most surgeons require only a one-night hospital stay.

Risks after surgery include scar tissue formation, infection, and increased risk of ectopic pregnancy. If the fimbriated end of the tube (the part that the egg enters from the ovary) is intact and your doctor believes that you have enough tube left to reconnect, your pregnancy chances after reanastomosis can be higher than IVF success rates. This is because with repaired fallopian tubes, the couple can "try at home" every month, whereas IVF is a one-shot deal.

A *tubal reanastomosis*, or tubal reversal, has some drawbacks. For one thing, it's expensive — around $10,000, about the same as an IVF cycle — and insurance usually doesn't cover the cost. For another, the success rate depends on how long ago your tubes were tied and how they were tied. Success rates can be anywhere from 20 to 70 percent, depending upon your individual situation.

Before you decide to have your tubal ligation reversed, consider these factors:

>> **Your age:** Are you in your late 30s or younger? If you're over 40, you may have other fertility problems related to age, and in vitro fertilization (IVF) may be a better option for you.

>> **Your partner:** If your partner has sperm problems, you may also be better off doing IVF rather than reversing your tubal ligation.

>> **How your tubes were tied:** If your tubes were blocked off or clamped with clips or rings instead of being cauterized or having a large section removed, your chance of success is higher. Studies show that you need at least 4 cm (about an inch and a half) of healthy tube to successfully conceive after having the tubes reconnected (the average length of fallopian tubes before sterilization is about 10 cm, or about 4 inches).

In today's world, IVF has become a very useful option. Consideration of costs and how many children you want to eventually have may influence which option to pursue.

Testing to Diagnose Structural Problems

Unfortunately, a quick exam isn't usually enough for your doctor to see that you have problems inside your reproductive organs that can prevent pregnancy. Fortunately, it's become much easier to diagnose tubal and uterine problems with new diagnostic tools, which we discuss in the nest sections.

Transvaginal ultrasound

Ultrasound has become the workhorse for evaluation of female anatomy. Ultrasounds can be done either abdominally or vaginally. In the early days of IVF, all ultrasounds were done abdominally, which meant that the woman had to have a full bladder. The water in the bladder helps to see the pelvic organs. Fortunately, an ultrasound device was developed for vaginal use that significantly changed the practice of IVF — making it a whole lot less uncomfortable and better diagnostically. Vaginal ultrasounds have now largely replaced the HSG and laparoscopy for the investigation of female pelvic anatomy.

Ultrasound can be used to count early egg units in the ovary (antral follicle count), to identify developing follicles, and to distinguish normal follicles from endometriomas; or, to measure the diameter of the follicle when monitoring stimulated cycles either with oral or injectable medication. Additionally, ultrasound can diagnose fibroids and many times can distinguish fibroids from *adenomyosis*. The uterus is composed of two main types of tissue: muscle (myometrium) and the glandular portion where the embryo implants (endometrium). A fibroid occurs when a muscle cell multiplies and divides and makes a ball of smooth muscle. Adenomyosis is when the endometrium invades the myometrium. Fibroids can be removed surgically if they need to be removed. Adenomyosis cannot, so making the distinction is critical for proper treatment.

HSG (Don't even try to spell out the word)

An HSG, or *hysterosalpingogram*, is an X-ray that outlines the inside of your uterus and fallopian tubes to make it easy to see where abnormalities may be keeping you from getting pregnant. (See Figure 11-3.) Dye is injected through your cervix to make the uterus and tubes easy to see on an X-ray.

Preparing for discomfort

HSGs can be uncomfortable, causing mild to severe cramping, but it is a valuable tool in diagnosing fertility problems you can't see. Some of the problems that can be diagnosed with an HSG are fibroids in the uterus, large polyps in the uterus, an unusually shaped uterine cavity, a septum (a piece of tissue dividing your cavity), or adhesions (scar tissue) in the uterus. If you know that you have fibroids, an HSG can show whether they're intruding into the inside of the uterus, where they may prevent implantation of an embryo.

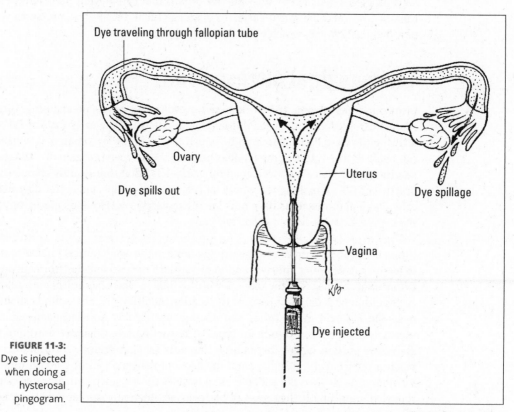

Dye traveling through fallopian tube

Ovary

Dye spills out

Uterus

Dye spillage

Vagina

Dye injected

Illustration by Kathryn Born

FIGURE 11-3: Dye is injected when doing a hysterosal pingogram.

The dye also outlines the fallopian tubes, so your doctor can see whether your tubes are normally shaped and, most importantly, whether your tubes are open, which your doctor can tell by noticing whether the dye passes through the tubes and flows into the pelvis. If dye passes through easily, your HSG report will say that the fallopian tubes "filled and spilled," meaning that the dye passed easily up from the uterus, all the way up the tubes, and out the end of the tube into the pelvis.

How uncomfortable is an HSG? That depends on your own pain tolerance and whether your tubes are open. If the tubes are slightly blocked with debris, your doctor may need to push the dye more forcefully to clear the block, which may increase cramping. Most doctors tell you to take ibuprofen or a similar pain medication an hour or so before your test to help head off any discomfort.

Looking at accuracy

How accurate is the HSG? If the test says the tubes are open, it is accurate more than 94–96 percent of the time. There can be rare instances where the dye appears to flow through the tubes, but the ovaries are surrounded by scar tissue and the tube can't get to the egg. The test is useful because, when normal, it says that procedures other than IVF may be successful.

What about when the HSG says the tubes are blocked? Here the test overall is correct only 40–45 percent of the time. One common finding is that the tubes appear on the HSG to be blocked just as they exit the uterus, which is called a *proximal occlusion*. Frequently if the test is repeated, the tubes will be open, meaning that the original test gave a false report that the tubes were blocked (called a false positive result). Here the person may be counseled to move to IVF when she may not need to. The other situation is that the blockage is at the far end of the tube where the fimbria are located (called a *distal occlusion*). Patient history can help distinguish whether the test is accurate or has falsely diagnosed blocked tubes. For example, a person may have undergone tubal surgery to repair damaged tubes or had a ruptured appendix. Here the HSG is much more accurate if it says the tubes are blocked. Some IVF centers will perform a blood test to determine whether the person has had a chlamydia infection by measuring chlamydia antibodies. Positive antibodies suggest that the HSG is correct if it says the tubes are blocked.

Other considerations

Schedule your test for the early part of your menstrual cycle, usually before Day 12 (before you ovulate), because both the dye and the pelvic X-rays can be harmful if you're pregnant.

Some doctors also do cervical cultures for gonorrhea and chlamydia and/or pre-treat with antibiotics before doing an HSG because pushing dye through the uterus and fallopian tubes can spread the infection and cause serious complications.

After the test, a small amount of bleeding is normal; you'll also leak a small amount of dye (which is clear, not colored) over the next day or so. You may be crampy for a few hours after the procedure as well. Take someone with you so that you don't have to drive yourself home.

WARNING

If you're allergic to contrast dye or shellfish, you may not be able to have the test done. Contrast dye and shellfish both contain iodine, and some doctors believe an allergy to shellfish means you have a higher chance of having an allergic reaction to the dye. No worries today, though — you may be a great candidate for a saline infused ultrasound — read on!

Saline infused hysterosonogram (SIS)

Saline infused sonograms (SISs) have increasingly replaced the HSG as the initial test for tubes being open *(patency)*. Devices have been developed that make tiny bubbles that reflect brightly on the ultrasound and thus can be followed through the uterine cavity and tubes. The SIS is not always easy to interpret, and at that point the physician may recommend moving to an HSG. The SIS is better tolerated than an HSG, there is no radiation, and there is no dye, which could elicit an allergic reaction. As with any uterine procedure, there is a small chance of infection. Some physicians choose to pretreat with antibiotics to try to lower the risk of an infection after the SIS. The test can be done in the doctor's office and requires no medication in most cases. The results are immediately available since the patient's own physician usually performs the test and can review the results as they are obtained.

Hysteroscopy (HSC)

Sometimes smaller polyps and fibroids are hard to see on an HSG. For a close-up look at the inside of the uterus, your doctor may want to do a hysteroscopy.

A diagnostic *hysteroscopy,* often done in the doctor's office, is a procedure in which a small tube is guided through the cervix into the uterus. The uterus is distended, usually with a saline solution, so that your doctor can clearly see the entire area, including any small polyps, adhesions, or fibroids. You may be given local anesthesia, such as a cervical block, or mild sedation for the procedure.

If the procedure detects polyps, scar tissue, or small fibroids in the uterus, your doctor may do an *operative hysteroscopy.* In this procedure, the doctor inserts small instruments through the scope to remove the abnormal tissue. Your doctor may perform this procedure in his office, or in the hospital if more extensive work needs to be done. You may have a nerve block, such as an epidural, or general anesthesia for an operative hysteroscopy done in the hospital.

There is controversy over the use of hysteroscopy for failed IVF cycles. Some doctors believe that it can uncover uterine pathology not seen on ultrasound, while others believe that if pathology did not show on an SIS then it is not clinically relevant. Hysteroscopy is relatively safe, so the decision on whether to do an HSC should be discussed between the patient and the doctor.

Laparoscopy (LSC)

A *laparoscopy* (LSC) involves placing lighted telescopes and other instruments through the abdomen. The incisions made are very small, about 1/2 inch or less, and the procedure usually involves one to three incisions. Endometriosis and scar tissue can be removed during a laparoscopy. Fallopian tubes that are dilated also can be removed this way.

A laparoscopy is usually done as an outpatient procedure in a hospital or surgical center. The most common problems after the surgery are pain (usually minimal) from the incisions and pain in the right shoulder from the carbon dioxide used to inflate the abdomen. The recovery period is usually short, less than a week. Before IVF, laparoscopy was an integral part of the infertility evaluation. However, since IVF, the use of a true diagnostic laparoscopy has declined to almost zero. If detectable pathology exists, such as fibroids, extensive endometriosis, suspicious ovarian cysts, or hydrosalpinges, an operative laparoscopy may be needed. A specialty called *minimally invasive endoscopic surgery* has emerged, and many REIs have chosen to refer surgical cases to specialists trained in minimally invasive surgery.

Checking for Endometriosis

More than 5 million American women have endometriosis, a common, complicated condition that affects 30 to 40 percent of all infertility patients. Despite its prevalence, it's often underdiagnosed and undertreated. (See Chapter 7 for more on getting pregnant with endometriosis.)

Endometriosis is the presence of endometrial tissue, which lines the inside of your uterus, in places it has no business being. Endometriosis can be found throughout the pelvis — around the fallopian tubes and ovaries — but it has also been found in the lungs, skin, and brain. No one is quite sure how endometriosis travels so far, but theories are that it travels through the circulatory system or the lymphatic system.

Because endometriosis is endometrial tissue, it reacts to hormone changes the same way your uterine lining does. So when you get your period or have midcycle spotting, endometriosis tissue also bleeds. Because this tissue doesn't have a handy exit point the way your uterine lining does, the blood stagnates, causing inflammation, irritation, pain, and eventually scar tissue.

WARNING

You may suspect that you have endometriosis if you have any of the following symptoms:

>> Chronic or recurring pelvic pain

>> History of ectopic pregnancy or miscarriage

>> Backache or leg pain

>> Nausea, vomiting, diarrhea, or constipation

>> Rectal bleeding or bloody stools

>> Blood in urine

>> Urinary urgency or frequency

>> Chest pain or coughing up blood, especially at the time of your period

>> High blood pressure

Because the symptoms are so broad and sometimes nonspecific, endometriosis may be confused with the following:

>> Appendicitis

>> Irritable bowel syndrome

>> Bowel obstruction

>> Ovarian cysts

>> Pelvic inflammatory disease

Endometriosis can be diagnosed by laparoscopic surgery or a laparotomy; endo-metrial lesions can often be removed at the same time.

Considering Ovulation Disorders: Symptoms, Diagnosis, and Prognosis

You can have all the right reproductive parts in all the right places, but if they're not functioning properly, pregnancy will never occur. Getting pregnant is dependent on the release of a healthy egg capable of being fertilized by a healthy sperm. If your menstrual cycle is messed up, your egg production and release may be, too. Your menstrual cycle is one of the first things your doctor will probably ask you about when trying to get to the bottom of fertility issues, so we go over the big three dis-orders here. (We take a closer look at other menstrual disorders in Chapter 2.)

Metrorrhagia — Irregular periods

Two terms are used by physicians to describe menses: metrorrhagia and menor-rhagia. *Menorrhagia* refers to menses that are heavier in flow and of longer dura-tion than normal. Menses with these characteristics can occur when the cycle is longer than usual. Many times, a long cycle is due to delayed ovulation, which allows the lining of the uterus (endometrium) to grow thicker. When pregnancy does not occur, there is more lining for the uterus to slough and thus the flow can be heavier, longer, and more painful than expected. This can be mistaken for an early pregnancy loss, but that is rarely true.

Metrorrhagia refers to cycles (Day 1 of one menses to Day 1 of the next menses) that have irregular lengths. Most cycle irregularity is caused by varying lengths of the first phase of the menstrual cycles — the follicular phase. This situation is seen most frequently in women with PCOS and results from the brain not telling the ovary what to do in a normal, regular fashion. Because the follicular phase is the phase of growth of the endometrium, irregular menses frequently can be heavy and painful. Cycles are considered regular and of normal length if they occur between 26 and 35 days apart and vary month-to-month by only a few days.

Some women can tell exactly when their menses will start, but for most women, cycle lengths vary. The more irregular the cycles, the more likely there is a problem that can reduce a person's chance of conceiving. Also, miscarriage rates seem to be higher for women who do conceive if they have irregular cycles. Consulting a physician, making a diagnosis as to why the menses are not normal, and correcting the problem increases the chance for conceiving and reduces the chance of miscarriage.

An area of concern when talking about cycle length is when a woman is aging and her cycle length is shortening. For example, a 38-year-old person, whose cycles previously ranged from 28 to 30 days but now vary from 26 to 27 days may be transitioning into the premenopausal state. Noting this and seeking medical help may allow that person to use technology to increase the chance of conceiving rapidly and thus take advantage of what may be a limited window of opportunity before age removes the chance for conception.

Amenorrhea — No periods

Amenorrhea is the absence of menstrual periods. If you've never had a period, undoubtedly, you've been evaluated sometime during your teenage years to see whether a structural problem, such as absence of the uterus, malformation of the vagina, or undeveloped ovaries, is the cause.

However, many women have periods at one time and then quit having them. This is called secondary amenorrhea. Secondary amenorrhea has many causes such as — well — pregnancy! Don't forget to check that first. Other causes include PCOS, severe thyroid disease, and increased prolactin secretion. Sometimes the cause is structural, as in Asherman's syndrome (see the earlier section "Addressing scar tissue") It goes without saying that if you've had periods previously and no longer do, have a checkup to see what the problem is.

Anovulation — Failing to ovulate

If you're not getting your period at all or if you're having irregular periods, you may not be ovulating, a condition known as *anovulation*. Many factors can cause anovulation.

Looking at your weight . . . or lack thereof

One cause of anovulation is weight gain or loss. Of course, most women don't want to look at their weight. But even a slight deviation — about 15 percent — either up or down may create menstrual irregularities and subtle infertility issues. After your weight falls within normal limits, your chance of getting pregnant without any other therapy may increase.

WARNING

In today's culture, where thin is in and "you can't be too thin" is a widely accepted standard, overweight women are far more likely to consider their weight a problem than the underweight. The fact is, however, that being underweight is equally as damaging as being overweight if you're having fertility problems.

Frequent, strenuous exercise can also cause anovulation if it causes the body fat percentage to drop to less than 22 percent, the amount needed to keep menstruation occurring.

Factoring in stress

TIP

The role of stress in causing infertility is another one of those controversial areas with devotees on both sides. Infertility and stress almost always go hand in hand but it's unclear whether stress plays a big role in abnormal periods. Much of the scientific literature suggests that infertility may cause stress, but stress rarely causes infertility. That does not negate the importance of stress as a symptom of infertility, nor does it suggest that treatment for stress is inappropriate. However, it does suggest that treatment may not improve the pregnancy rate. Lowering stress levels is easier said than done, but if you're under severe stress, you may want to consider therapies such as working with a mental health professional to find methods to decrease stress. (See Chapter 10 for more on stress and infertility.)

REMEMBER

Waiting a year to meet the definition of infertility under your insurance plan is generally not necessary when menses are irregular, abnormal or absent. Early evaluation and treatment may help get you to a successful pregnancy.

test results

» **Checking for physical problems**

» **Dealing with functional issues**

» **Seeing how his history affects your fertility**

Chapter 12

Your Turn, Honey! Back to the Boys

You always knew men were different — but you may not have known *how* different! When it comes to reproduction, everything about men is different — from the way they let it "all hang out" to the way they produce gametes (both eggs and sperm are called *gametes*.) In this chapter, we hang out with the boys, examining their reproductive organs, their sperm-producing mechanisms, and the ways things can go awry in the sperm production department.

What is Male Factor Infertility?

Anything associated with the male that reduces the chance for conception is technically male factor infertility. Some men cannot ejaculate while others can't ejaculate when having intercourse but can ejaculate through masturbation. Some men experience anxiety-provoking erectile dysfunction due to the stress of having to perform at a specified time. However, male factor is primarily diagnosed using the semen analysis. The prevalence of male factor based upon the results from the semen analysis depends upon the group of people being considered. For women over the age of 38 with regular cycles and men who have fathered a pregnancy even if it did not go to term, the percentage of couples diagnosed with male factor is small. For women under the age of 35 with irregular menses and diagnosed with

PCOS, the percent of men diagnosed with male factor is small, but some studies have suggested that in couples where the female has PCOS, as many as 20 percent of the men have an abnormal semen analysis. Finally, when the woman is young with regular cycles and the male has never fathered a pregnancy, the percent of males with an abnormal semen analysis may be greater than 50 percent.

REMEMBER

Before we get to male factor as a diagnosis, we have to do a bit more investigating. Just as you are being evaluated upside down and sideways, your partner needs to be evaluated as well to get the full picture. The following sections help fill in the background that may lead to a better treatment plan.

Sizing Up the Semen

Much has been said about the semen, and considerable reliance has been placed upon the results of the semen analysis. But just how was the semen analysis developed and what do the numbers mean? There is considerable debate about the usefulness of the semen analysis, so it is important to understand how it was developed and what clinical value it has.

How does the sperm make it to the oocyte and fertilize it? The sperm are produced in the testes, mature as they travel through the epididymis, and are stored in the tail of the epididymis. At orgasm, a portion of the stored sperm move into the ejaculatory ducts where fluid is added, and the semen is expelled into the vagina. The fluid *(seminal plasma)* coagulates for 30–40 minutes while sperm escape the fluid and enter the cervix. From there the sperm travel through the uterus and enter the fallopian tubes. Once the sperm are near the oocyte, they can bind to the shell of the egg *(zona pellucida)*, and release enzymes that digest a pathway through the shell. One sperm binds to the cell membrane of the oocyte, which then ingests the sperm, while at the same time enzymes are released by the egg, changing the oocyte so that other sperm cannot fertilize it. From the 40 million of sperm in the ejaculate, only about 100 to 1,000 actually make it to the fallopian tube. So why does any of this matter? The semen analysis counts live, motile sperm — period. It says nothing about how many sperm, if any, will reach the oocyte. It says nothing about the ability of the sperm to actually fertilize the oocyte. Please do not misunderstand — numbers matter — but many questions about male fertility are not answered by the semen analysis.

Obtaining a high-quality specimen

Semen analysis (SA) can be done at your doctor's office, if he has the proper tools, or in a laboratory. In fertility clinics, they have specially trained personnel called *andrologists* who are responsible for all semen testing. There's no special preparation for a semen analysis There are two schools of thought when obtaining the first semen analysis. One says that the male should produce the sample at home with no specified time frame for abstinence. This may be a better reflection on the true status of the male. The other school of thought says to follow the recommendations of the World Health Organization (WHO) for the first semen analysis, which requires abstinence (no ejaculation) for two to five days.

Usually, semen samples are produced on-site; some clinics or offices may provide "visual aids" to ejaculation such as magazines or movies. Can you "help" with production? Only if you promise to use no lubricants or saliva, which can mess up the sample!

If it's absolutely impossible for your partner to produce on-site, you can bring in a sample produced within the last hour. The specimen needs to be kept warm in cold weather.

Most any laboratory can do a "screening" semen analysis. However, the determination of *morphology* (proportion of "normal" forms), especially by the criteria of Kruger, takes a high level of expertise, and is generally only available at a bona fide fertility program.

REMEMBER

The semen sample must be collected in a sterile container (just like the samples used for IUI that we discuss in Chapter 14). So, no makeshift containers allowed. If you're bringing in a semen sample, keep it at next-to-body temperature — holding it under your armpit is ideal. Make sure that the lid's on tight!

Development of the semen analysis and what the numbers mean

Male factor infertility has been recognized as a problem for a long time. However, there was no standardization concerning the performance of the semen analysis until 1980 when the WHO published the first manual on the performance of the semen analysis. The purpose of the manual was to standardize the technique of performing the semen analysis. The manual has been updated three times with the latest version published in 2010. The WHO also established normal values for the test — and here is where the rub is. The data for establishing the normal values used information gleaned from the semen analysis of men where the couple had had a pregnancy within the last year. The WHO calculated the lowest 5 percent of the values and said this was abnormal even though all of the values were from fertile men. For the latest version, the data was derived from 1,953 men and from five studies in seven countries on three continents. There was no data from Asia, Africa, the middle East, or Latin America. The general impression is that the semen analysis is not a very accurate test, especially if the values are only slightly abnormal. In general, the more abnormal the test results, the greater the chance that there really is male factor. At the very least, the semen analysis can alert a couple that therapies for male factor may increase the chance for conception. Home semen kits are available that may help couples identify where further evaluation is needed.

Given the inadequacies of the semen analysis, more accurate tests are needed that better identify couples who would benefit from therapies for male factor infertility. Recently, it has been suggested that the total motile number of sperm is a more accurate indicator of a decreased chance of spontaneous conception. The study divided the groups into those where total motile sperm (TMS) was < 5 million, 5–20 million and > 20 million. If the TMS was > 20 million, there was no reduction in the chance for conception. If there was < 5 million, there was a significant reduction in the chance of conception, but some people did conceive even if the TMS was 1 or 2 million. For couples trying to conceive where there are no other abnormal fertility factors and the woman is < 38 years old, conservative management may be warranted. However, most pregnancies require ART (Assisted Reproductive Technologies, which includes intrauterine insemination and in vitro fertilization). The overall success rates for ART used for male factor are high when there are no other infertility factors present.

TECHNICAL STUFF

The WHO has set standard parameters for a normal semen specimen. Your physician should review these results along with their clinical significance.

>> **Volume:** Should be 1.5 to 5 ml, or somewhat less than a teaspoon.

>> **Concentration:** Should be greater than 15 million sperm/ml, or a total of greater than 40 million per ejaculate.

>> **Motility:** More than 40 percent of the sperm should be motile or moving.

>> **Morphology:** More than a certain percentage of the sperm should be normally shaped, as determined by the lab technician. If the lab is using the WHO criteria, the normal cutoff is 30 percent. If the lab is using Kruger criteria, which are stricter, the normal cutoff is 4 percent.

>> **Forward progression:** Motile, non-progressively motile, and immotile.

>> **White blood cells:** < 1 million/ml.

>> **Hyperviscosity:** Should gel promptly but liquefy within 30 minutes after ejaculation.

>> **Ph:** Should be alkaline, to protect sperm from the acidic environment of the vagina.

There are some other tests that the doctor may order, although these are no longer considered routine diagnostic tests and would only be ordered under special circumstances. These include:

>> **HOS, or hypo-osmotic swelling test:** When semen samples have no or very little motile sperm, the question arises as to whether the sperm are dead or just not moving. One way to test for this is to do a viability assay on the raw specimen by adding a dye to the semen and seeing if the dye is absorbed by the sperm. Alive sperm keep the dye out.

>> **Antisperm antibodies (ASA):** A normal semen sample contains no antisperm antibodies. Antibodies cause problems if they're attached to the sperm tail, because they interfere with movement, or to the head, where they may make it difficult for the sperm to penetrate the egg.

>> **DNA-fragmentation assay:** Sperm are essentially DNA bullets. Their purpose is to insert the male genetic material into the egg. For normal embryo formation, the DNA needs to be undamaged. Some circumstances cause the DNA to be fragmented, and thus these sperm can't form a normal embryo. Diagnostics tests have been developed to measure what percentage of the sperm in a semen sample are damaged.

REMEMBER

It takes three months for sperm to properly develop, so if your partner was sick, taking medication, or had anything else unusual going on three months ago, his specimen may be abnormal.

Interpreting the SA Test Results

With some of the test results back, you may be even more confused than you were before. If your partner's semen analysis comes back with some results askew, he may be too embarrassed to ask what the results mean. Sometimes it's easier to look up the problems in a book, so here you are!

Semen samples can vary from month to month, or even day to day. That's because it takes about 72 days for sperm to develop. Unlike eggs, which are present from your embryonic days, sperm are replenished all the time.

REMEMBER

Because men are constantly producing new sperm, one "bad" semen analysis should be followed up with another in a month or so to see if the problem was a temporary one. An illness, injury, or medication or drug used a few months before may make one sample not so superior, but checking again a month later may show an improvement.

Making too few sperm

Sometimes a semen analysis shows a very low number of sperm, less than 15 million/ml, a condition called *oligospermia.* While 15 million sperm may sound excessive — why isn't one or two million enough? — large numbers of sperm are needed in the ejaculate because many sperm are abnormal even in a good sperm sample, and it's a long way to the ovulated egg, so many don't make it all the way.

There are many causes of oligospermia, ranging from varicoceles (see "Correcting Varicoceles") to lifestyle issues (check out "Making Lifestyle Changes to Improve Sperm Production"). Other causes may be:

>> Hormone imbalances, which can be checked by a simple blood test

>> Chromosomal abnormalities such as a congenital deletion of part of the Y chromosome

>> History of lymphoma or testicular cancer or chemotherapy (see Chapter 7 for more about fertility and cancer treatment)

>> Diabetes

>> Sickle cell disease

>> Kidney disease

>> Liver disease

TIP

You can get pregnant without fertility treatments if your partner has oligospermia, but your chances of pregnancy are higher if you do one of the following:

>> **Intrauterine insemination (IUI):** The sperm are concentrated and "washed" so that the best sperm are used for insemination. (See Chapter 14 for more on IUI.)

>> **In vitro fertilization (IVF):** This treatment allows fertilization to take place in the lab, where a high concentration of sperm can be put in with the egg. If the sperm are especially abnormal, the lab may need to utilize intracytoplasmic sperm injection (ICSI), the insertion of a sperm directly into an egg. The procedure is done by an embryologist under a high-powered microscope. (See Chapter 17 for more information on ICSI.)

DOES HAVING TOO MANY SPERM MATTER?

When men have high sperm counts, they are usually told they can fertilize a nation or something to that effect. Maybe yes, maybe no. Normal functioning in any area of physiology means conforming to the normal. So while it is easily understood that a low count can impair fertility, it is not as intuitive that a very high count can impair fertility. Questions to be asked are whether the male ever created a pregnancy even if it ended in a miscarriage or abortion, and whether there are female factors that could explain the infertility. However, if there seems to be no other cause of infertility and the man's count repeatedly remains high, then that may be a cause. As with many male factor problems, this one could be treated using IVF with ICSI as long as the sperm can function properly.

When there's no sperm in sight

If no sperm are seen, it's called *azoospermia*. About 1 percent of males have azoospermia. If your partner has azoospermia, you won't be able to get pregnant conventionally. Different factors can cause azoospermia; either the production of the sperm or the delivery of the sperm can be at fault. Sperm production problems can be caused by the following:

>> **Sertoli cell only syndrome:** In this condition, the germ cells that produce sperm in the testes are absent. There is no way for a person with this syndrome to father a child.

>> **Anabolic steroids:** Their use may cause irreversible shutdown of the sperm production.

>> **Abnormal hormone levels:** Low levels of LH, FSH, or testosterone can cause low sperm production. This problem can be treated with hormone injections, pills, or transdermal patches.

If the problem is obstruction, in general, the sperm production is normal, and the sperm simply can't get to the ejaculatory duct. In these cases, your partner will need a surgical procedure to extract the sperm from the testicle (discussed in the nearby sidebar "If you need a sperm aspiration"). This procedure must be done in conjunction with IVF because the sperm need to be injected directly into the egg. Obstructive problems include the following:

>> Absence of the *vas deferens,* the tube that delivers sperm to the ejaculatory duct and the prostate

>> Previous vasectomy

>> Previous infection that causes scarring and obstruction of the epididymis

>> Obstruction from prior surgery

Mechanical problems with getting the sperm where they need to be include the following:

>> Retrograde ejaculation, in which the majority of the sperm go into the bladder

>> Spinal cord injury that prevents ejaculation

>> Previous injury from trauma

>> Previous injury from surgery, such as hernia surgery

>> A disease such as diabetes

IF YOU NEED A SPERM ASPIRATION

Sperm can be aspirated from either the epididymis, which sits on top of the testes, or from the testes themselves. There are four different types of procedures, each with advantages and disadvantages:

- **MESA (microsurgical epididymal sperm aspiration):** This procedure can be done only for obstructive azoospermia, because men with nonobstructive azoospermia rarely have sperm in the epididymis. A small incision is made in the scrotum, and then a dilated tubule in the epididymis is cut open and examined through a lighted microscope. Fluid is collected from the tubule and examined for sperm. This procedure can be done in the doctor's office. You may be given a spermatic cord block and sedation during the procedure. You can generally return to work the following day.

- **PESA (percutaneous epididymal sperm aspiration):** This procedure is done in the office. A blind needle stick into the epididymis is used to extract sperm. Local anesthesia and sedation may be given.

- **TESE (testicular sperm extraction):** A small incision is made, and a piece of testicular tissue is removed. Testicular sperm doesn't freeze or thaw as well as epididymal sperm but may be the only sperm found in men with nonobstructive azoospermia.

- **TESA (testicular sperm aspiration):** This procedure is done in the office, using a blind needle aspiration of the testicle.

Considering the sperm's shape and movement

After checking how many sperm are available, the andrologist will look at what shape the sperm are in and how they are moving — kind of like a test to see if they are "in condition" for conception. The terms you'll see on the report are the *morphology* (shape) and the *motility* (how they swim).

Morphology

There are hundreds of papers written about the shape of sperm. The concern has to do with the ability of sperm to navigate the female reproductive tract to get to the egg in the fallopian tube at the correct time. There are many barriers to this; the cervix with its protective mucus is the primary obstacle. Putting sperm beyond the cervix through the use of intrauterine insemination is based upon the fact that the cervix keeps many sperm from entering the uterus. So while the cervix can act as a storage place for sperm, it can also prevent sperm from moving forward. The theory is that sperm need a specific shape to get through the cervical mucus (see Figure 12-1). Sperm with an abnormal shape may be filtered and not able to move forward. Both IUI and ICSI correct for this problem. But sperm have another issue. Once they reach the egg, they need to penetrate the shell of the egg. Sperm penetrate the shell by binding to the shell and releasing proteins that digest a pathway through the shell. If the sperm do not have these proteins, you could place a bazillion near the egg and they could not penetrate the shell.

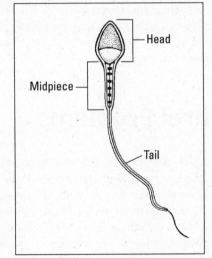

FIGURE 12-1: A normal sperm.

Illustration by Kathryn Born

In the early days of IVF, before ICSI, sperm and eggs were simply placed in a dish. Fertilization had to be done by normally functioning sperm and eggs. It became apparent that some men had sperm that were incapable of fertilizing an egg, but there was no highly reliable test to determine this before the IVF procedure. That meant that couples could go through IVF only to find out that they had no embryos. One school of thought suggested that the shape of the sperm may give an indication about the ability of the sperm to fertilize an egg. To that end, they developed a very detailed process for determining if a sperm had a shape that suggested that the sperm could fertilize the egg. Originally called the Kruger method, the term *strict scrutiny* is now used to identify that this detailed methodology is being used to determine the percentage of sperm with the desired shape. Labs vary in what they consider normal, but in general anything < 5 percent is abnormal, from > 4 percent to 14 percent may be an indication of a reduced fertility potential, and above 14 percent is normal.

Motility

In the sperm world, it's swim or die. Sperm must traverse the female reproductive tract to get to the egg. Any reduction in motility reduces the number of sperm that even have a chance to get to the egg. Like morphology, a reduced motility may sometimes also indicate that the sperm lack the ability to penetrate the shell of the egg. Normal percentages for motility are > 40 percent motile and 32 percent forwardly motile. Sperm lose their motility if they remain in semen too long, and this is why andrology labs needs the specimen within an hour of collection. Also, cold conditions, such as a cold car seat in the winter, can artificially lower the motility. Another condition that can result in lower motility is the thickness of the semen (viscosity). After ejaculation, semen coagulates just as blood does. Over the next 30–45 minutes, it liquefies. Some men have conditions that create either super thick semen (increased viscosity) or failure to liquefy. Both of these may reduce the fertility potential for the man.

Checking for Structural Problems

As with the ladies, a lot of information can be gained by doing a thorough examination of the male reproductive organs. The physical exam of the male can identify a number of reasons why a male may have an abnormal semen analysis. Most physicians will check to see if the male has a hernia. Examination of the penis can identify problems where the opening of the penis is lower on the shaft. Examination of the scrotum can identify the presence of a varicocele (we talk more about this in the following section). It can also identify the presence of cysts in the scrotum. Examination of the prostate by a rectal exam can identify infections of the prostate.

While some fertility specialists will do these exams themselves, many will refer you to a urologist for a complete examination. Once there, the urologist may suggest other tests to help determine whether there are any structural problems that are reducing your potential fertility.

Correcting Varicoceles

A varicocele is an abnormal dilation of the spermatic vein. Varicoceles are more common than you may think; about 15 percent of men have them. However, 40 percent of males with an abnormal semen analysis have a varicocele. The majority of men with a varicocele are fertile, but the varicocele is the most frequently diagnosed problem for infertile males. More varicoceles are found on the left testicle than the right — around 90 percent, in fact. The effect of varicoceles on male fertility is controversial because there is no irrefutable evidence that varicocele repair improves fertility. However, some doctors feel that they are a leading cause of male infertility.

Varicoceles have been theorized to lead to decreased fertility in the following ways:

>> Increased temperature in the testes

>> Stagnation of blood around the testicles

>> Hormonal alterations

>> Decreased sperm production and motility

Varicoceles can be corrected in one of two ways:

>> **Surgery:** Done as an outpatient; a small incision is made just above the groin, and the offending vein is located and tied off. Recovery time is a week to ten days, but heavy lifting should be avoided for a month or so. Surgical risks include infection, nerve injury, and *hydrocele formation* (a collection of fluid around the testicle).

>> **Radiographic embolization:** Also an outpatient procedure; advantages are immediate recovery with no restrictions on lifting. A small catheter is threaded through the femoral vein in the groin; dye is injected to show exactly where the problem vein is, and then the vein is blocked, or occluded, so that no blood flow can reach it.

In the past, varicocele repair was a very common procedure. Most recently, varicocele repair has become controversial because studies designed to demonstrate improvement in fertility after the surgery have not been able to show the degree of improvement that was anticipated. Only very large and obvious varicoceles tend to be repaired these days. It can take up to four months for an improvement in sperm count to be seen after a varicocele repair. But, while an improvement in sperm count is a desired outcome for the surgery, the purpose of the surgery is to improve the chance for conception. It may take one to two years after a repair before a conception occurs. After that, conceptions occur at the same rate as if the repair had never been done and are very unlikely to occur.

Since most pregnancies actually occur in the first year after surgery, if a conception has not occurred, IVF with ICSI is a reasonable form of treatment. The opinion of ASRM is that surgical repair of large varicoceles in men with abnormal semen values and a negative evaluation for young females is an acceptable form of treatment. Many women over the age of 38 have a reduced ovarian reserve, so for these women moving to IVF offers a better option than having a varicocele repaired.

Looking for Clues in Your Blood

Just when your male partner thought he was safe, the clinic's resident "vampire" ushers him into the lab to draw his blood, too! If we can learn things about your fertility from your blood, why can't we do it with your guy? Well, we can. Just like the female, the male should be tested for infectious diseases as we discuss in Chapter 4, but there a few other tests that can help put the puzzle pieces together and get everyone on the right track.

Testosterone

Testosterone is a steroid hormone. Both males and females make testosterone, but females convert it into estrogen. Males produce considerably more testosterone than females, which creates the usual features of maleness. Testosterone is responsible for a normal libido and ejaculatory function. Men with low testosterone may see a decrease in libido and a failure to achieve an erection. Performance anxiety can also produce these symptoms, and the routines involved with infertility treatment can create a lot of stress. Therefore, it is important to distinguish the cause of the decreased libido so that the proper treatment can be implemented. Obesity in males can also lead to low testosterone because the fat changes the testosterone to estrogen. Finally, aging can reduce the testosterone levels. It may seem logical that if the problem is low testosterone, then testosterone treatment should improve the problem. And if erectile dysfunction is the problem, that logic holds true. But it turns out that testosterone suppresses the brain's stimulation of sperm production by the testes. Low testosterone in males who are experiencing erectile dysfunction (unable to obtain or maintain an erection) can be treated by the use of medication such as Viagra or Cialis to help maintain an erection or by Clomid if there is also a low sperm count.

Other strategic hormones

Men have follicle stimulating hormone (FSH), too — who knew! Males and females have many similar hormones. In males, FSH reflects how well the testis is working. Testicular failure, just like ovarian failure, causes the FSH levels to rise. If a man has a low sperm count and the FSH level is high, the diagnosis is testicular failure. Knowing this tells a patient that using hormone therapy such as Clomid will not help. The treatment option becomes either IUI or, more frequently, IVF with ICSI. However, if the man has a mild/moderate male factor and normal FSH levels, then Clomid may be helpful.

Some other hormones to consider measuring in the male partner include the following:

>> **LH (luteinizing hormone):** LH is as important to men as it is to women. LH stimulates cells in the testicle to make testosterone. A man can have no sperm but because he has cells (Leydig cells) that make testosterone, the man will develop as a male with normal male sexual functioning.

>> **TSH (thyroid stimulating hormone):** Males can have thyroid disease, which can affect sperm production. Thyroid disease is much less frequent in males but does occur.

>> **Prolactin:** *Yes!* Males do make prolactin — no, they don't use it to breastfeed. Some men have a growth in the pituitary *(pituitary adenoma)* that can produce very high levels of prolactin. These high levels affect normal reproductive functioning and can lead to impotence. If an adenoma is suspected because of high prolactin levels, an MRI of the brain can describe the size of the adenoma. Treatment consists of oral medications such a Parlodel or Dostinex, and frequent prolactin testing assures that the treatment is effective and that the adenoma is most likely not enlarging.

Considering Potential Functional Issues

Abnormal sperm may be a problem you both can deal with. Problems with ejaculation or the ability to sustain an erection, however, may be so difficult to address that you may have difficulty in bringing it out into the open. Yet issues with being able to function are common: Ten percent of men between the ages of 18 and 59 have experienced erectile problems in the last year, and 10 percent of men between the ages of 40 and 70 have complete erectile failure.

Plenty of medical-related conditions can cause problems with erection and ejaculation. The following list gives examples of what can cause such problems:

>> **Medications**

- Antidepressants
- Antiulcer medications
- Certain blood pressure medications
- Cholesterol-lowering medications

>> **Diseases**

- Diabetes
- Heart attack (myocardial infarction)
- Hypertension or other vascular disease
- Hypothyroidism or hyperthyroidism
- Leukemia
- Liver cirrhosis
- Renal failure
- Sickle cell anemia

>> **Surgeries**

- Abdominal perineal resection
- Proctocolectomy
- Radical prostatectomy
- Transurethral resection of prostate

Radiation, trauma, heavy alcohol use, and neurological damage from surgery, stroke, epilepsy, or multiple sclerosis can also cause erectile dysfunction.

Help for erectile dysfunction

Erectile dysfunction (ED) is a complex problem that can have many causes, some very benign and some serious. Therefore, ED needs to be addressed and evaluated to make sure that the cause is not a serious harm to the man. ED is defined as the inability of the man to maintain an erection sufficient for satisfying sexual functioning. ED is common in men where the couple has an infertility diagnosis, occurring as frequently as one out of every six men.

Less commonly addressed is the lack of ejaculation (the act of ejecting semen from the body), but this occurs in one out of ten men. ED may be due to the stress of infertility and having to perform on demand at the proper time. This does not place the man in harm but does create problems when trying to conceive. One way to avoid this is to have the man produce specimens on his schedule and then freeze the semen so that the semen can be used at the proper time if the man is unable to perform. Some men have never been able to have intercourse because of ED. Again, if the man can ejaculate on his own time, then the semen can be frozen.

When ED is present, the man needs to be evaluated further. The evaluation looks at both the general health of the man and also at the hormonal status of the man. The causes of ED are numerous including heart disease, vascular disease, diabetes, and obesity, to name just a few. Other causes include alcoholism, surgery for prostate disease, sleep disorders, and certain prescription medications. The approach to the treatment of ED depends upon the cause of the ED. Most ED can be addressed with proper treatment. But for those circumstances where ED is persistent, sperm can be surgically extracted from the testes and used in IVF with ICSI.

Intervention for retrograde ejaculation

Retrograde ejaculation (RE) is when the semen goes into the bladder and not into the penis during orgasm. The physical symptom is that a man has an orgasm and very little or no semen comes out of the penis. Most people are amazed at how little semen is consider a normal volume, especially when faced with a semen collection container. Consider that a teaspoon equals 5 ml and a normal ejaculate volume is > 1–1.5 ml — so not even a teaspoon. Yet less than 0.5 ml is considered too little and suggests the diagnosis of retrograde ejaculation (RE). In its journey from the testis to the end of the penis, semen is faced with a fork in the road: One fork goes out of the penis and the other goes into the bladder. Usually, the fork in the road is constructed to favor the semen going out of the body. However, some conditions change the favored road signs and, since the distance is much shorter to go into the bladder, the semen makes a wrong turn and ends up in the bladder. Common causes of RE are surgery, some prescription medications, or nerve damage as a result of medical conditions such as diabetes, Parkinson's disease, or spinal cord injury. Sometimes sperm can be collected by having the man empty his bladder, ejaculate, and then collect the urine (where the sperm are) and quickly process this to isolate enough sperm to do intrauterine inseminations for the female. This process can also be used in the IVF/ICSI setting. Finally, the ultimate form of treatment can extract sperm from the testes to be used in IVF with ICSI. (This involves the procedures talked about in the section "When there's no sperm in sight" earlier in this chapter.)

Undoing a Vasectomy: Is it Worth It?

About 500,000 vasectomies are performed each year. As with tubal ligation, many men regret their decision and decide to have the surgery reversed. Vasectomy reversal surgery is often successful in that sperm will be found in the ejaculate in the majority of cases, but the number of sperm may be too small to make pregnancy likely.

Your chance of pregnancy after sterilization reversal depends on several factors. Consider carefully whether reversal will be more cost effective and offer a better chance of success than IVF, in which tied tubes can be bypassed or sperm can be removed directly from the testicles via sperm aspiration. Of course, personal preference plays a great role in this decision. The principal appeal of vasectomy reversal is that pregnancy can occur naturally. The main disadvantage is that it may not work, and if it doesn't, IVF will be needed anyway.

Analyzing the Effects of Age and Lifestyle

For years, it's been considered unfair that men, unlike women, had no age limit placed on their fertility. While new dads in their seventies still make the news from time to time, studies have shown that age may play a part in male fertility as well as female fertility. Some studies suggest that older men produce fewer mature sperm. Immature sperm are slower moving and lack the strength to "go the distance" to the egg. Decreased testosterone production in older men may lead to erection difficulties and a weaker ejaculation.

A recent study showed a possible link between older men and the incidence of autism in their offspring; similar studies have shown an increase in offspring with schizophrenia born to older dads. A Canadian study showed abnormalities in DNA in sperm of men over age 45 — in fact, men over 45 had double the number of abnormal sperm found in men aged 30.

Of course, you can't change your age, so if you're attempting pregnancy over age 40, the best thing you can do is maintain a healthy lifestyle to make sure you're producing the best sperm possible. Many lifestyle issues can impact sperm production in a big way; consider the following and change what you can:

>> **Weight:** As with women, overweight men have decreased fertility, according to some studies. If you're overweight, reducing may help increase your sperm count — and give you more energy to chase after your future bundle of joy!

>> **Smoking:** Cigarette smoking can decrease sperm count, increase the number of abnormal sperm in a semen sample, and some studies suggest that smokers are more likely to be impotent (unable to sustain an erection) than nonsmokers.

>> **Marijuana:** Marijuana use in men can lower the amount of seminal fluid produced and can result in decreased sperm production. There is considerable controversy about the effect of marijuana use on the pregnancy rate, which hopefully will be addressed as more and more men will be using marijuana since legalization in many states has taken place.

>> **Alcohol:** Alcohol, in large quantities, increases the number of abnormally shaped sperm, can change male hormones, and leads to impotence.

>> **Cocaine:** Cocaine use is associated with subfertility. Duration of cocaine use and how recently the use was are associated with lower concentrations and increased abnormal forms in the semen analysis.

>> **Anabolic steroids:** Anabolic steroids suppress testosterone, resulting in small testes, possible impotence, and severe decrease in sperm count, or even a total absence of sperm.

>> **Chemical exposure:** Working with chemicals such as pesticides, chemical compounds, or inhalants can result in a decreased sperm count and/or an increased number of abnormal sperm in the ejaculate.

>> **Medications:** Many prescription drugs used to treat high blood pressure and depression have negative effects on fertility; if you are dealing with a low sperm count or impotence, be sure to discuss any prescription medications you're taking with your doctor.

>> **Bicycling:** Cycling seems like a great way to burn calories and stay in shape — and it is. However, studies have shown that competitive (not recreational) cyclists are more likely to have fertility issues.

>> **Antioxidants:** Many studies suggest that taking antioxidants improves semen values and conception rates.

Chapter **13**

Riding the Roller Coaster of Early Pregnancy Loss

As upsetting as it is not to get pregnant, getting pregnant and having the pregnancy end in loss is even more devastating. Why do so many pregnancies end early, and what does it mean for future pregnancies? And how can you avoid personal feelings of failure when a loss occurs? In this chapter, we discuss how and why pregnancies are lost in the first 12 weeks, and we offer advice on how to pick yourself up and try again if this happens to you.

Defining What Being Pregnant Really Means

You've been through your treatment cycle, and you are waiting for the magic words — "you are pregnant." But how do you know if you are really pregnant or not? In pre-modern times, you'd have to wait until your tummy started to swell and you felt the baby moving. Thank goodness you don't have to wait that long anymore. There are easier (and earlier) ways to know if you are successful, which usually occur in a stepwise progression to confirming those magic words.

Taking a home pregnancy test

Even though your doctor probably told you not to take a home pregnancy test, you are going to do it anyway. We know, you can't help it, but we want you to be a little cautious. These tests are good indicators of pregnancy if your hormone levels are at a certain point, but not so good if your levels are low. More tips on this in Chapter 18.

Getting a blood test

Ahhh. Now we are getting somewhere. If you're under treatment by a fertility doctor, you may be asked to do a blood pregnancy test, called a beta–HCG (this stands for the beta subunit of the HCG molecule, the hormone of pregnancy produced by the implanting placenta, or "beta" for short), about two weeks after ovulation or embryo transfer. Discussed more in Chapter 18, when this hormone comes back at a certain level (usually double digits) and rises appropriately (almost doubles within 48 hours), you can claim the "pregnant" pennant.

Scanning the uterus

This is the penultimate pregnancy test! At approximately 5–6 weeks, your doctor can do a vaginal ultrasound to see the fetus. This procedure not only confirms where the fetus is growing (we hope, in the uterus) but also gives an indication of how good the pregnancy is by measuring the size of the fetus and identifying whether there is a visible heartbeat.

Being "A Little Bit" Pregnant: Chemical Pregnancies

Most of you have heard that there's no such thing as being "a little bit" pregnant. This statement is true in one sense, but at times, you do feel that you're "almost" pregnant . . . and you may be right.

Understanding chemical pregnancies

Even after embryos successfully implant, a large percentage (depending on the age of the mother) stop developing before they develop a heartbeat. Many of these early miscarriages, up to 30 percent, take place before the time when you would notice any signs of pregnancy. If this happens, you may have no pregnancy symptoms at all, not even a missed period. Or you may have very early pregnancy signs, such as breast tenderness, which suddenly disappear. These signs may be followed by a slightly late, heavier-than-normal period, which is actually the passing of a very early pregnancy. You may pass more clots than normal (for you), or you may feel crampier than usual. You probably wouldn't even realize that you had been pregnant unless you did a sensitive early pregnancy test, such as a blood test (a beta-hCG). Your beta number may be positive (most labs have a sensitivity of 5, meaning that anything over 5 is considered positive; some labs have a sensitivity of 2, or even 1.5) but very low when first tested, and it may be negative a few days later, at the second test. Your doctor may say that you had a *chemical pregnancy* if this happens.

Testing for possible fixes

At least 50 percent of the time, chemical pregnancies are caused by the implantation of a chromosomally abnormal embryo, but other factors can also cause very early miscarriage. Your doctor may do tests, such as checking your progesterone level, to see whether there are other reasons why the embryo isn't "sticking." In a normal pregnancy, the *corpus luteum*, or leftover "shell" of the ovulated egg, produces a hormone called *progesterone.* Progesterone is necessary for the implantation and growth of the early embryo. If your progesterone is lower than normal, the embryo may not be able to grow properly.

A simple blood test can check your progesterone levels. There is a distinct difference between a progesterone test done in the nonpregnancy state to test for adequacy of ovulation and one done during the early part of an established pregnancy. The progesterone level during an early pregnancy may reflect a problem with the pregnancy if it is low. Some studies suggest that a progesterone level of less than 12 ng/ml has a 70 percent chance of resulting in a miscarriage. The majority of these miscarriages are due to a pregnancy that has the wrong number of chromosomes. This raises the issue of possibly saving a pregnancy by using progestogen once a person is pregnant. There is some controversy over this, and many gynecologists will add progesterone if the level is low. There is very little evidence that this will make a difference for the outcome of the pregnancy, and certainly for the majority of these pregnancies, the fact that they have the wrong number of chromosomes means that there is really nothing that can be done to save the pregnancy.

REMEMBER

So even though people may say that you can't be a "little bit" pregnant, the truth is that a pregnancy can start to implant and then stop before you even miss a period. You may not realize this is happening to you without a very early blood pregnancy test. If your doctor suspects that you're having chemical pregnancies, he or she will order further testing to identify a problem that might be corrected.

Suffering a Miscarriage

A *miscarriage* is a pregnancy loss that occurs after you know you're pregnant but before the fetus is *viable*, or able to live on its own.

REMEMBER

Miscarriages are very common: About one in four women has a miscarriage during her reproductive years. But knowing that miscarriages are common events and not likely to recur doesn't make them any easier to deal with.

The vast majority of miscarriages occur in the first 12 weeks of pregnancy. Based on this fact, many couples decide not to shout the news to friends and relatives before this time has passed.

Understanding the language of loss

Doctors call all miscarriages *abortion*; that term doesn't have the same meaning as what you're used to. There are different types of miscarriages, and they're tied to the type of symptoms you have:

>> **Threatened abortion:** The first sign of possible miscarriage is usually spotting. But because spotting is common in pregnancy (occurring in one in five women), doctors don't always take it as a dire sign. If spotting and cramping stop quickly, the chances are excellent that the pregnancy will carry to term. Most doctors restrict sex and heavy exercise if some spotting has occurred. Your doctor may call cramping and spotting a *threatened abortion.* Bleeding can be caused by implantation of the embryo or by the sloughing off of the lining around the area where implantation has occurred. An ultrasound done around six weeks will show whether a fetus is in the uterus and may show a heartbeat. A heartbeat *should* be seen by vaginal ultrasound by seven weeks at the latest.

>> **Inevitable abortion:** If your cervix has started to open, or *dilate,* and you're bleeding, you'll almost certainly miscarry. Your doctor may call these symptoms an *inevitable abortion.* An ultrasound may show no fetal heartbeat. Your doctor will want you to watch for signs of infection, such as a temperature over 100-101 degrees or a foul-smelling discharge. Hospitalization isn't necessary in most cases of miscarriage. Save any tissue that you pass so that your doctor can send it to a pathologist, and in some cases the tissue can be tested especially for the number of chromosomes for the pregnancy. Recently developed tests can evaluate the chromosome number even if the tissue has been passed at home. You'll probably continue bleeding for seven to ten days.

>> **Missed abortion:** A *missed abortion* occurs when the pregnancy stops progressing but there are no signs of miscarriage, such as bleeding or cramping. Your pregnancy blood levels may be lower than expected, and the ultrasound shows no fetal heart activity. A missed abortion may require a

dilation and curettage, a minor surgery, to remove the tissue. More and more of these unfortunate outcomes are being treated medically using vaginal inserted prostaglandins.

Knowing if you need a D&C

You may need a D&C, or *dilation and curettage*, if you don't pass all the pregnancy tissue on your own. This procedure involves opening the cervix and scraping the uterus with a blunt instrument called a curette, or with a plastic tube with an opening connected to suction vacuum, to make sure that no tissue is left, because leftover tissue can cause an infection. This surgery is done under light sedation, usually as an outpatient procedure. Your doctor may tell you not to take tub baths, use hot tubs, douche, or have sex for a week or two. You may be asked to return for a follow-up visit to make sure that you're healing normally. There won't be any stitches to remove after a D&C.

Don't be upset if your doctor calls your miscarriage a *spontaneous abortion*, or SAB. This is the medical term for a miscarriage.

Recognizing possible causes

REMEMBER

More than 50 percent of miscarriages are due to chromosomal abnormalities. In these cases, no amount of rest or anything else that you do — or don't do — will prevent them. There is no good news about a pregnancy loss. However, one positive to note is that the vast majority of these are considered random and non-recurrent, which means that the next time you get pregnant, there is no reason to think the same thing will happen. However, sometimes the miscarriage is a sign of poor egg quality. For example, a miscarriage for a young couple who conceived easily probably does not predict a problem and they will be able to conceive and have a child easily. But a miscarriage for a 38-year-old who had tried for more than six months is a symptom of a reduced ovarian reserve and needs further evaluation.

Blighted ovum

A blighted ovum is the most common outcome (other than a chemical pregnancy) of a conception that has a chromosomal error. *Blighted ovum* occurs when the placenta and amniotic sac develop and put out pregnancy hormones, but the fetus itself doesn't develop. So you may test pregnant, but there is no fetus. You and your doctor may discover this fact when you start spotting and the doctor tests for fetal activity and finds no fetus. Since most fertility doctors perform routine ultrasound testing of all pregnancies, a blighted ovum (or "empty sac") may also be picked up at the time of a routine evaluation. The most frustrating part of a blighted ovum is that the HCG is produced by the placenta, and therefore may be quite high, with associated pregnancy symptoms — morning sickness, breast tenderness, tiredness — and yet there is no baby.

Molar pregnancy

TECHNICAL STUFF

Another, somewhat rare type of chromosomal anomaly is called a molar pregnancy. Molar pregnancies, also called a *hydatidiform mole,* occur in one in a thousand conceptions in the United States. *Molar pregnancies* result when the egg is abnormal; it has no chromosomal content to pass on, so there is no fetus, only a placenta. The placenta usually grows very quickly; you may show signs of pregnancy very early and have unusually high beta levels.

Molar pregnancies are treated with a D&C to evacuate the abnormal cells. In some cases, the cells can transform into *choriocarcinoma,* a rare disease that behaves like a cancer in that it can spread to other parts of the body. In these cases, you may be given methotrexate, a chemotherapy drug, to stop the abnormally fast cell division. After a molar pregnancy, you will be advised to avoid another pregnancy for 6 to 12 months to be sure that no abnormal cells remain in the body and that a choriocarcinoma does not develop.

Other common causes of miscarriage, such as abnormalities of the uterus, lack of progesterone support after ovulation, or vaginal infection, can be evaluated before you try to get pregnant again.

Factoring in age

As in most fertility issues, age is a definite factor in miscarriage rates. Consider these numbers:

>> If you're under 35, the miscarriage rate is about 6 percent.

>> If you're pushing 40, the miscarriage rate increases to 14 percent.

>> If you're just over 40, your chance of miscarriage is 23 percent.

>> If you're around 43, the rate goes up to nearly 50 percent.

>> After age 45, 87 percent of all women are infertile, so pregnancy is rare, making miscarriage rates more difficult to gather. Also, periods are more irregular, so what appears to be a late period could be a miscarriage.

These statistics reflect the increased number of chromosomally abnormal eggs still left as you get older; your "best eggs" have already been ovulated. We discuss age-related fertility issues more in Chapter 1.

WARNING

You should know, though, that regular cigarette smoking can increase the rate of miscarriage by 30 to 50 percent, so cutting down drastically or stopping smoking is a good idea if you want a successful pregnancy.

Evaluating chromosomes

Today pregnancy tissue from a miscarriage can be tested to see if the loss resulted from a pregnancy with the wrong number of chromosomes. If the pregnancy had the wrong number of chromosomes, then that was a result of a damaged egg and may warrant further investigation. Certainly, if someone has had two miscarriages, it becomes important to test the pregnancy tissue on the second loss to try to determine if the issue is the egg or the uterus. Two losses with normal chromosomes suggest the issue is the uterus.

Testing products of conception

Even though most miscarriages are caused by chromosomal abnormalities, don't expect your doctor to always be able to prove this. This can be so very frustrating, especially if you have had a D&C and the tissue (also called *products of conception* or PCC) has been sent for special testing. The tissue may be sent for analysis, but the cells may not grow (the cells must be viable and divide in the lab in order for the chromosomal testing to be done). Other times, the mother's own cells may overgrow the cells of the placenta, and the chromosomal analysis simply confirms that the mother was normal (46 XX); this is called *maternal contamination.* As has been mentioned, newer testing no longer requires the ability to grow pregnancy cells to test. Furthermore, the mother's blood can be matched to the genes of the pregnancy tissue so that a test that returns the female XX can be identified as either maternal or fetal.

Chromosome testing of the parents

Whereas the vast majority of chromosomally abnormal conceptions are caused by random errors and are non-recurrent, some mistakes are caused by rearrangements in chromosomes that are passed on by the parents. Even if you have the right number of chromosomes (46), two of them, or parts of two of them, may have gotten "stuck" together. Now imagine what happens when you try to make an egg (or a sperm) and put half of your chromosomes into the gamete (remember you only get to contribute half of your chromosomes, and your partner provides the other half). If two of your chromosomes are "stuck" together, instead of contributing 23 chromosomes, you may only be able to contribute 22, or 24. Any pregnancy that occurs will always have the wrong number of chromosomes.

DEALING WITH LOSS WITHOUT BLAME

Are you feeling guilty about your miscarriage because you once sneaked a cigarette, had a glass of champagne at a wedding, had sex, or went skydiving during your pregnancy? Maybe you've been depressed or had an abortion when you were 17. Whatever, now you blame yourself and your careless ways for the miscarriage. Don't. Although some of these actions may not have been the best decisions, the truth is that almost certainly *none* of them caused this miscarriage.

Remember: Most miscarriages are caused by chromosomal abnormalities in the embryo — not by anything the mother did or didn't do!

Your doctor will recommend chromosomal testing, also called *karyotyping*, if you have had two or more miscarriages or if the chromosomal test on one of them revealed a translocation. Chromosomal abnormalities fall into one of several categories:

>> The wrong number of chromosomes — either too many or too few

>> Translocations, or rearrangements, of chromosomes

>> Data added to or subtracted from certain chromosomes

We talk a whole lot more about chromosomes and your genes in Chapter 3.

Navigating an Ectopic Pregnancy

An ectopic pregnancy is a different type of miscarriage. In an *ectopic pregnancy*, the embryo may be developing normally, but it's growing in the wrong place, usually in the fallopian tube. Like a miscarriage, an ectopic pregnancy ends your hopes for a baby *this time*, but it can cause other problems as well.

Ectopic pregnancies aren't rare — 1 out of 100 pregnancies is ectopic — and the percentage has been rising over the last 30 years. With an ectopic pregnancy, the fetus may be normal but attaches to tissue outside the uterus, usually in the fallopian tube, and begins to grow there. The fallopian tube is much smaller than the uterus, and the baby can't grow beyond a certain point, usually around seven weeks, before rupturing the tube, causing severe complications. Ectopic pregnancy is the leading cause of maternal death in the first trimester of pregnancy.

Recognizing the signs of an ectopic pregnancy

WARNING

Any time you have severe one-sided pain, severe shoulder pain, or a feeling of lightheadedness and weakness a few weeks after missing a period, you *must* go to the emergency room to make sure that you don't have an ectopic pregnancy. A positive pregnancy test and an ultrasound showing no fetus in the uterus can suggest an ectopic pregnancy. If you have no physical symptoms, an ectopic pregnancy may be suspected if the beta hCG is lower than it should be; rarely, the pregnancy test can also be negative. An ultrasound will show nothing in the uterus — no sac, placenta, or fetus.

Calling your doctor: NOW

An ectopic pregnancy is a medical emergency that will not resolve without medical treatment. If you have a suspected ectopic, you will have frequent follow-up appointments and be cautioned to contact your doctor with any of the known warning signs. Treating an ectopic pregnancy involves either dissolving the developing pregnancy with a drug called methotrexate, the same drug used for molar pregnancies (see the section "Molar pregnancy," earlier in this chapter), or removing the pregnancy through surgery. Surgical removal of an ectopic pregnancy can also cause more infertility problems; the fallopian tube may need to be removed, and adhesions or scar tissue may develop after the surgery. An ectopic pregnancy can be a life-threatening event. If the fetus gets too big, the fallopian tube will burst, and you could be in danger of bleeding to death.

Nonsurgical treatment

For ectopic pregnancies that meet certain standards, the most common treatment is a medication called methotrexate, which is given as intramuscular injections by trained medical professionals (you will not give this at home). Methotrexate causes the pregnancy to dissolve by stopping the rapid cell division necessary for a fetus to grow. Before you get the medication, you will have blood drawn to check blood levels for your liver function and blood count. Methotrexate is a chemotherapeutic drug that when given in higher doses, has serious side effects. While you will receive very low doses, you will need to be monitored. Four percent of women taking methotrexate have diarrhea, mouth soreness, or stomach irritation because these cells are also fast-growing and affected by the disturbance in cell division. Serious side effects, such as liver toxicity or lung problems, are rare.

WARNING

Stop taking folic acid while on methotrexate because it may interfere with the action of the methotrexate.

Methotrexate successfully dissolves an ectopic pregnancy 90 percent of the time, but it must be used before the fetus grows larger than 3.5 cm (a little over an inch). After that, surgical removal is necessary.

Surgical treatment

If surgery is required, it is generally done laparoscopically (the so-called Band-Aid surgery) in an outpatient setting so that you will most likely go home the same day. In some cases, your doctor may try to save the fallopian tube if possible. If the fallopian tube has to be removed, you can still get pregnant. An egg can even be released from the right ovary and find its way to the left tube if the right tube is gone.

TECHNICAL STUFF

Can the pregnancy be moved somehow from the fallopian tube to the uterus? The plain answer is "no." Because the placenta and the tissues involved with growth are "dug in" to the tube, removing the fetus from the tube and reattaching it to the uterus are impossible at this time.

Understanding why ectopic pregnancies happen

Although anyone can have an ectopic pregnancy, ectopic pregnancies are more likely in women who have any of the following risk factors:

» If you have a swollen, dilated fallopian tube, called a *hydrosalpinx,* you're six to ten times more likely to have an ectopic pregnancy. Hydrosalpinx is frequently caused by pelvic inflammatory disease (PID), often associated with a chlamydia infection. (See Chapter 4 for more on chlamydia.) Even if you have IVF, in which the embryo is placed directly in the uterus, it may migrate back up into the hydrosalpinx and implant there!

» If you smoke, you're one and a half to four times more likely to have an ectopic pregnancy.

» Have you had a previous tubal surgery? You have a 15 percent chance for an ectopic pregnancy. If you've had a prior tubal sterilization reversed, the risk is about 5 to 10 percent (it's less than after surgery for diseased tubes because, in most cases, tubal ligation is performed on healthy tubes, and they should be healthy again after the reconnection).

» Previous use of an IUD slightly increases the chance of an ectopic pregnancy. (If you currently have an IUD and you get pregnant anyway — not likely if you're reading this book, by the way — the risk that the pregnancy is in the tube is about 20 percent.)

» Current use of progestin-only birth control pills also increases the chance of an ectopic pregnancy.

- » If you've had a previous ectopic pregnancy, your chance for another is 20 percent. Your chance of being infertile is about 30 percent.

- » Some older literature suggests that if you douche regularly, at least three times a week, you're more likely to have an ectopic pregnancy.

Other origins of ectopic pregnancies

Most infertility treatments are associated with a higher rate of ectopic pregnancies. In fact, just being a patient in an infertility doctor's office increases your risk of ectopic pregnancy! Twin, triplet, and other multiple pregnancies can be associated with ectopic pregnancies; in some cases, one fetus may implant in the uterus and another in a tube, a condition called a *heterotopic pregnancy*. Heterotopic pregnancies are quite uncommon, but they pose a very real danger. Usually if a pregnancy is found in the uterus, not much further imaging is done to determine whether there is also one in a tube. At an early stage of pregnancy, seeing a pregnancy in the tube is difficult. So many of these pregnancies declare themselves when they rupture, which is a medical emergency. Frequently, the removal or rupture of the tubal heterotopic pregnancy does not cause the intrauterine pregnancy to also miscarry.

Experiencing Recurrent Pregnancy Loss

One to two percent of all couples suffer *recurrent miscarriage (RPL)*, which is the loss of three or more early pregnancies. The American Society for Reproductive Medicine (ASRM) defines RPL as two or more failed clinical pregnancies. A clinical pregnancy is a pregnancy that is seen on ultrasound or by pathology of the pregnancy tissue. Biochemical pregnancies are not considered a clinical pregnancy for this definition. Extremely vexing is the fact that for 50 percent of the people with RPL, no cause will be defined. For people with unexplained RPL, after three losses, the chance of a fourth loss increases to 45 to 50 percent.

Exploring common causes

The risk of a subsequent loss increases with each additional loss. However, the chance for repeat loss can be influenced by the reasons for the RPL if a reason is known. What causes this repeated heartbreak? There are several known reasons:

- » Uterine problems, such as fibroids that intrude into the uterine cavity, scar tissue in the uterine cavity (Asherman's syndrome), or malformations of the uterine cavity shape, can result in a miscarriage Between 15 and 20 percent of recurrent miscarriages are caused by uterine problems. (We discuss this topic in depth in Chapter 7.)

>> Chromosomal abnormalities in either you or your partner cause 5 percent of recurrent miscarriages. Chromosomal karyotyping, performed as a blood test, on you and your partner can be used to diagnose chromosomal abnormalities. (Chapter 3 tells you a lot more about this.)

>> Immune problems, including diseases such as lupus, may be a factor in a miscarriage. Antibodies called antiphospholipid antibodies, which cause clotting problems, and many other possible immune deficiencies are currently a hot topic in fertility workups. (See Chapter 7 for more information about immune issues.)

Answering the question, "Why me?"

One of the hardest parts of pregnancy loss is trying to understand why. Why did this happen to me? In her nursing career, coauthor Lisa had countless patients ask what happened and how they could make it better. Finding out what caused the loss seemed to give some patients comfort, so she always suggested sitting down with the doctor to discuss the loss and what to do next. However, others just needed time to grieve and encouragement to keep trying.

REMEMBER

Pregnancy loss is an issue of biology, not morality. Fertility problems are not a punishment for anything; they're the result of biology gone awry.

Suffering insensitive remarks

What's worse after a miscarriage than friends who become pregnant? Or friends who continue to be pregnant when you're not? How about relatives who try to jolly you out of depression with stories of how miscarriage was probably a blessing and that you should be thankful for the children you have? Or what about women who regale you with stories of their own miscarriages?

REMEMBER

Everyone has her own way of dealing with people who can't be avoided. Some women politely ask that it not be discussed. Other women not so politely ask the offender to please shut up. Yet other women agree and pretend that they're feeling better. Try to remember that people are feeling awkward and don't know what to say, but they're trying to make you feel better because they care about you. Spouses may be having an equally difficult time because few men discuss miscarriage with their friends; if they do, they may find little sympathy for an early loss. They may also feel out of the loop and uninformed about exactly what happened and may not want to question you for fear of upsetting you more. If you can bring yourself to talk about it, a little conversation goes a long way toward making your partner feel more like a partner and less like a hindrance during this difficult time.

Knowing what to do next

As hard as it is to contemplate trying again, your doctor will want to talk with you about taking the next step. Sometimes, it is just a matter of repeating the treatment that got you pregnant in the first place — especially if the POC showed chromosomal abnormalities. However, there may be some additional measures that you can take to get more information and, hopefully, improve your chances of not repeating a loss.

RPL-specific testing

RPL testing is specifically outlined by the American Society of Reproductive Medicine. The testing is based upon known causes of RPL. Remember, even after a thorough evaluation as recommended by ASRM, 50 percent of the time, no known cause will be identified for your pregnancy losses. A starting point is your history to identify possible environmental, occupational, or personal habits that may increase the risk for RPL.

Both partners can have a karyotype done to determine whether one of the partners has a structural problem with one of their chromosomes. Anatomic issues can be evaluated using any one of a number of imaging studies, for example, hysterosalpingogram, saline infused sonogram, 3D ultrasound, MRI, hysteroscopy, or laparoscopy. Hormone testing includes testing for prolactin and thyroid functioning with a TSH level. Antithyroid antibodies are not recommended. Evaluating the metabolic state with a hemoglobin A1c is recommended. Immune testing is a highly controversial area and seems to change frequently. Recommended autoimmune testing includes anti-lupus antibody, anticardiolipin antibody (IgG and IgM) and anti-beta 2 glycoprotein.

Not recommended are circulating NK cell levels. There are newer tests using an endometrial biopsy, but these are considered experimental.

Considering immune therapy

Maybe you've heard that there are some drugs that can actually prevent a miscarriage — is this a miracle or a misperception? ASRM guidelines are clear: "Immunotherapies reviewed in the present document are either not associated with improved live-birth outcome in IVF or have been insufficiently studied to make definitive recommendations." [ASRM 2018] Okay, so not so clear. And not to keep repeating — you need to know the underlying reason for the pregnancy loss to even consider these therapies.

If a person has antiphospholipid antibody syndrome (APS), the recommended treatment is heparin and low-dose aspirin. APS is present if there have been vascular thromboses (clots) or various types of pregnancy problems and abnormal lab values such as lupus anticoagulant antibody or anticardiolipin antibodies. Suffice it to say that this is quite uncommon.

All recommendations emphasize that general use of immunotherapy for RPL is not indicated. However, for some groups the use of these treatments, such as prednisone (a steroid commonly used for serious allergies or asthma) may be useful. Routine use of *Intralipid* (a fat solution) or *IVIg* (intravenous immunoglobin: helpful antibodies isolated from multiple serum samples) are not indicated. Again, there may be RPL patients where these make sense.

Finally, there is no current indication for the use of *adalimumab* (Humira: an anti-inflammatory antibody) in RPL. The best that can be done now is to seek the expert medical advice from one of the very few REIs who specialize in the immunology of RPL.

How is Recurrent Implantation Failure Different?

Recurrent implantation failure (RIF) is a problem that could only exist after IVF was established as a treatment. It is very different from RPL, which occurs after a pregnancy is established. In general, RIF is just what the name implies — no evidence of any embryo implanting — after a number of embryos have been transferred in IVF/FET cycles. Experts disagree about how many embryos need to be transferred before the definition applies, but some suggest that three IVF cycles with the transfer of one or two high-quality embryos per cycle meets the requirement to diagnose a patient with RIF. Recent advances in the ability to test embryos for chromosome number may alter this definition. One reason for RIF is age and the effect that age has on increasing the number of abnormal embryos that are created in older women. However, if the embryos are known to be chromosomally normal, then the emphasis is on the uterus.

The actual number of times RIF occurs is low. Most of the time, no cause can be identified, especially if the embryos have undergone preimplantation genetic testing for *aneuploidy* (abnormal number of chromosomes). Possible causes include anatomic abnormalities of the uterus including fibroids, autoimmune factors, infection of the lining of the uterus, or a shift of the implantation window (the very narrow time frame that an embryo can implant in the uterus). There is also the possibility that genetic factors and the production of certain proteins may be involved. Treatment depends upon the reason for the RIF, but since most cases are undiagnosable, treatment options are limited.

Picking Yourself Up after a Loss

As if you haven't heard it enough, your body needs to heal after a miscarriage. However, also remember that miscarriage is a common event and is a part of reproduction. Women have been having miscarriages for millennia.

Your doctor may recommend waiting up to three months before trying to conceive again. However, a recent study evaluated the risk of another miscarriage in women who conceived in the first month after a miscarriage — without a single intervening period — and found no increase in a second miscarriage as compared to women who waited longer. Therefore, there is no reason to wait longer than one month before trying again. This is especially important if you're over 40. Remember, time is not your friend!

REMEMBER

If you're still bleeding after a miscarriage (or a D&C), your cervix may still be open, and your body is telling you that it is not yet ready for conception. So you probably want to avoid intercourse until the bleeding stops. After that, you should be fine. If you bleed for longer than two weeks after a miscarriage (or a D&C), call your doctor and get an ultrasound. There may be some tissue left behind.

Time truly does heal, or at least dulls the pain. Each passing day will help to make your next pregnancy a joyous experience completely its own, not a shadow of the fear and doubt of your early pregnancy loss.

REMEMBER

Even the most optimistic of you will experience those times when your hope button is stuck on "off." This phase is a temporary, albeit painful, condition. Rebooting your emotions can go a long way toward resetting your physical condition as well.

What to do while you're waiting

TIP

Just like your body needs to repair itself, your spirit needs some help as well. As you count the days until you can begin trying again, consider using this time to help your future child in another way. Here's your to-do list:

>> **If you have already been blessed with a child or children, take a moment to appreciate them.** A hug from your precious one can right many of the world's wrongs.

>> **Allow yourself the time to grieve.** Trying to pretend that you're back to normal when you're not may make you feel temporarily better. In the long run, however, covering up grief rather than expressing it and working through it will cause it to resurface again, possibly during your next pregnancy, in the form of resentment or guilt. Take the time to heal.

>> **Do something wonderful for yourself.** Whether it's a special purchase, a dinner out with your partner, or an ice cream sundae, indulge a whim.

>> **Do consider professional help if your sadness is debilitating or lasts longer than three months.** A counselor can help guide you through the minefield of emotions that you're facing.

REMEMBER

You and your partner are allies, not enemies, no matter how differently you process the stress and grief of your loss. Helping your partner deal with their emotions will help you come to terms with your own feelings as well. This experience can make you a stronger team if you work together.

What not to do

TIP

Taking care of yourself during this time and allowing others to care for you should be your first priority, if not your only one. Part of this task, which may seem daunting enough, is to keep in touch with your own feelings and stay in touch with those who care about you. To help accomplish this, here's our list of things to avoid:

>> **Don't force yourself to do anything that you don't feel up to.** You may need to decline an invitation to a friend's baby shower, christening, or family gathering, and that's okay. This time is about getting better, emotionally and physically. Don't do anything to compromise your recovery.

>> **Don't go into hiding.** You'll want to skip some events, but don't completely isolate yourself. Your community of friends and family can help you heal. Although pain is unavoidable, suffering, particularly alone, is optional.

>> **Don't redecorate the nursery or wander through baby stores.** These types of behaviors are similar to picking at a scab. The temptation to do these things is great, and you can talk yourself into believing that these actions will be cathartic. In actuality, they'll most likely cause you more pain and prolong your healing process.

REMEMBER

An early pregnancy loss does have somewhat of a silver lining. It confirms that you can conceive, which can often be more than half the battle.

4

Moving from No-Tech to High-Tech Conception

Find out your lower-tech options and whether they can work for you.

Discover the ins and outs of in vitro fertilization (IVF).

Understand what you're in for when beginning an IVF treatment.

Get a glimpse at what happens in the IVF lab.

Gain some advice for getting through the treatment process and the two-week wait.

Look at what all the data gathered during your treatment means to you and your fertility.

Chapter **14**

First: The Lower-Tech Options

S tarting a stimulated medication cycle or an *intrauterine insemination* (IUI) cycle is a big step up from just trying to figure out when you're ovulating and planning to have sex accordingly. IUI cycles involve monitoring blood and ultrasound results, and often involve injecting hormone stimulators called gonadotropins.

There are several roads to travel when seeing a fertility doctor, and on which one Dr. Specialist places you depends on the reason for your infertility. (See Chapter 8 for more on how to find the right Dr. Specialist.) If the problem is diagnosed as mild male factor, Dr. Specialist may suggest doing an IUI to give the sperm a "leg up" on getting where they need to be. If you're not producing an egg or not releasing an egg, you may be prescribed stimulating medications to increase egg production. Even if your partner's sperm is fine, you're ovulating, and your tubes have been tested and found to be open, you may still be faced with so-called "unexplained infertility." Many studies have shown that couples with unexplained infertility have substantially higher chances of pregnancy if the woman takes fertility medications and the sperm are placed in the uterus with an IUI.

In this chapter, we explain how stimulated cycles and IUI work and discuss some of the testing involved and the medications you may be taking.

Seeking Personalized Fertility Treatment

The search for the best treatment options begins with making a diagnosis. Thus, the journey usually begins with two parts: first, diagnostic testing to make a diagnosis and then a treatment phase.

Discussing options with your fertility specialist

Exploring options begins with a discussion about the need to begin the fertility journey at all. Many times, this will have taken place with the gynecologist who then recommends consulting a fertility expert. The REI (reproductive endocrinology and infertility specialist) will explain what testing needs to be done and why it is important. The reality is that there are only three things needed to work — sperm, eggs, and structure — so this discussion can be short and to the point. However, once a diagnosis is made, treatment options can be presented with a discussion about what they involve, how successful they are, how long it takes, what the risks are, and finally what it costs.

Deciding what's more likely to work for you

Deciding what will work best for you has many components. At the core are the predictions based upon statistics, but you don't have to be a statistician to understand and use this information. The information comes in two predictions:

>> **The treatment-independent pregnancy rate:** In other words, what is the chance of achieving pregnancy and a healthy baby if you do nothing? This is a very critical prediction because if you are going to do something, you want to make sure it is worth doing. For patients with infertility, this rate may be quite low, but this information exists, and the REI can review it with you.

>> **The treatment-dependent pregnancy rate:** Since some people will get pregnant no matter what they do, it is important to know the success rate if you actually do something.

Once you have these two predictions you can start to consider what it is you really want to do. Deciding what to do is a combination of the information about the success of the options and the social conditions. For example, some women choose not to do IVF because they fear that if it does not work, they have no other option. Some people have a distrust for technology so that making a decision to use the technology of ART (assisted reproductive technologies) is just not possible. Others have religious reasons for making a specific decision.

The point is that most people do not make a decision about what to do based strictly upon the statistics. All decisions involve subconscious, subjective elements. The guiding principle is what you can live with in ten years if you don't get what you had planned. Remember that REIs are people, and they have biases just like you. So just because your REI thinks something is perfect for you does not make it so.

Jump-Starting Your Ovaries

Frequently, physicians will prescribe medications to "jump-start" the ovaries. That may be progesterone for people who don't get periods or oral fertility medications to regulate the cycles. However, the ovaries are always functioning — just not always in a regular, fertile manner.

The ovaries have a fixed number of eggs determined prior to birth. Each month the ovary recruits a large number of eggs out of the resting pool, which for a young woman may be as many as 1,000 eggs per month. Over at least 5½ months, the ovary develops the eggs. The ovary allows only a single egg to survive this developmental stage and actually systematically kills off 999 eggs. But in the last two weeks of this period, the developing egg units must be exposed to FSH, which rescues them. Otherwise they suffer the fate of all eggs and are destroyed. The FSH allows only a few of the remaining egg units to continue to develop. One egg unit takes the developmental lead and becomes a dominant follicle that is eventually ovulated while the other egg units die.

Assuming a woman has eggs, lack of menses or irregular menses are due to the failure of the pituitary to release FSH in a timely, cyclical fashion. So proper release of FSH is the critical element for normal menstrual cycles. The brain decides how much and when to release FSH by measuring estrogen. If the estrogen is low, the brain thinks the egg unit is not developing, and so it increases the release of FSH. If the estrogen is high, the brain thinks the egg unit is developed and reduces the amount of FSH it releases, and when the amount of estrogen reaches a critical level, the brain releases LH causing the ovary to ovulate. Virtually all fertility treatments using fertility drugs are based upon this basic physiology.

"Take two Clomid and call me in three months"

Remember Dr. Basic from Chapter 8? Well, your basic M.D. may have given you a prescription that says "Clomiphene citrate 50 mg qd X 5 days, #10. Refills 3." Or it may simply say "CC 50mg qd d 3-7." What does this mean?

WHAT ABOUT LETROZOLE?

Letrozole use is rising, and it's prescribed much like Clomid, so it's taken the same way. Usually a patient starts with one pill a day (2.5 mg) on Day 3–5 after the start of a menstrual cycle. If you don't get pregnant, or there are other factors, your dose may increase up to 7.5 mg per day. Monitoring and IUI are also possible additions to this treatment. Possible side effects are also like Clomid's and can present as hot flashes, headaches, breast tenderness, fatigue, and leg cramps. Your doctor needs to know about any symptoms you have while on this drug, so be sure to keep them informed.

We note earlier that Clomid can help you release more eggs every month. To get that started, you have to take the pills — but when? Normally, you take Clomid for five days. Some doctors start you on it on day three of your cycle, and others start you on day four or five. The exact timing isn't important; the point is to start it before your ovaries start to develop one dominant follicle.

Usually doctors give you one pill a day the first month or two and then move up to two or three tablets a day if you still don't seem to be ovulating regularly. Clomid comes in 50 milligram tablets, so if your doctor starts you at a higher dose, 100 to 150 milligrams per day, you'll need to take more than one. Sometimes (and if you are using Clomid at a fertility clinic) your doctor will order a blood test after ovulation to check your progesterone level. If you are not pregnant, the result can help adjust your Clomid dose on the next cycle. After you stop taking the pills, you can check for ovulation by using your old friend, the ovulation predictor kit, or your doctor may do ultrasound monitoring. (See "Using an ovulation predictor kit" in Chapter 6.)

TECHNICAL
STUFF

Most pregnancies from Clomid occur in the first three to six months, so if you're not pregnant by that time, your doctor will want to investigate why you're not getting pregnant.

Clomid or letrozole are great drugs for the proper diagnosis. Clomid is approved for certain ovulatory disorders, unexplained infertility when combined with intrauterine insemination, and some forms of mild male factor (yes, some men may benefit from Clomid therapy). These medications work best for those whose ovaries are capable of functioning normally but need a little tune-up.

Using Clomid or letrozole for other causes of infertility will not increase the chance of achieving a pregnancy, and for some problems many physicians feel they may actually decrease the chance for pregnancy.

Comparing Clomid and letrozole

Clomid or *Serophene* (brand names for clomiphene citrate) and *letrozole* (generic for Femara) are two oral medications that reach the same endpoints in your ovary but approach it from opposite directions. The goal is to increase the release of FSH by the pituitary. Both Clomid and letrozole cause the brain to release more FSH. Clomid does this by blocking proteins, called receptors, within cells in the brain that measure estrogen. So, if you block these receptors the brain thinks there is not enough estrogen and it increases the amount of FSH released. Letrozole works by blocking the production of estrogen so that the actual levels of estrogen decrease. But is Clomid better than letrozole? Some evidence suggests that letrozole is slightly better than Clomid for PCOS but not for unexplained infertility. One common misperception is that these medications will help you make a better egg. That is not true. They do not alter the basic structure of the egg, and it is this structure which is critical for a successful pregnancy.

Side effects of oral stimulation meds

Clomid (and letrozole) have a few drawbacks, including the chance for multiple births. Between 5 and 10 percent of all Clomid pregnancies are twins, 1 in 400 is a triplet pregnancy, and 1 pregnancy in 800 results in quadruplets. Obviously, you may be delighted to have a twin pregnancy, but triplets or quads may not be so thrilling. Higher-order multiples (triplets and above) have a very high rate of premature delivery and significantly higher than normal maternal and infant complications. Multiples result from Clomid working too well and stimulating more than one follicle to grow. Some doctors monitor you with ultrasounds while you're on Clomid to be sure that you're not making too many eggs. If you're making a large number of eggs, you may develop ovarian hyperstimulation syndrome, which can cause a very high estradiol level, making hospitalization necessary. If you're on Clomid and feel very ill, with a sudden weight gain, severe bloating in your abdomen, or abdominal pain, call your doctor immediately. This is a rare side effect of Clomid.

Clomid also has some less serious side effects, some annoying, some potentially detrimental to pregnancy. For example:

>> Because your body has been fooled into thinking that it doesn't have enough estrogen, you may have some of the same symptoms women have when they enter menopause and their estrogen drops: hot flashes, headaches, nausea, or blurred vision. Some doctors may give you estrogen to decrease your symptoms.

>> Clomid and letrozole interfere with your production of cervical mucus because it blocks all the estrogen receptors, including those in your cervix, so they don't make mucus in response to rising estrogen levels like they normally do. Clomid and letrozole also cause the lining of the uterus to be thinner than in a normal cycle. Some physicians suggest adding estrogen to the cycle or using

IUI because of the thick cervical mucus. There is no compelling evidence that this makes a difference in the pregnancy rate, so many REIs do not use these additions to the treatment cycle.

Will oral meds work?

So how successful are letrozole and Clomid? It depends upon the diagnosis. For women with PCOS, 80 percent will respond to the Clomid and of those, approximately 50 percent will achieve a pregnancy within the first three cycles. Extending Clomid or letrozole to six months or even a year raises the overall success rates to about 70 percent and by some estimates even more. If there is no male factor, then initially adding intrauterine inseminations (IUI) is not necessary. After multiple failed cycles, many REIs will suggest adding IUI. If the diagnosis is unexplained, then after three cycles of either clomid or letrozole and IUI, approximately 25–30 percent of the couples will be pregnant. Extending the use of Clomid often doesn't improve the success rates, and other treatment options are needed.

Deciding whether to monitor

Many REIs prefer to monitor Clomid/ letrozole cycles with ultrasound and blood studies. Most gynecologists, who frequently prescribe Clomid as a first-line treatment for PCOS or infertility, do not. Which one is right? Well, the snarky answer is the one who got you pregnant. But being more realistic, if you have tried Clomid and it hasn't worked, then referral to an REI and monitoring will probably result in a better chance of conceiving. But for initial treatment, monitoring may not be necessary.

Checking out your eggs

Ultrasound of the ovaries has become a mainstay in the management of treatment. The ultrasound measures the developing egg unit (follicle) because as the egg develops it surrounds itself with fluid. The more mature the egg, the larger the follicle, and experience has demonstrated that when the follicle is > 18 mm the egg is mature enough to be released. So frequently, people will say they are monitoring the egg thinking that black circle on the ultrasound screen is the egg. Eggs are microscopic and can only be seen with a microscope. But more importantly, a mature egg may not be a normal egg. So, following the developing follicle and seeing it increase in size does not say the egg is normal.

Monitoring your hormone levels

Monitoring blood levels of hormones is sometimes done, but the usefulness of extensive monitoring is questionable. Some REIs use both ultrasound and hormone levels of LH, FSH, estradiol, and progesterone to decide when to "trigger" ovulation. Other REIs use a progesterone level obtained 6–7 days after ovulation, either spontaneous ovulation or trigger ovulation, to determine whether the dose of the medication is sufficient. There is no one agreed-upon progesterone level but one source suggests a progesterone of over 15 ng/ml. If the progesterone is low, the dose may be increased. However, once the dose has been determined to be the correct dose for that person, further increases in dosage are generally not helpful, and considering Clomid was originally discovered while looking for an oral contraceptive, for some people the increase is harmful. Once the dose is correct, the strategy is to hang in there and give it sufficient time to work, which may be as much as 6–12 cycles of treatment.

Getting a "trigger" shot

In a normal menstrual cycle, somewhere around midcycle, the egg is mature, and the follicle has reached an optimal size. Two things need to happen. The final stages of development of the egg need to occur and the follicle needs to open and release the egg. Both of these functions are accomplished by a surge in the release of LH. This surge needs to last up to 48 hours to be effective and reach a certain level. If neither of these happen (the surge is either not present or inadequate), then the egg may not complete its maturation or it may not be released. Fortunately, we can help you "push" ovulation.

Injecting hCG to mature your eggs

When the egg is ready, hCG can be used to "trigger" ovulation by injecting a dose of hCG. This has a number of advantages. First, hCG is actually a stronger hormone than LH, so it will adequately complete ovulation. Second, ovulation is set when hCG is used, so, if you are doing IUI, you really only need one! Really? Yes! We know that the approximate time of ovulation is 36-42 hours after hCG.

hCG helps the eggs in the follicles to mature and complete the cell division needed before they can be fertilized. It is made by several companies (Novarel and Pregnyl are two brands) and is usually given intramuscularly; however, a newer laboratory-created hCG called Ovidrel can be given subcutaneously.

It works the same way but comes already prepared with its own syringe so is easier to use. As to whether using a trigger actually results in a better pregnancy rate, the evidence is not compelling. One subtle advantage of hCG is that it lasts a lot longer than LH. The effect of this is to promote progesterone secretion well into the second half of the cycle. A successful pregnancy requires a normal egg and proper follicle development, so extra progesterone in the second half of the cycle may not really be necessary since a properly formed follicle will secrete sufficient progesterone.

Boosting progesterone with an hCG "booster" shot

Progesterone is absolutely required for proper implantation and pregnancy development. It's just how much is necessary that is the issue. Early work suggested that for people using FSH to treat cycles, added progesterone may have increased the pregnancy rate. Progesterone has become standard in IVF and frozen embryo transfer cycles. But for Clomid, maybe not so much. The chances for pregnancy are determined in the first half of the cycle: structurally normal eggs directing a properly constructed and functioning follicle. If that happens, then extra progesterone or a booster of hCG (a second intramuscular injection given after ovulation) to increase the progesterone should not be needed. However, there is little evidence that the booster or extra progesterone is harmful. The choice about using a boost is up to you and your doctor.

Considering Artificial Insemination

Artificial insemination may sound like it's a fake procedure, but it's the real thing. *Artificial insemination* (another term for "insemination," which in today's day and age means *intrauterine insemination* or IUI) means simply that sperm is placed into the uterus to give it a "leg up" on getting where it needs to go, which is to your egg. Eggs are fertilized in the fallopian tube. A normal ejaculate will have > 20 million total motile sperm, but of this number, when having intercourse, only as few as a couple of hundred to a few thousand make it to the tube where the egg needs to be fertilized. So placing sperm beyond the major filter, which is the cervical mucus, tremendously increases the number of sperm in the fallopian tube.

Comparing your options

Two things factor into the choice of either using intercourse (IC) or IUI: the diagnosis for the female, and the presence of male factor. If there is a severe male factor, then neither IC nor IUI hold promise for success, and IVF with ICSI becomes the treatment of choice. Okay, there may be a third factor — money. While many insurance plans cover IUI, there are some that don't, and then you have to factor in the cost of the sperm prep and procedure in making your decision. (More about that later in this chapter.)

Practical considerations

For most people, IC is the more convenient method for achieving a pregnancy. However, some males experience erectile dysfunction and cannot ejaculate when having IC. Some women find IC so painful that they cannot tolerate it. Some couples have schedules that keep them apart when the need to be together to have IC. So there are some practical considerations where IUI is better.

Comparing success rates

The success rates vary depending upon the diagnosis. For PCOS with a normal semen analysis, IUI does not improve the success rate. For mild male factor, IUI does seem to improve the success, but the addition of Clomid to these cycles, which is usually done, may not be necessary. For unexplained infertility, the addition of IUI does seem to make a difference, so the combination of Clomid with IUI is commonly the first treatment of choice in these instances.

Although statistics reported for IUI seem to vary widely, most studies have shown about a 10 percent per month success rate for women under age 35 using clomiphene plus IUI, with decreasing success as your age goes up. Injectable medications produce more follicles per month, and thus, the per-cycle success rate with their use along with IUI is a little higher, about 15 percent for women under 35. Many experts believe that your chance of getting pregnant after three to six failed IUI cycles is slim unless you do in vitro fertilization.

Weighing the costs

When IC will suffice, adding IUI is expensive because it usually adds at least one ultrasound. However, when indicated, the improvement in success rates outweighs the most common other option, which is IVF. Three cycles of Clomid with IUI is usually much cheaper (still not cheap) than one cycle of IVF, and many times the success rates are the same. However, more than three cycles raise the cost, with very little if any improvement in success rates.

Collecting and prepping the sperm

When your partner is directed to produce a semen sample in a cup, you may have a mental picture of a little paper drinking cup. Of course, no clinics use paper cups to collect sperm — at least, we hope they don't. Clinics give the guys a plastic sterile container for this purpose. You may be surprised at how little volume there is to the ejaculate. Most ejaculates have volumes of 1–5 ml (5 milliliters = 1 teaspoon), which doesn't seem like much when you see it in this seemingly large collection cup.

Semen collection and concentration are a big part of IUI. Several methods are used both to collect and to concentrate the sperm:

>> **Clean container collection:** A *sterile* container is used to collect the sample obtained through masturbation. (Your clinic will give you the right container. If you lose it [oh no — but it happens!], please do not use any container you have at home. No pill holders or Tupperware. You can usually buy a sterile urine container at most pharmacies — ask the pharmacist.)

>> **Condom collection:** A special condom containing no lubricants or spermicides is used if the semen sample has to be collected during intercourse. This method is useful for those whose religious beliefs prohibit masturbation. This method is not as good as masturbation, because less of the specimen is collected, plus contact between the semen and the penis inevitably introduces bacteria into the specimen.

>> **Withdrawal:** Other men who cannot masturbate may be able to ejaculate as a result of intercourse and withdraw at the last minute to collect the specimen into a sterile cup. This takes a certain presence of mind! This method is also not as good as masturbation for the same reasons as the condom collection method, but it may actually result in a slightly better collection and a slightly cleaner specimen than the condom method.

REMEMBER

Don't be insulted if the andrologist (the person who deals with sperm) asks whether there was any spillage. This isn't a comment on your general clumsiness or the look of your sample! The first part of the semen has the highest concentration of sperm, so if any was lost, your semen sample may not be as good as it should be.

WARNING

Sperm need to be "washed" before they're ready for IUI. Washing must be done because the unwashed semen specimen contains not only the sperm, but also the seminal plasma. This liquid, which originates in the prostate gland, is designed to protect the sperm from the acidic environment of the vagina. It is alkaline, forms a sticky clump to keep the sperm in the vagina, and contains large amounts of prostaglandins, chemicals that cause smooth muscle contractions. None of these qualities are favorable for a trip directly into the uterine cavity. If a large amount of semen — more than 0.2 ml — is injected unwashed into the uterus, the prostaglandins can cause severe cramping at the least!

Two points about the IUI process: It does not make better sperm, and it does not increase the total number of motile sperm. Sperm are either structurally normal and have normal fertility or they don't. Isolating damaged sperm does not make them better. After the sperm are washed, only the motile sperm are collected, and this can give a false sense that somehow immotile sperm were made to move. Don't be misled if the post-wash specimen has a motility that is significantly higher than the pre-wash specimen. After all, if all you are collecting are motile sperm, then the percent of motile sperm should be high — the total number of sperm, however, will be lower.

Getting the timing right

REMEMBER

Timing is all-important when doing IUI because washed sperm don't seem to live as long as sperm ejaculated into the vagina. At best, washed sperm are thought to live in the woman's reproductive tract 24 hours, while ejaculated sperm can live up to three days normally, and as long as five days in optimal mucus. What this means is that IUI timing has to be well coordinated, with egg release and sperm placement timed so that the short-lived sperm can get to the egg at the right time. This is why you don't always get a choice of appointment dates and times when "it's time."

Considering a few risks of IUI

The main risk of doing IUI is the risk of infection, which is quite low. Estimates of infection rates are usually < 1 percent. Nonetheless, if you had an insemination and you start to feel sick, call your clinic immediately. Symptoms of an infection include lower abdominal pain, sweating, nausea, and a foul-smelling cloudy vaginal discharge. Your doctor will usually ask you to come in for a pelvic exam, check your temperature, and take blood to see if there seems to be an infection. During the pelvic exam, the physician will inspect the cervix with a speculum exam to see if there is any abnormal discharge (pus) coming from the cervix. The physician will then perform a bimanual (internal) vaginal exam and will move the cervix. If this movement causers pain on both sides of the lower abdomen, called *cervical motion tenderness* (CMT) it implies that the tubes are infected. If an infection even remotely seems to be present, most doctors will treat this aggressively with antibiotics. A tubal infection after an IUI can cause tubal damage and add another factor causing infertility. Aggressive, early antibiotic treatment minimizes this risk.

Checking out the Controlled Ovarian Hyperstimulation Option

Clomid or letrozole are usually the first drugs given to start your follicles growing because it can be given orally and has fewer side effects than injections. If they aren't working for you after a few months, your doctor may suggest moving up to the big time: injecting gonadotropins, a technique called *controlled ovarian hyperstimulation,* or COH for short. We talk about gonadotropins in the section "Defining gonadotropins," later in this chapter.

Understanding the need for injections

With COH, the goal varies: If you are not developing a follicle, then COH is used to promote the development of a follicle. For other situations, the pregnancy rate can be increased by increasing the number of eggs released and COH can accomplish this.

Obviously, taking injections is a big step. Not only do you have a possibility of making too many follicles when taking injectable stimulating medications, but you also have to deal with the logistics of COH, including going in for frequent blood tests and ultrasounds and finding someone to give you your injections. A few

clinics may offer to give the injections, usually for a fee, but most want your partner or someone else to come in and learn how to give the shots. Fortunately, with
newer formulations of the gonadotropins, many can be given subcutaneously
(called "subq" or "SQ" for short); it means that the shot is given with a small
needle just under the skin, much like an insulin shot that may be taken by a diabetic.

Getting injections from your partner

Believe it or not, most partners do very well giving injections — after the first few
times, that is. Giving shots is a learning experience, and unfortunately, *you* are the
learning tool in this experience.

Your clinic will probably show you and your partner how to give injections, and it
may send you home with lots of backup, like a CD or written instructions or —
better yet — online videos! You'll refer to these frequently in the first few days.

TIP

If at all possible, insist on doing your first injection in front of someone at your
clinic, so a person skilled in this procedure can critique and give pointers. Also,
after you and your partner have done it once, your partner is less likely to pass out
the first time you do an injection at home.

Giving yourself shots

If you know that you'll be doing your own injections, ask your doctor if he can give
you subcutaneous gonadotropins. These are injected with a very tiny needle —
like a diabetic needle — and can be used in the top of your leg, in your stomach,
or in the back of your arm, although this latter site is a hard place to inject yourself. Subcutaneous gonadotropins are *recombinant* or *purified,* so they can be
injected subcutaneously without causing a rash. The medication your doctor
orders depends primarily on personal preference, since there are no studies prov-
ing the superiority of one medication over another.

TIP

If you end up taking intramuscular injections (called "IM" injections), such as
Repronex, made from human urinary proteins, standing in front of a mirror when
you give them may be helpful. Or ask your clinic if you can inject them into the top
of your leg.

Your doctor may recommend that you take all medication intramuscularly if your
body mass index (BMI) is over 30, so that the medications will be absorbed better.

REMEMBER

Subcutaneous injections can be given anywhere on your body where you can
"pinch an inch" of skin. In intramuscular (IM) injections, the needle should go in
at least one inch. All injections hurt a lot less if you do two things — make sure
the bevel of the needle is face up and inject with a firm and steady darting motion
to get through the top layer of your skin.

TIP

The injection mantra is **swab** (clean the area), **dart** (inject the needle), **push** (the plunger) and **pull** (withdraw the needle). Also, many manufacturers have made it even easier to take these drugs by supplying them in an injector pen that does a lot of the work for you.

Defining gonadotropins

Gonadotropins are stimulating medications, meaning that they make follicles grow. Each follicle contains an egg, so making five follicles each month rather than one or two may give you a better shot at getting pregnant.

Gonadotropins contain either all follicle-stimulating hormone (FSH) or a combination of FSH and luteinizing hormone (LH). Some doctors prefer that you have a little LH because they feel it aids stimulation, while others prefer a pure FSH product. Urinary products are cheaper and some need to be injected intramuscularly, although most of the newer medications are injected subcutaneously.

Some doctors have definite preferences about which type and brand of drug you should take. The reality is that studies that have tried to compare the various medications have consistently failed to demonstrate the superiority of one medication over another.

The advent of IVF has dramatically reduced the use of COH. COH carries a higher risk of high-order multiple pregnancies and ovarian hyperstimulation syndrome (see below). Don't be surprised if your physician discussed both COH and IVF but prefers IVF.

Exploring the side effects

WARNING

Because these drugs are hormones (which stimulate your ovaries to make more hormones), you can expect to be more "hormonal" when taking them. The most common side effects are headache, bloating, weight gain, and mood swings. Obviously, the hormone changes are going to be a big part of making a stressful situation worse for some people.

Deciding which medication to use

All gonadotropins are purified in the laboratory from a raw protein product. This product can be either the urine of menopausal women or the product of a cell culture that has been bio-engineered to make gonadotropins. The cells used for this are Chinese hamster ovary cells that have had the DNA for the gonadotropins injected into them. When the cells grow, they make FSH, LH, or HCG, depending on which DNA is in the cells. The choice between medications depends on several things:

>> With which medication does your doctor feel most comfortable working? If your doctor has a preference, ask him why. He may have done or read studies that have influenced his opinion that one is better than the other.

>> Do you have drug coverage? Which medication will it cover? If your prescription plan covers only one type of injectable, that's probably what you'll get. If you have no drug coverage, you may want to go with what's least expensive.

>> How needlephobic are you? If you're extremely needlephobic, you'll need to go with subcutaneous medications (see the section "Giving yourself shots," earlier in this chapter) or risk being a wreck for two weeks, dreading each shot.

>> Do you have someone to give you your injections? If you'll be doing most of your shots yourself, you'll probably want to do subcutaneous injections.

>> Have you taken one or the other in the past? How did you respond? If you've taken stimulating medications before, you have some kind of track record. Did you do well on that medication? If not, you'll probably want to try something different. If you did well, you may want to do the same, because changing to something else may change your results.

Injecting hCG to Mature Your Eggs

Whether you are using oral medication or injectables to stimulate your ovaries, you may have a final injection to take called hCG to mature your eggs and help them release from their follicles. We talk about this medication more at the beginning of this chapter. The hCG injection will be given exactly the same way if you use Clomid, letrozole, or gonadotropins in your cycle.

REMEMBER

The hCG injection is usually necessary with a gonadotropin cycle. Most of the time, when you take gonadotropins, this affects your ability to release LH at the right time and in quantities sufficient to induce follicle release. For this reason, hCG is given as a substitute LH surge. However, in some cases, LH release does take place. The risk is that your IUI may be timed on the basis of the hCG injection, and if you have already ovulated on your own, the timing will be wrong. Therefore, some fertility clinics ask the patients to monitor their LH surge with a urinary ovulation kit, and others instruct the patients to have intercourse every other day during stimulation "just in case."

WARNING

Don't take nonsteroidal anti-inflammatories such as aspirin, Motrin, or ibuprofen during the middle part of your cycle. They may inhibit prostaglandin production, which may keep you from ovulating.

Ensuring Proper Monitoring throughout Your Cycle

If you're taking stimulating medications of any kind — injectables or Clomid — your clinic may want to monitor you to make sure that you're not making too many eggs. Some centers will cancel your IUI or insist that you do in vitro fertilization if you're making a lot of eggs because the risk of hyperstimulation and getting pregnant with triplets — or more — is increased.

WARNING

Ovarian hyperstimulation syndrome (OHSS) is a serious complication that can land you in the hospital. It starts when you take injectable stimulating medications and make a lot of follicles. If your estradiol rises over 1500, OHSS may occur; it's more common with IVF but can also occur with IUI cycles. Some symptoms of OHSS are the following:

>> Difficulty urinating

>> Difficulty breathing

>> Sudden weight gain of ten pounds or more

If you have OHSS, your clinic may want to monitor your blood count, liver function, weight, and urine output. OHSS may not resolve itself for several weeks, and symptoms may worsen if you're pregnant.

REMEMBER

OHSS isn't the only complication of taking gonadotropins or Clomid; multiple pregnancies of five or more babies are usually the result of stimulating medications. Albeit rare (there's a reason why they make the evening news!), these high-order multiples are more often the result of COH than IVF because IVF can control the number of embryos put back into the uterus, whereas COH can't. The number of follicles you have is the number of babies you could end up with!

Deciding When to Pursue Higher-Tech Options

Because statistics vary so much on how many cycles get you to a pregnancy, it can be difficult to know when to say "enough." You may also notice that every doctor has a different take on your odds for success. Although most doctors quote you numbers that reflect their *own* success with any given process, they may also alter them a bit to better reflect your age or your response to treatment so far.

Many doctors have you try a particular method three times and then move on to something else if that approach doesn't work. Others point out that if a particular protocol hasn't worked by (for example) the fourth try, the odds of success are greatly diminished.

But, regardless of whether you're on IUI #1, 4, or 40 (which rarely happens anymore), after a while, it *all* becomes a bit too much.

Growing sick of getting stuck

Perhaps you grew sick of waiting when the first home pregnancy test read negative. But even if you're more patient, what if a month, or two or three, of nightly injections of hormones is just about all you can handle?

First off, be assured that your impatience and irritability aren't a reflection of your winning personality, but more likely the side effects of the drugs you're taking. Most women find that acknowledging that their moods or mood swings are largely chemical in nature does lessen the burden. If you haven't confided in a friend about your fertility struggles, perhaps now is as good a time as any. You'll find that friends or relatives in the know will treat you with kid gloves right about the time that you're ready to pull out the boxing gloves.

REMEMBER

Another thing to remember is the numbers game that is human reproduction. One of our favorite stories is that of a professional basketball player who smiled and clapped every time he missed a free throw. When asked about this odd behavior, he responded, "With every miss, I'm one shot closer to success." Consider *your* shots the same way.

Being sensitive to your partner's feelings

Just as you may find the fertility rituals to be all-consuming, your partner may be sharing your views, more than you know. The partner being treated may feel that he or she is undergoing the lion's share of discomfort and disappointment. But remember, even if your partner isn't experiencing every needle stick or test result, that person is watching you go through it. "Big deal!" you scoff. Well, it can be. Watching another person experience pain or sadness can be as difficult as going through it yourself. The silent partner also must suffer with feelings of inadequacy and powerlessness in being unable to relieve your discomfort. Partners of terminally ill patients often need their own support networks as well. And, studies show, fertility patients, due to the sometimes-long nature of their treatment, share some of the same issues faced by the chronically and terminally ill.

TIP

Encourage your partner to share their feelings with friends, family, or a professional. Although you may feel as though you're losing your sanity, your partner may feel as though they're losing you.

Chapter **15**

Going High-Tech: Welcome to the In Vitro Fertilization (IVF) Club

I n vitro fertilization (IVF) and the other *assisted reproductive technologies* (ARTs) represent the top of the high-tech mountain of infertility treatments, so naturally, you may be a bit nervous about moving into an invasive, expensive, no-guarantees treatment. Everyone knows it's a club you do not want to belong to. The good news is that high-tech fertility has come a long way and is no longer a shot in the dark. Pregnancy rates can approach or even exceed 50 percent per attempt in good prognosis situations, and even if you are not under 35, IVF still represents your best chance for fertility even if all simple treatments have already failed. So being an IVF club member is not necessarily a bad thing!

The term *in vitro fertilization* means fertilization (the joining of egg and sperm) that occurs in the laboratory; that's where the term "test tube baby" comes from. Before you get to the fertilization point, you have to develop eggs in the ovaries with the help of stimulating medications called gonadotropins and retrieve them from the follicles they grow in during an egg retrieval procedure.

Twenty years ago only a handful of clinics performed IVF. Now more than 400 clinics offer this service in the United States and Canada, never mind the hundreds of clinics around the world, and IVF has become a big (and lucrative) business. In the early days of IVF, a pregnancy rate of 5–7 percent was considered great, and if a center did three to five cycles a month, it was busy. Now success rates for some patients are over 60–70 percent, and centers report on hundreds of cycles per month. At last count (2018) it was estimated that over 6 million children had been born worldwide from IVF, and in the United States 1–2 percent of all deliveries were from children conceived through ART.

In this chapter, we help you evaluate different IVF clinics, decipher the confusing statistics about IVF success rates, and give you some help in deciding whether IVF is the next step for you.

What IVF Means for You

For those of you who just basically need to know when to show up at the clinic, here's the scoop on IVF:

>> IVF is expensive.

>> IVF is time consuming.

>> IVF is unpredictable.

>> IVF does not guarantee success.

>> IVF involves injections.

>> IVF requires frequent ultrasounds and blood work.

>> IVF can be frustrating; you will scream at the IVF nurses at least once during your treatment.

>> IVF can make your whole life stressful; you will scream at your partner at least once, and then *he'll* scream at the IVF nurses.

Sounds very discouraging. If there ever was a time to keep your eye on the ball, it is when you go through IVF — the goal is to resolve your issues about fertility. While not everyone will achieve a successful pregnancy, the overall story is encouraging. For couples willing to use multiple cycles of IVF, over 85 percent of women under the age of 35 will achieve a successful pregnancy and 40–50 percent of women 35 and older will achieve a pregnancy. Obviously, age is a critical factor for the success of IVF. IVF can help women discover what their true age-related fertility is by evaluating the outcome of IVF. A 44-year-old female who has done cycles of IVF and tested the embryos for chromosome number may find that her eggs have never made a normal embryo. That knowledge may help her deicide to pursue other avenues, such as donor eggs.

REMEMBER

Perhaps the most intimidating part of IVF is the notion that you're at the end of the technologic line, the top of the fertility treatment mountain in your quest for a biological baby. While part of you may feel enormous excitement anticipating that you've finally found the magic path, the other part may fear what will happen if IVF doesn't work. If it fails, you may find yourself going back to less-technological methods, or you may move forward to other means of creating a family, such as donor eggs or adoption. Think of IVF as a beginning and taking you one step closer to your dream, however it may be attained.

Getting real about what it costs and the chances for success

Although IVF gets a large share of publicity when it comes to infertility, the fact is that only about 2 percent of infertile couples actually end up doing IVF. In 2003, when the first edition of the book was written, approximately 122,000 IVF cycles were done in the United States. In 2017, there were 255,968 cycles of IVF done in the United States. Worldwide in 2015 over 800,000 IVF cycle were performed resulting in the birth of 157,449 children. By 2018 over 8 million IVF cycles had been done since that first birth over 40 years ago. Because the techniques used and the ethical issues are still considered cutting edge, media coverage of IVF far exceeds that of, say, intrauterine insemination. So, it may seem that way more people are doing in vitro than really are.

Publicity for every celebrity IVF baby may also make it seem like IVF is a surefire success method, but of course, media coverage is almost always oversimplified. However, the national statistics for live births per initiated IVF cycle are about 35 percent — and that's for women under age 35. The national statistics break down this way (SART data 2017):

>> **Under age 35:** A 46.8 percent chance of a live birth per IVF cycle

>> **Ages 35 to 37:** Approximately 34.4 percent chance of a live birth per IVF cycle

>> **Ages 38 to 40:** A 21.0 percent chance of a live birth per cycle

>> **Ages 41 to 42:** A 10.1 percent chance of a live birth per cycle

Ages 43 to 44: A 3.1 percent chance of a live birth per cycle

>> **Over age 45:** Virtually no chance of pregnancy unless you use donor eggs

TIP

If you want to see all the national statistics for ART, check out the following website: www.sart.org/.

The cost of one IVF cycle can vary from about $8,000 to over $20,000 including medicine and ancillary procedures such as genetic testing of the embryos. It generally includes monitoring, which means ultrasound tests; egg retrieval; embryo culture; and embryo transfer. Most centers charge extra for additional laboratory procedures, like intracytoplasmic sperm injection (ICSI). Of course, these items may not be covered by insurance. We talk more about insurance coverage and covering the costs of IVF later in this chapter.

Looking at the preceding success rates, you can see that it may well take two or more cycles to get pregnant with IVF, and the cost equals or exceeds a new car. Plus, you have no guarantees of success. The cost of IVF can limit a person's chance of ever resolving their fertility issues. The chance for success may drive people to spend all of their resources on a quest for which there is no happy ending. It is important for people embarking upon IVF to set a limit and then stick to that limit. Remember, keep your eye on the goal: resolution of fertility-related issues.

Looking at the risks of IVF

Although IVF has become a familiar and accepted way of dealing with infertility, it's not entirely without risk. Some risks are well established, and others are not as clear-cut. Before you decide to move on to IVF, consider these factors.

REMEMBER

There are also risks for a woman related to the egg retrieval process. These include the risk of anesthesia, bleeding, and infection. Usually, antibiotics are used to reduce the risk of infection. Internal bleeding is possible but rare. The anesthesia used is IV sedation, which has a very low chance for risk such as an allergic reaction to the medications. However, one area of rising concern relates to the fact that patients weigh more now than they used to. Increased weight adds the risk for breathing difficulties during IVF. Overall, the risk of any serious complication for IVF is <1 percent — reassuring but definitely not zero.

High rate of twins or triplets

Traditionally, the best documented risk of doing IVF was the high rate of twins or triplets. Because more than one embryo, usually two to four, was placed into the uterus at one time, the risk of getting pregnant with more than one baby was high. In the normal population, twins occur a little over 1 percent of the time, or about 1 in 90 births in the United States.

Previously, about 25 percent of IVF births were twins! You may see this as an advantage — two for the price of one — but almost every risk for mothers and babies is increased for twin or triplet pregnancies. No parent would want to purposely put their child at risk. The risk has changed dramatically since the success of IVF has increased. The reason so many embryos were transferred in the past is that the chance of any one embryo making a baby was a low as 5 percent. Today, for embryos that have been tested and are known to have the correct number of chromosomes, pregnancy rates for each embryo are near 50 percent, and in some centers have been higher.

Because the problem with multiple pregnancies was so significant, ASRM established guidelines about how many embryos to transfer. The goal was to reach the ability to transfer a single embryo (commonly written as SET — single embryo transfer) and still have a good chance of success. If the embryo is known to have the correct number of chromosomes, ASRM suggests that only one embryo should be transferred regardless of the woman's age. If the embryo has not been tested, then both age and other factors are considered. For women 37 and under with favorable conditions transferring a blastocyst embryo, the recommendation is to transfer only one. For favorable conditions and a woman 38–40, two or fewer is the recommendation, and for a woman 41 or 42, the recommendation is to transfer three or fewer embryos. For cycles that are less favorable, the recommendation is to transfer two or fewer for women 37 and under and three or more for women over the age of 37.

WARNING

About one-half of twins are born prematurely (before 35 weeks gestation) or with a low birth weight. Up to half have a lower than expected birth weight, compared to 10 percent of single babies. One-half or more of twins are delivered by cesarean section, as compared to about 30 percent of the normal population. (Of course, for reasons that are not clear, the cesarean section rate after IVF, even for singletons, is substantially increased. It may be that after all that work getting pregnant, more women are likely to simply schedule their delivery and accept the cesarean as part of the deal.) Mothers of twins are twice as likely to have preeclampsia (high blood pressure and fluid retention, factors that can lead to preterm delivery and in extreme cases can cause maternal seizures).

WARNING

Neonatal deaths are rare these days. Nevertheless, premature infants in general are three to six times more likely than full-term infants to die in the first year of life. Premature babies also have a higher risk of vision problems, cerebral palsy, and learning difficulties. And you thought that getting pregnant was the only thing you had to worry about!

Ovarian hyperstimulation syndrome

Previously, *ovarian hyperstimulation syndrome* (OHSS) occurred in 1 to 5 percent of all stimulated cycles in which gonadotropins, medications that stimulate growth of follicles, were taken. Today, newer methods for doing IVF have significantly reduced the risk of persistent serious OHSS. OHSS is different from controlled ovarian stimulation (COH). Everyone who takes any fertility-enhancing medication that causes more than one egg to develop has COH. OHSS occurs after the ovary is exposed to the pregnancy hormone hCG or LH. IVF uses hCG when the eggs are mature because hCG is required for the egg to complete the last stages of maturation and to allow for the successful retrieval of eggs. If hCG is never given, the cycle is aborted, but OHSS does not occur.

Unfortunately, some people will have gone through almost the entire cycle and yet not have a retrieval due to the risk of severe OHSS. However, once hCG is given and an egg retrieval is done, there is no going back. At that point, OHSS can generally be managed with fluids and pain control, but in extreme cases can cause serious maternal illness, including blood clots and pulmonary emboli. Your doctor will monitor you for the development of this serious complication, whether you are doing COH for IUI or for IVF. When the risk of OHSS is high, pregnancy is intentionally avoided by freezing all of the embryos and allowing the ovaries to return to normal size before trying the embryo transfer. Surprisingly, the pregnancy rate is higher for the cycles using the frozen embryos.

More recently, it was discovered that the use of a long-acting GnRH agonist (Lupron) could reduce or eliminate the need for the hCG shot. By using Lupron as a "trigger" and freezing all embryos, the risk of OHSS has been reduced even further, and if it occurs, it is usually less severe. Also, the use of a medication that had previously been given for women with high prolactin levels seems to reduce OHSS. Finally, if a significant amount of fluid builds up in the abdomen, that fluid can easily be removed. OHSS causes the blood system to become "leaky," and fluid accumulates. Your circulation is affected by your blood becoming concentrated. This increases the risk of clotting issues, but many times medication can be used to reduce the risk of clotting and subsequent pulmonary embolism or stroke. If you have OHSS, keep in touch with the doctor's office. Serious complications have been reported after severe OHSS, including stroke.

Birth defects

An increase in the rate of birth defects is a controversial and as yet unproven possibility in IVF. Some studies show an increase in birth defects in IVF pregnancies, while other studies don't support this claim. This may be because babies born after IVF tend to be scrutinized more than the general population. It's also not clear whether an increase in birth defects is associated with IVF or simply with infertility. Much more research will undoubtedly be done in this area as IVF children become older.

WARNING

It's logical to expect that men who need to do ICSI for male factor issues may pass the gene responsible to their sons, who will most likely also need to do ICSI (or whatever the equivalent technique is) 20 or 30 years from now.

Switching Doctors: Will a Change Really Matter?

The clinic you've been going to for IUI or monitoring may also perform IVF. And if you're comfortable with the staff and the doctors, know the routine, and have all your insurance coverage set up there, you may decide to stay with that clinic.

REMEMBER

You should, however, think about it and do some reading before deciding to stay with your current center. More than 400 U.S. clinics do IVF, and they range from little more than the "weekend dabbler" that does maybe 30 to 40 egg retrievals a year to the megacenters that do more than 1,000 or even 3,000 egg retrievals a year.

Bigger isn't always better, but when it comes to high-tech procedures such as IVF, success rates are highly dependent on the quality of the IVF lab. It stands to reason that a small center doing 30 or 40 retrievals a year may not have the same lab setup as a center doing 1,000 a year. (This is why many small centers actually use a lab that is associated with a large IVF center. You need to ask and find out what the individual setup is.)

TIP

You can evaluate centers by

>> **Comparing their statistics and what they offer via the Society of Assisted Reproductive Technology (SART).** SART is the professional society for doctors and clinics performing IVF. At the very least, you should be sure that the center with which you work belongs to SART. A condition of membership is that every center sends all of their IVF data to a central organization, which compiles and publishes them. Since member clinics also voluntarily agree to have their data audited periodically, SART is, in effect, the statistic watchdog of IVF. We describe in detail what it monitors and how the statistics are compiled in the section "Sorting through SART statistics," later in this chapter.

>> **Talking to patients who are currently doing IVF there and to your doctor or the nurses.** Sometimes the nurses are more candid about whether you should stay or move on, especially if they've gotten to know you, like you, and want what's best for you. If the nurse slips you a little note about another clinic a few towns away, pay attention!

Choosing the Best Clinic for You

Sometimes the decision to move on to another clinic is easily made. For example, if your current clinic doesn't take your insurance, you don't like the staff, or its hours aren't convenient for the more intensive monitoring of IVF, you know you need to switch doctors. Or maybe you need or want specialized treatment that your present clinic doesn't do, such as sex selection, preimplantation genetic diagnosis (PGD), or sperm aspiration. Luckily for you, Dr. Magic most likely has a website, a good place to start looking for your IVF doctor.

Surfing IVF websites

Most medium to large IVF clinics have an extensive website, and even the smaller centers have an online presence so you should check them out to learn what you can "from their perspective." At the very least, the website should tell you the following information:

>> How many egg retrievals the clinic does in a year

>> How many embryo transfers the clinic does in a year

>> Pregnancy rates for all age groups, broken down per egg retrieval and per embryo transfer

>> Whether it freezes embryos

>> Whether it does ICSI

>> Whether it transfers three-day embryos or blastocysts (see Chapter 12)

>> How many doctors do IVF

>> The educational level of the doctors and whether the doctors are reproductive endocrinologists

>> Whether the clinic has a donor egg or embryo program

TIP

You may have other concerns pertaining to your own situation. If you can't find the answer on the website, you may be able to call the center and ask to speak to a patient representative or even an IVF nurse. Usually they're happy to answer any questions you have about their program, and you won't feel as committed as you might after talking to a doctor. (You don't have to give your real name, either!)

Sorting through SART statistics

The Society of Assisted Reproductive Technology (SART) is an organization affiliated with ASRM (American Society of Reproductive Medicine), the organization for healthcare professionals involved with reproductive medicine. SART's members are the approximately 430 IVF clinics in the United States that submit the following information to SART for publication each year:

>> The number of cycles they do

>> The types of infertility their patients have

>> The outcome of their cycles

>> Pregnancy rates

>> Multiple pregnancy rates

>> Miscarriage rates

>> Cancellation rates

In short, the clinics provide information on just about anything and everything concerning their patients' IVF cycles.

SART takes the information and compiles a booklet of information about every one of the 437 clinics and distributes it to its members; it also publishes the data on *its* website. SART data is also found with other data from the Centers for Disease Control and Prevention (CDC).

Clinics that are members of SART can be audited and their data checked for accuracy. The amount of information required by SART is astounding: Your age, Social Security number, infertility type, and type of cycle are reported to SART for every IVF cycle that you do.

SART confirms clinic-reported data by visiting a number of clinics each year and auditing selected patients' charts to make sure that the submitted information is accurate.

REMEMBER

Individual clinic statistics presented on their websites can be difficult to read because not all clinics report their numbers in the same way. For example, one clinic may report pregnancy rates per retrieval, and another may report per transfer. One advantage of the SART data is that it does allow you to compare apples to apples. But remember that statistics don't tell the whole story. For example, SART statistics don't tell you anything about the clinic population except for its breakdown by age. A center dealing with only the crème de la crème of patients, the place everyone else calls the "Mecca," certainly has higher pregnancy rates than the center that treats everyone, including patients rejected at the Mecca. Further, some clinics have chosen to bypass SART and report their statistics directly to the CDC. This does not mean that they are "bad" clinics by any means — they have just chosen a different route to get required information to the public.

Looking for a clinic

Although SART statistics make interesting reading and may help you decide which clinic to use, they don't tell the whole story. You also need to check into the following information:

>> The clinics that are nearest to you. Long-distance IVF is possible but complicated.

>> The clinics that are accepting new patients.

>> How much clinics charge if you don't have insurance.

>> Whether the clinics take insurance — not all do!

>> Whether the clinics treat patients like you, an important consideration if you're over age 40 or have been turned down by another clinic.

>> The kind of feeling you get from the clinic. For the answer to this question, you'll probably need to make a consultation appointment with a doctor. The clinic usually charges for this appointment. However, compared with all of the other costs associated with fertility treatment, the cost of the initial consultation is a relative bargain! Before deciding on the clinic with which you are going to work, you should seriously consider visiting two or three that you've picked out. You will find that this is a worthwhile investment of time and money.

REMEMBER

You don't need to commit to a program at your initial consultation. It never hurts to go home and think everything over before you go any further. Remember, also, that if you're at one of the big-name clinics, you're also being sized up as a candidate for its program, and you could be turned down for treatment if you don't fit the clinic's criteria. Some centers don't want to give you false hope if they don't believe that they can help you.

TIP

Whether you need or want to know everything about a clinic before you go there depends on your personality. You may be happy to go wherever it was that your best friend went, or to go where your insurance tells you to go, or to go to the clinic around the corner. There's nothing wrong with trusting your instincts and other people's personal experiences.

Evaluating a clinic's personality

IVF clinics have personalities just like people do, and just as with individuals, you may find your personality is a better fit at some clinics than at others. Usually, but not always, the head honcho or main doctor at the clinic sets the tone for the whole office. Sometimes instead of one main doctor, a clinic has a team of fairly equal doctors, all of whom leave their impression on the way the clinic functions.

Whether you seek out the "razzle-dazzle" office that is selective and expensive, or the "neighborhood go-to" because it's close to you and where your friends went, you need to consider whether any office is a good fit for you. If the environment makes you feel good, the doctor and staff confidently answer your questions, they have good references, and their success statistics measure up, go for it! You're like Goldilocks and have found the "just right" office.

Addressing the High Costs of IVF

Why on earth does IVF cost so much? Although supply and demand may have a bearing on costs — in other words, doctors respond to market pressures — the fact is that IVF costs are high because IVF is a high-tech procedure and high tech costs money. An IVF lab costs over a million dollars to set up, and you will see lots of employees — doctor(s), nurses, lab personnel, ultrasound techs — when you go for your consultation. This makes IVF a very hands-on, time-intense process — for you and for your medical team.

Fortunately, as fertility procedures become more routine, many insurance plans cover the costs. In the next sections, we help you get every penny out of your insurance company to which you're entitled to help pay for your IVF cycle.

Figuring out what your insurance plan really covers

Even if you have insurance coverage, you may be amazed to see that you may still be responsible for some (or most) of the IVF bill. Some insurance plans cover only monitoring, meaning the frequent blood draws and ultrasounds. Because these can run well over $2,000 per cycle, this coverage is a help. Other plans cover only the medications, which (again) is a help, but not by any means relief from the total cost. In 2010, the Patient Protection and Affordable Care Act (ACA) was enacted to help provide insurance coverage for what were deemed "essential health benefits." While many hoped this was a boon to infertility patients (because who wouldn't see infertility as "essential?"), the industry soon learned that it was up to each state to determine what was essential. The bottom line is that there is no federal law that requires insurance plans to cover the cost of infertility treatment.

REMEMBER

In some cases, it's not easy to decipher your insurance plan. Check out your plan *before* you start treatment. Some plans may cover only diagnostic testing or only certain parts of fertility treatment. Even if you live in a state with mandated coverage, your particular employer plan or insurance carrier may still be outside the mandated coverage such as employer plans that are self-funded or plans that cover less than the required number of employees. Finding out you're not covered at the pharmacy you usually use the night before your cycle is supposed to begin isn't a good way to start treatment.

The best way to start finding out what applies to you is by reading your policy (okay — not so easy!) If you need more help, go to your employer's human resources department or call the insurer's customer service number. Bonus: Some fertility clinics have patient navigators that will help you with this task!

TIP

Many insurance companies require preauthorization even if you do have coverage — and we mean *require!* Preauthorization can take more time than you think to complete (including providing previous medical records), so don't leave this step until the last minute!

You may be covered only if you go to an "approved" clinic. But what if you don't want to go to this clinic? Maybe it doesn't offer treatments you want or it doesn't have high success rates. In that case, you'll be forced to make an unpleasant choice: Will you go for care that costs you less but may not succeed, or will you pay more for a higher chance of success? These decisions would have had even King Solomon, the master of wise decisions in the Old Testament, in a quandary.

Changing jobs or changing insurance to get infertility coverage

People have been known to change jobs to get better insurance, or to drop insurance at their place of employment and pick up coverage under their spouse's policy, even if it costs more per month. Lisa has seen patients pursue both of these options (and others) to cover the high cost of IVF cycles. It can work, but you have to do your homework before you make the leap.

INSURANCE 101: THE DIFFERENCES BETWEEN TYPES OF INSURANCE

You may be confused over whether your insurance is public or private, group or individual. Public insurance is paid for, at least in part, by the government. Medicaid, for those on public assistance; Medicare, for those over age 62 or disabled in some way; and CHAMPUS, for military families, are public insurances. Private insurances are paid for by you, either directly or indirectly. If your employer pays the costs for you as part of a benefits package, you have group insurance. If you pay the entire cost yourself, you have an individual policy, which is usually quite expensive.

>> You may be able to choose a different employer-offered plan where you currently work. Some companies offer a choice of plans — even if it costs you a bit more money. Maybe that HMO plan you didn't want when you signed up last year is more attractive because it covers IVF even if you have to switch primary care providers to get it.

>> Switching to your partner's insurance (if you are eligible) may also work. Some plans allow a spouse or partner to pay for coverage that may come out to less than the IVF bill.

>> Taking a lesser-paying job to cover IVF costs? If the drop in pay isn't too much, it may be worth it. Three or four IVF cycles can certainly cost you more than $40,000 over a year or so.

>> You may even consider adding a part-time job as another way to gain insurance coverage. Some companies offer insurance to part-timers (20 or more hours a week).

WARNING

Don't cancel old policies before you are sure of your new policy's coverage limits. Any change in policy may also mean you have to observe a waiting period before the coverage kicks in (which means you will not be able to start your IVF cycle as soon as you want) and you may have alterations in which providers you can see.

REMEMBER

Some companies allow you to change insurance only at certain times of the year; this is usually called *open enrollment*. Check out your choices ahead of time so that you can have your insurance in place before you need to start using it.

It's the Law! States That Mandate Fertility Coverage

There is no federal law that compels insurance coverage for infertility treatment. It is all left up to the states. Furthermore, in many states that do have mandates, the law targets the employer — not the insurance company. So, the benefit accrues to the patient only if the employer meets the mandate's requirements. The employer then must find insurance companies and a plan within that company that provides the required coverage. So, changing insurance companies may not help if the employer is not caught under a state mandate.

Today, 16 states mandate some sort of reimbursement for in vitro fertilization. No consensus exists between states on how coverage should be applied or who has to offer it. This coverage is still a mixed bag for the average patient; even if your state mandates insurance coverage, your employer may be exempt from offering coverage if he meets certain requirements such as:

>> The employer is self-insured (so does not have to follow the state law mandate).

>> There are fewer total employees than the number that triggers mandated coverage, which is usually 25 or 50.

>> The policy is written in another state that does not have a mandate.

REMEMBER

State mandates affect the states where your employer/corporation reside — or, where the insurance plan originates. So, even if you are a sales representative living in a covered state, if your employer is based out of a noncovered state, your insurance may reflect the laws of your employer's domicile (state), not yours. The opposite applies as well. You may live/work in a state that is not mandated but your company headquarters are in a state that is. (For example, you live in Delaware, but your company's headquarters are in Virginia.) Don't just assume. That's what human resource departments are for — to help you determine what is covered.

States that currently have some infertility coverage mandates are Arkansas, California, Connecticut, Delaware, Hawaii, Illinois, Louisiana, Maryland, Massachusetts, Montana, New Jersey, New York, Ohio, Rhode Island, Texas, Utah, and West Virginia.

TIP

While 16 states are listed, more consider coverage for many health benefits every year. You can check on whether your state is considering infertility coverage by going to their government website and querying "pending bills" and "fertility," for example.

Here are more details on state insurance mandate requirements as of this writing:

>> **Arkansas:** Requires coverage for infertility if maternity benefits are offered, including IVF and cryopreservation, up to a lifetime cap of $15,000; HMOs and self-insured employers are exempt.

>> **California:** Employers must make available a policy covering infertility treatment, excluding IVF but covering gamete intrafallopian transfer (GIFT), a type of IVF in which the egg and sperm are placed in the fallopian tube before fertilization takes place. This avoids the religious/ethical difficulty of having embryos in the lab, but adds a laparoscopy to the mix, which adds cost and invasiveness to the procedure; religious organizations and self-insured employers are exempt.

>> **Connecticut:** Must offer a policy covering infertility, including IVF; lifetime maximums apply on number of cycles (for example, two IVF cycles); religious organizations and self-insured employers are exempt.

>> **Delaware:** Comprehensive coverage is required for up to six egg retrievals per lifetime (but there are age limits); experimental services are prohibited; religious organizations and self-insured employers are exempt.

>> **Hawaii:** Requires individual and group insurers to cover infertility, including one cycle of IVF; spouse's sperm must be used to fertilize eggs; self-insured employers are exempt.

>> **Illinois:** Requires coverage of diagnosis and treatment of up to four IVF cycles (two more allowed after a live birth). Employers with fewer than 25 employees, religion-affiliated organizations, and businesses that follow federal guidelines for benefits (ERISA) are exempt.

>> **Louisiana:** This one is a little different. It prevents excluding coverage for a correctable medical condition solely because it results in infertility; self-insured employers are exempt.

>> **Maryland:** Requires coverage for IVF after certain conditions are met up to three IVF cycles per live birth and $100,000 lifetime maximum; companies with fewer than 50 employees, self-insured employers, and religious organizations are exempt.

>> **Massachusetts:** Requires comprehensive coverage without any exclusions on treatment or lifetime caps; self-insured employers are exempt.

>> **Montana:** Requires HMOs to cover infertility services as part of basic health services; self-insured employers are exempt.

>> **New Jersey:** Requires coverage, including up to four cycles of IVF (with an age cut-off); employers with less than 50 employees, employers who are self-insured, and religious organizations are exempt.

>> **New York:** Requires coverage of diagnosis and treatment as part of a correctable medical condition in group policies (usually 100 or more employees) but not individual or small policies; maximum of three IVF cycles; exempts self-insured employers.

>> **Ohio:** Requires HMOs to cover infertility when it is medically necessary under "basic healthcare services." This may include IVF, but it is not required; self-insured employers are exempt.

>> **Rhode Island:** Requires comprehensive coverage if an insurer or HMO provides pregnancy benefits but allows a 20 percent co-pay; $100,000 maximum; self-insured employers are exempt.

>> **Texas:** Requires group insurers to offer coverage for IVF only but does not require an employer to pay for it; religious organizations and self-insured employers are exempt.

>> **West Virginia:** Requires HMOs to cover infertility under "basic health services"; self-insured employers are exempt.

REMEMBER

Many of the state laws set a definition of infertility that you must meet before any coverage is triggered. This is generally a time frame for unprotected intercourse, or, perhaps, a list of certain conditions that lead to infertility. After you get past what is and isn't covered, in some states, you still may not get your insurance plan to pay for infertility treatments if

>> The company you work for has fewer than a certain number of employees — usually 25 or 50.

>> The company doesn't cover maternity care.

>> You haven't done at least several cycles of intrauterine insemination (IUI) before moving to IVF.

>> You've had a vasectomy or tubal ligation.

>> You're over a certain age.

>> You haven't had the required number of years of documented infertility.

TIP

If you are still unsure of your state's policy, you can always contact your local RESOLVE chapter (www.resolve.org) to find the information for your area.

REMEMBER

State mandates are always an issue under consideration in the legislature. If you are feeling particularly motivated or vocal in trying to get your state covered for infertility, there are groups who work hard to get these laws enacted. You can contact your local RESOLVE chapter or the Academy of Adoption and Assisted Reproduction Attorneys. They are generally on the front lines when it comes to advocacy in this area. They can let you know "what's on the table" and how you can help.

Fighting City Hall: Insurance Appeals

Insurance appeals need to attack one of the three basic reasons insurance companies give for not covering infertility treatments:

>> Infertility is not an illness.

>> Infertility treatments are not medically necessary.

>> Infertility treatments are experimental.

You need to address one of these issues to win your claim. In some cases, your doctor may write a letter of "medical necessity" for some of your treatment.

A policy with vague wording may be easier to appeal than coverage that specifically excludes infertility treatment.

Take it up the ladder. Don't just settle for a "no" from the first person who gives it, particularly if you feel that there is a legitimate "yes" that should apply instead. Generally, decisions or reversals get made at a higher level. Keep asking for a supervisor's name (and their supervisor, and their supervisor, and so on). If you're going to get turned down, put up a good fight, and besides, you just might win after all!

Coauthor Dr. R cautions that benefits are determined by the negotiation between the purchaser of the policy — which is usually your employer or yourself — and the insurance company. The benefits are described in the policy, and this is considered a contract. Your doctor is not a party to this contract and cannot add benefits to the contract. So while having your doctor write a letter of necessity or do a peer-to-peer review is possible, my experience is that it's usually unsuccessful.

When Having Insurance Doesn't Help

You can have the world's most comprehensive infertility insurance that can end up being worth nothing to you if your clinic is not on the preferred provider list. This is why the best kind of insurance is the type that pays a certain amount, regardless of where you go. Why would a clinic choose not to contract with an insurance company? For one thing, the amount the insurance offers isn't enough to cover clinic costs. Insurance contracts are convoluted, may require the doctors to fill out special forms, and the insurance company may refuse to pay for a given treatment because some procedure was not followed correctly, they deem it "unnecessary," or for some other reason. Because the contract is between the clinic and the insurance company, this is not your problem, but it may be a serious enough problem for the clinic to cancel that particular insurance contract.

Some clinics take your insurance amount but require you to pay the rest of the bill out of pocket. If a clinic is a preferred provider for that insurance, it's generally required to accept the amount offered as payment in full. If a clinic doesn't want to accept the amount offered, which is usually quite a bit below what most clinics charge for high-tech treatments (such as IVF), it may simply refuse to take the insurance at all. But this is not allowed if the clinic is on the preferred provider list! So, double-check the list and contact the insurance company if you see the clinic there.

Getting Creative When You're Out of Other Options

If you don't have insurance or if your insurance doesn't pay anything toward IVF treatment, you may need to get creative. There are ways to have your IVF cycle paid for if you meet certain requirements and are in the right place at the right time!

Donating eggs to reduce costs

A few clinics have innovative donor egg programs that let you donate half your eggs to another couple in return for treatment. The recipient of your eggs pays for your medications and your IVF retrieval and transfer. You need to pay for your own pretesting (such as infectious blood work and a hysterosalpingogram), blood and ultrasound testing, and the cost of freezing any excess embryos you have. ASRM cautions that this situation may lead to problems with coercion, especially if the donors are given a discount on their own cycle.

REMEMBER

Usually, you must meet certain requirements to be an egg donor. Generally, you must be under 35 years old and have a normal follicle-stimulating hormone (FSH) level. Usually a donor list is sent out every month or so by the clinic, and you need to be picked by a recipient to be able to do a retrieval cycle. The donors and recipients need to be matched ahead of time so that their cycles can be synchronized, thereby ensuring that both the donor and the recipient can have a fresh embryo transfer.

Your chances of getting picked are highest if you meet the following requirements:

» **You're young, preferably under 30:** The younger you are, the better the chance that you'll make a lot of eggs.

» **You're of normal weight and height:** Overweight donors aren't usually a first choice. Recipients may worry that obesity is hereditary and also may be concerned that they may have infertility problems, such as polycystic ovaries, a condition in which many eggs are made but the egg quality may be lower than normal.

Very short donors may also not be picked as quickly because, given a choice, more people choose to have a taller donor (and hopefully taller children).

» **You have proven fertility:** If you have children already, you're more likely to be picked as a donor.

>> **You have a male-factor issue:** If your only fertility issue is male factor, you may be picked because you don't have any fertility issues yourself.

>> **You have a good family background:** You have lots of brothers and sisters with lots of children, no genetic diseases, and no mental illnesses. These factors make you a prime candidate.

>> **You're a nonsmoker:** Evidence exists that smoking can damage eggs, plus nonsmokers are perceived as healthier people who take better care of themselves.

>> **You complete all FDA requirements to be accepted as a donor.**

REMEMBER

Egg recipients are often looking for someone whose blood type matches theirs and who has certain physical characteristics or racial background, so you may be selected faster if you have what a lot of people are looking for a common blood type, or a rare one if someone on the list is looking for that.

Your savings as a donor could equal between $8,000 and $12,000, but you need to be comfortable with the idea that your genetic child could be growing up with another family, or that the recipient could get pregnant with your egg and you may not. Only you can say whether you can accept the emotional repercussions of donating eggs to another couple.

Some women say that they don't feel a genetic connection because their egg isn't being fertilized with their partner's sperm, so the child created isn't the same as the offspring from their own relationship. Other women become very angry when their recipients get pregnant and they don't. This is another one of those times where "know thyself" is of the utmost importance.

Joining a drug study

Some doctors' offices are well connected to certain drug companies and do frequent drug studies for compensation. The compensation may be made to the office as well as the patient. Patients may receive anything from a free cycle of medication to an entire paid IVF cycle, including blood work, ultrasounds, and egg retrieval costs.

Some studies have very specific requirements for age, weight, and infertility problem. Others are less strict with their requirements and let the clinic select patients whom they feel are suitable.

REMEMBER

In most studies, a new drug not yet approved by the FDA is being tested. If you sign up for the study, you need to understand that you may get fewer eggs or less fertilization than you would from proven drugs. Most studies require that you sign a document stating this. You may also have to keep a journal of all side effects and have frequent interviews with the person running the study.

Centers selected to run drug studies are usually the larger centers, so you may want to check and see whether the clinics you're considering ever participate in drug studies.

Getting Your Medications for Less

As any smart shopper knows, it's always best to avoid paying the retail price. Instead, look for outlets, sales, and other bargains that can help you get the same product for less money. In this section, we discuss some of the "deals" available when purchasing fertility medications.

Shopping at mail-order pharmacies

Many doctors suggest that you order your medications from one of the mail-order pharmacies now specializing in fertility medications. These pharmacies carry all fertility medications, can ship quickly, and often offer the best prices. In addition, they may provide 24-hour access to nurses or pharmacists who can answer questions for you and websites that address common concerns. Many mail-order pharmacies offer overnight shipping at no additional cost with a minimum order. Many mail-order pharmacies also provide booklets, tapes, and hotlines to provide you with information any time of the day or night.

Another added benefit is virtual anonymity. You won't risk standing next to a nosy neighbor who's certain to share your fertility battle with the neighborhood, if not the world. Mail-order pharmacies are subject to the same Food and Drug Administration (FDA) regulations as your corner drugstore and are completely safe to use.

Making a quick trip over the border

For those adventurous types who would rather use the drive-through to get low-cost medications, should you consider a trip over the border? Mexico and Canada are both sources for lower-cost medications, and for some people, they're only a car ride away, but this practice is illegal under federal law. In addition, the standard for drug quality in the United States, set by the FDA, is quite rigid, and you have no guarantee that other countries will employ the same quality controls. The more Westernized a country, the more likely it is to maintain standards similar to those of the United States. But if you want the security of homegrown products, the only option is to stay home!

REMEMBER

When we speak of going over the border to buy medications, we're not referring to scoring fertility drugs from the guy on the corner. Your only source should be the local pharmacy. Some individuals and couples join forces and elect a representative to travel across the border and fill prescriptions for the group.

Scoring freebies from the drug companies

With the growth of the infertility industry and the volume that the participating drug companies realize, some have taken an extra step to help educate and even finance their clients' efforts.

EMD Serono, Ferring, and Merck, three of the larger infertility drug companies, have started services manned by health professionals to answer basic questions on infertility (but don't expect them to give you recommendations on your particular protocol, lay odds on your success, or adjust your meds!). Another interesting facet of these services is the financial aid that they have developed by donating cycle medicines to patients who are in need and have limited resources to pay for the drugs that they require. This "scholarship program" is run on a case-by-case basis, and you must contact the company directly to find out the requirements and how to apply. Be aware that you may need to show proof of income such as an income tax return, which may be more information than you want to have to supply.

Shopping for "sales"

Clinics and drug companies can also be helpful when financing IVF is an issue. The following deals may appeal to you!

Going for the money-back guarantee

Some clinics try to overcome resistance to the high cost of IVF by offering a money-back guarantee. This offer sounds good, but it does have a few catches.

Some centers call these "shared risk" programs. The specifics vary, but usually you pay an up-front fee, such as $15,000, for one or two IVF cycles. If you get pregnant in any of the cycles, the clinic keeps all your money. If you don't get pregnant at the end of the last cycle, you get your money back (or at least a large part of it). You must pay extra charges for intracytoplasmic sperm injection (ICSI) or using an egg donor or gestational carrier.

Patients must meet certain requirements for acceptance into the programs; usually, you must be under a certain age and have a normal uterine cavity and normal baseline blood test results.

Are these programs a good deal? That depends. Obviously, they try to hedge their bets somewhat by selecting patients they feel have a good chance of success. If you get pregnant on the fourth try, you'll have gotten a good price per try. If you get pregnant on the first try, you'll have spent a great deal of money for one cycle, far more than you needed to. But if you get pregnant on the first try, will you care about the cost? Only you know the answer.

If you're able to look at a pregnancy on your first try as an incredible blessing and not count the cost, this program may be for you. After two cycles, the clinic begins to break even on you.

Taking 'em up on a twofer

REMEMBER

ASRM (the American Society for Reproductive Medicine) has supported shared risk programs as a way to decrease costs to patients if they don't get pregnant. If you do get pregnant on the first try, you're basically subsidizing other people's third and fourth tries.

Ask your doctor whether his or her practice offers this type of quantity discount (or any discount at all for that matter). For specific information on networks of physicians who offer this type of pricing, visit your local search engine on the internet. One such organization is www.arcfertility.com, but other such networks are available as well.

Going overseas for IVF

As you may have heard, the terms *medical tourism* or *cross border reproduction* now describe a new type of travel, one that can certainly benefit those pursuing lower cost infertility treatments.

South Africa, South America, Mexico, and certain parts of Europe have infertility programs that provide higher-tech options such as IVF and donor egg at lower prices, with some clinics quoting IVF cycles under $10,000, inclusive of travel, and donor egg cycles under $15,000, inclusive of travel. Before you rush to make your reservations or shudder at the thought of a back-alley operation, keep a few things in mind:

>> While not FDA regulated, many countries have their own federal board of standards that requires that certain conditions be met to insure safety and efficacy. When researching a clinic abroad, you may want to directly contact one of the regulatory agencies in the region. South Africa has SASRSS (South African Society of Reproductive Science and Surgery) and the South African Department of Health; European countries may be regulated by ESHRE (European Society of Human Reproduction and Embryology). If you're not sure what agency to contact, start with the country/government Board of Health. You can also contact the local docs at ASRM (American Society of Reproductive Medicine) to get the latest on which countries or clinics are the best regulated.

>> For donor egg programs, you want to be assured that the donors are being screened for infectious diseases and/or sexually transmitted diseases as well as basic genetic mutations.

Make sure that the price(s) that you are being quoted are inclusive of all necessary medical services. Is anesthesia extra? You may want to know. Some programs include the price of air travel in their package. Make sure to find out what the travel arrangements are and verify that they meet your needs.

Lastly, take some time to enjoy the scenery! One of the benefits of "infertility tourism" is the tourism part. Ask the clinic to recommend good hotels and/or activities that you may enjoy.

Chapter **16**

Ready, Steady, Go! Starting Your IVF Cycle

I n vitro fertilization (IVF) is the high-tech method of getting pregnant. During an IVF cycle, you take stimulating hormone medications called gonadotropins so that your ovaries are willing to develop more than one or two eggs. Then you go through an egg retrieval, a minor surgery to take the eggs out of the follicles in which they grow. After that, the eggs are fertilized in the lab and then can either be put back into your uterus so they can grow or frozen for a transfer in the future to the uterus.

The treatment sounds complicated, and it is — but not so complicated that you can't understand the basic idea and walk into your clinic confident that you know what to expect.

In this chapter, we discuss how to get through an IVF cycle with the least amount of frustration, explore what egg retrieval involves, and explain how your best friend's cycle may be completely different from yours and why you shouldn't worry about it.

Preparing for a Roller Coaster Ride of Emotions

In vitro fertilization is a complicated process. It involves injecting medications with possibly serious side effects for several weeks, taking time out of your schedule to have blood work and ultrasounds done, and undergoing surgery, albeit minor, to retrieve your eggs. And that's just the beginning! Every step of the way through IVF is crucial, and every day brings news that will either thrill you or bring you to your knees in despair. Is it any wonder that you're feeling scared?

Experiencing the emotional ride

Even though you're scared to death, you're also excited. You've probably been through a lot to get here, you've spent buckets of money, and you have high hopes that high tech will not fail you.

Behind the excitement may be depression. This is where you've ended up. You've tried all the simpler methods of conception, and they failed. This may be your last shot, and it may seem that there's nowhere to go from here. Before you got to IVF, you always knew you had one last thing to try. Now you're trying IVF, and if it fails, you don't know what you'll do next. Don't lose sight of the fact that IVF is also diagnostic. If nothing else, you are going to find out a whole lot more about you and your partner's reproductive potential.

REMEMBER

From the emotional side, you will have a lot of support from your clinic's staff. Take it from Lisa (who has been there with many patients!). IVF nurses and other clinical staff spend a great deal of their time just helping their patients understand the IVF process and deal with the emotions it stirs up. You can also rely on that support network that you've been building. With the growth of IVF as a fertility treatment, many of your friends and family know about IVF and are right there with you. Some women find "cycle buddies" in chat room sites, in Resolve meetings, and in mind-and-body classes, literally other women going through IVF (or any of the lower-tech measures) at the same time. You can check with your clinic for other support group options as they often have their own programs or keep a list of nearby services you may want to consider. You may find comfort in sharing your experiences, good and bad, with someone else who is going through the same thing at the same time (even some of that IVF staff — many of them have done exactly what you are doing now!). Remember, though, to share and not compare! You're not in competition with anyone. You're trying to have *your* baby.

And try to get your partner to read this chapter, because they are going to be bewildered by the roller coaster ride. Your partner is experiencing much of the IVF process secondhand. You're the one dealing directly with the physical discomfort, the scheduling madness, and the emotional ups and downs, so your partner will likely relate to the experience much differently than you do.

Looking at your protocol and dealing with schedules

When you first sit across the desk from an in vitro fertilization specialist, he'll probably give you a stack of papers that you'll promptly file in your fertility notebook — you know, the notebook that every patient seems to carry around with her. One of those undecipherable papers is probably your protocol. A *protocol* is nothing more than a blueprint or schedule of how your cycle will be done. It includes the medications you'll be taking, instructions on how to take them, and the procedures you need to follow throughout the cycle.

Reading your protocol

TIP

So, it's time to take out your protocol. **Step Number 1: Read the protocol!**

You would think this would go without saying, but it doesn't. Read the protocol!

Now, your cousin Mary out in Duluth may be going through IVF too, so you call her up and start comparing your protocols. Even though you're only four months apart in age, and everyone says you're more like sisters than cousins, you have two completely different protocols! How can this be? Relax. Doctors rely on a few standard IVF protocols (we list them in Table 16-1), and most doctors prefer to use one over the other. Here are some possibilities:

>> If you're under 35 and your baseline hormone levels are normal, your doctor could choose to start you on a down regulation cycle, starting leuprolide acetate (which has the brand name Lupron) a few days after you ovulate. (Some clinics like to start birth control pills on the third day of your menses, and then overlap the pill with the Lupron shots; this takes a little longer, but you avoid having to monitor your ovulation.)

Lupron shuts down your normal hormone allowing for control of the cycle. The drug also keeps you from ovulating before retrieval. Before there was Lupron, almost one-third of women ovulated just prior to the procedure and the procedure had to be cancelled. Imaging how disappointing it was to have gone through all of that work only to have the cycle cancelled. You may start your hormone-stimulating drugs when your period starts. Some centers call this a "long Lupron" cycle, and others call it a "down regulation" cycle. Lupron is a GnRH (gonadotropin-releasing hormone) agonist; it shuts down your normal growth of one dominant follicle by suppressing your pituitary gland. This prevents the development of only one follicle like you would normally do, and allows an entire group of follicles to be developed.

>> Your protocol may use a drug called ganirelix, a GnRH antagonist (with the brand name Antagon), or cetrorelix (with the brand name Cetrotide) in conjunction with follicle-stimulating medications; this drug also suppresses your LH surge so you won't ovulate before your egg retrieval. (The difference between the GnRH agonists and the antagonists is that the agonist must be started sometime before ovulation would normally happen in order to prevent its occurrence, whereas the antagonists work right away and prevent ovulation on the same day that they are given.) The antagonist protocol may also be used for women at risk for developing OHSS. For women at risk for OHSS, spontaneous ovulation is suppressed by the antagonist but the agonist is then used for the trigger.

>> If you're over 35, you may be given a "microdose Lupron" protocol, in which Lupron is diluted in normal saline so that only a minute amount is given each day; this protocol is used for women who didn't stimulate well in a previous cycle or those who have an FSH (follicle-stimulating hormone) level above normal (10.0 to 15, depending on your lab's values). In this case, the Lupron is used for its stimulatory properties, as opposed to its suppressive properties (as in the long Lupron protocol).

>> You could also be doing a natural protocol, with very little or no medication.

The core of the IVF procedure is the use of FSH to promote the development of more than one follicle. There are numerous preparations of FSH, which allows the REI to tailor the amount of FSH to your situation., FSH is required for developing follicles to reach maturity. Many follicles in differing stages of development are always progressing in the ovary. FSH permits some of the developing follicles to continue to develop but the number that can be rescued is determined by the ovary. The point of using FSH is to obtain more eggs, but FSH will not repair an egg that is structurally damaged.

REMEMBER

Your doctor will prescribe the protocol and medications he feels most comfortable using for your particular case. Try not to compare what you're getting to what anyone else is using.

Birth control pills may be used in association with any of these protocols to help cycle scheduling or to suppress the occasional ovarian cyst. The duration of birth control pill treatment is quite variable and is not included in the table. Multiple reviews and meta–analyses have revealed that there is not one perfect protocol in spite of what each physician may believe. If there was a perfect protocol, everyone would be using it. The fact that there are so many variations on the types of protocols proves that there is no perfect protocol. Consequently, if a person has to do more than one cycle of IVF, the physician may change the protocol to get a more favorable outcome. So, don't be surprised if the second cycle of IVF has a different protocol.

TABLE 16-1

Common IVF Protocols at a Glance

Protocol	Used For	Average Days on Medication	Vials of Medication Needed
Long Lupron	Women under 35; good responders	21+ days total, including at least 10 on Lupron alone	About 40, plus one 14-day Lupron kit (for one cycle)
Antagon or Cetrotide	Patients of any age or patients at risk for OHSS	10 days on stimulating medications; start ganirelix on day 6 of stimulating medications	About 30 to 40 vials of stimulating medications plus 5 to 6 prefilled syringes of Antagon or Cetrotide
Microdose flare	Poor responders; women over 35	10 to 12 days of microdose Lupron and stimulating medications	60 vials of stimulating medications; one bottle of microdose (diluted) Lupron
Modified long Lupron (also called stop Lupron)	Women over 35; poor responders	10 days of Lupron; then approximately 10 days of stimulating medications	60 vials of stimulating medications; one 14-day Lupron kit

Reviewing your protocol

Most IVF centers have some sort of orientation, usually with a nurse or an IVF coordinator, who reviews the protocol, injection instruction, finances, and other issues surrounding the IVF cycle. Having your partner inject medications is one of the scariest parts of IVF — for you *and* for your partner. Make sure that you get very clear instructions on how to do this. While you may receive excellent, specific instructions through the orientation session, remembering all of that is almost impossible. IVF centers provide written material, but there are also a number of videos on the internet that can help with the IVF process.

REMEMBER

One further point is to make sure you actually have the medication you will need. Trying to get these very unique medications in the middle of the night is almost impossible. Because of how insurance coverage works, you may need to get meds through the mail, and when they arrive, there are more meds than you can imagine. Time taken to ensure you have the correct meds at this point is time well spent. Whatever else you may do, make sure you have the medication that will be used for the trigger: either hCG or Lupron (or maybe pure LH for newer protocols). Almost all other medication issues can wait, but the timing of the trigger is the most critical aspect that you will be asked to do correctly. If in doubt about your trigger, page the doctor on call or wait until morning.

If your IVF center is large, designated nurses probably take care of only IVF patients. If your program is smaller, the nursing staff may take care of both non–IVF and IVF patients. Some programs have only one IVF nurse with whom you deal throughout your cycle; others have so many nurses you can't tell who's who without a scorecard!

TIP

Try to figure out how your center works and to whom you should be talking before your cycle starts. In many centers, the IVF nurses draw blood and also do your ultrasounds; larger centers have a separate staff that draws blood and ultrasonographers who do the ultrasounds. Make sure that you talk to the right person when you have a problem or need help.

Some protocols use less stimulating drugs and develop fewer follicles by design. The reasons for using a low-stimulation protocol may include the following:

>> Less cost to the patient

>> Less risk of hyperstimulation, or OHSS (see "Is hyperstimulation avoidable?")

>> Less chance of producing more embryos than you can ever use, along with the ethical considerations that accompany an overabundance of embryos

Dealing with a disappearing doctor

After your initial consult appointment, you may wonder where your doctor went. In smaller centers, doctors may do callbacks with your blood results; some also do their own ultrasounds. In larger centers, you may feel as though your doctor has vanished from the face of the earth because all your instructions come from the nurses. This system of patient communication can be upsetting if you came to a center specifically to deal with a particular doctor.

Rest assured that your doctor *is* reviewing your callbacks and instructing the nurses on what you should do next, but in bigger centers, doctors simply don't have the time to do more than 50 callbacks a night. Some centers have even gone to a system where you don't talk to *anybody:* Your instructions are left on a message tape you can access.

If your center has more than one doctor doing IVF procedures, you may also feel like you've lost the doctor you came to see. Many centers rotate doctors through IVF on a one- or two-week cycle; you may never see the doctor with whom you had your consultation again! Sometimes you can request that a certain doctor do your procedure but granting that request may not always be possible.

TIP

The doctor you saw on your initial visit to the clinic may not be the doctor who is managing your IVF procedure. Try to find out what your center's policy is for scheduling doctors and whether you can request the doctor of your choice.

Taking your medications without having a nervous breakdown

Suppose that you had your injection class a week ago, and on this beautiful bright Sunday morning, you're ready to begin taking your medications. Your partner, with shaking hands, opens the first vial to mix your first injection. "No, no!" you scream, as he proceeds to draw up the liquid. "That's not how she said to mix it!" He stops, and both of you stare dumbfounded at the boxes, the needles, and each other. In one week you've forgotten every word the nurse said. You look at the film you were given on giving injections again, read the colorful pieces of paper that tell you how to mix and inject, and still feel confused, scared, and totally out of control. And it's a Sunday. What on earth are you going to do?

First, take a deep breath. Of course, giving yourself injections is hard to do. Most people are scared the first time they give a shot or mix a medication. Your reaction is normal.

Second, and you are not going to believe this — go to Doctor Google. As we mention earlier, there are wonderful, clear, and concise injection instructions at your fingertips. Many IVF centers have their own online instructions just for situations like this. Or, you can find specific medication injection instructions on "fertility" websites and even generic instructions on various websites. This is when you can thank your lucky stars that you are not the first person to forget how to give a shot.

TIP

If no one is there, you can call the answering service and ask for the doctor on call. Some centers also have nurses who "take call" so they can answer questions when the office is closed. If you got your medications from a large mail-order pharmacy, it may have a nurse on call who can also give you instructions. Call the main number and ask. Remember that medication confusion (dosing, mixing, injecting) is considered a bona fide "emergency" at a fertility center. Do not hesitate to call!

If you can't get anyone, take a little break, compose yourself, and then go back and try again. The procedure probably won't look quite as overwhelming the second time.

TIP

Fertility clinics really do need to know if you did not take your medication as directed (you were "short" so took half a dose) or you took your medication at the wrong time (hCG was scheduled at 1 a.m. but you overslept and took it at 3 a.m). This is not the time to pull the blanket over your head and deny a mistake — 'fess up! These types of changes compromise the outcome of your cycle and, more importantly, they can be usually be accommodated in most cases to still make things go well. So tell your doctor or IVF coordinator as soon as possible (yep, call them first thing in the morning!) so that they can work on fixing the slip.

Monitoring your progress (more poking and prodding)

After a few days of injections, you'll start to feel like a pro, your partner will have his injection techniques down pat, and your protocol will start to make sense to you. It's time to find out how well this is working. It's time to have blood drawn and do an ultrasound.

Most centers monitor you every few days to see how you're responding to the medication. The purpose of the monitoring is to obtain the eggs at the proper point of maturation. Immature or postmature eggs don't work. In general, there needs to be two or three egg units (follicles) that reach a diameter on ultrasound of 16–20 mm (physicians vary on what diameter they prefer) all on the same day. The blood tests measure estrogen and progesterone. The estrogen gives information about the state of maturity of the eggs and also the risk for OHSS. The progesterone should remain low but, in some cycles, it will start to rise. This interferes with the coordination of the lining of the uterus and the stage of development of the embryo and reduces the pregnancy rate. This can be overcome by freezing the embryo and then doing a frozen embryo transfer on a more controlled, unstimulated cycle. If your follicles are growing nicely and your estradiol is rising, your medications will probably not be changed. If you're stimulating too well, or not stimulating well enough, your medications may be decreased or increased.

Is hyperstimulation avoidable?

WARNING

Stimulating too well can be another example of too much of a good thing. The goal of IVF is to have a number of follicles grow so that more than one egg can be retrieved. With some women, especially those who have polycystic ovaries (see Chapter 7 for more about this condition), hyperstimulation can get way out of hand very quickly. If your estradiol rises too fast, or if you make too many follicles, you run a risk of developing OHSS, or ovarian hyperstimulation syndrome. Patients with OHSS can be very ill after egg retrieval, with fluid buildup in the pelvis and in the lungs. Some women become sick enough to require hospitalization. In the past, a few patients have even died from severe OHSS, which causes fluid volume shifts through your whole body and can make your blood very thick and prone to clotting.

Because OHSS is so potentially serious, most centers watch patients on stimulating medications quite closely, monitoring their blood and ultrasound results every few days. If your clinic thinks that you're in danger of severe OHSS, you may have to freeze all your embryos after retrieval and not do an embryo transfer. OHSS becomes worse if you become pregnant, due to the rising hormone levels from the pregnancy. Some centers may not do egg retrieval at all and simply cancel the cycle, because the hCG trigger given before retrieval also makes OHSS worsen.

On the other hand, you may not be stimulating well, and your clinic may be increasing your medication to see whether you can do better. This situation also requires closer monitoring because your medications may require frequent adjustment. See Table 16-2 for a typical IVF stimulation cycle, but remember that your cycle may vary.

TABLE 16-2   **A Typical IVF Cycle — Yours May Vary**

Day of Cycle	Monitoring	Medication	Time Taken
2	Blood and ultrasound	FSH/hCG (stimulating medications)	2 vials a.m./2 vials p.m.
3		Keep taking medications	No change
4		Keep taking medications	No change
5	Blood and ultrasound	Adjust according to monitoring results	Change if clinic tells you to
6		Keep taking medications	No change
7		Add Antagon/Cetrotide	Add Antagon/Cetrotide in a.m.
8	Blood and ultrasound	Keep taking medications	No change
9		Keep taking medications	
10	Blood and ultrasound	Take morning medications/hCG	Morning medications: no change; hCG at exact time clinic tells you
11	Blood work only	No medications	
12	Egg retrieval		

As a rough guide, you'll probably be on stimulating hormones ten to twelve days before you're given hCG to mature the follicle for your retrieval. During those days, you'll probably have blood work and ultrasounds done four times, or maybe more or less depending on your circumstances. Some centers insist that all your blood work and ultrasounds be done at their facility; others allow patients to be monitored at outside facilities closer to their homes. You need to find a place capable of doing same-day reports and willing to fax results to your clinic.

Getting your next-step marching orders

It's going to happen. By phone, text, or email, your clinic will be sending you information about how you are doing. Regardless of the method of communication, your whole world stops for a second, as you try to decipher from the tone of the message whether it is good news or bad news.

Setting up your callback instructions

Blood and ultrasound callbacks consume a huge part of your life after you start IVF. You find yourself leaving whole volumes of information on how to reach you that day (portal, email, text, cell phone, home phone, don't leave a message with the babysitter, partner's number, don't call before 6, don't call after 6, don't leave a message, I really need to talk to you) on your callback sheets, because this call, whether good or bad news, is the highlight of your day.

REMEMBER

Most clinics have specific methods for reaching their patients with next-step instructions during their IVF cycle. This is designed to ensure that you get the info that you need. The best thing you can do to stay sane is to follow those instructions! Understand that test results won't get to the clinic until the afternoon and then the IVF coordinators need to talk to the doctor, get new orders and *then* contact their patients. Checking for calls, texts, or emails before that happens will leave you frustrated.

TIP

If your clinic has a lot of staff, try to cultivate a good relationship with one or two nurses with whom you feel comfortable. It doesn't hurt to ask to speak with that nurse when you call. Most nurses are happy to call you if you personally ask for them. Also, if you get to know one or two people well, you won't have to explain all the ins and outs of your case every time you call in.

TIP

You may find it easiest to have the clinic call you on your cell phone, and some clinics prefer that you give them your cell number as your primary source of contact. That way, you can have it with you at all times and don't have to feel tethered to the office phone, home phone, and so on. And what if you have to go to the bathroom! Many centers also use a portal system with their electronic medical record so that you can access the information 24/7.

Knowing what to do if you don't get along with the IVF coordinator

The first question is "Is the problem the process or the person?" The IVF process is extremely stressful. It requires you to give up your time, your routine, and your privacy, and it means you must have frequent contact with the healthcare personnel. This can sometimes lead to uncomfortable interactions. What if the clinic has only one nurse and you just don't get along? Try to make it easier for both of you by talking about the elephant in the room. Many times, just confronting the issue will help identify the problem and clear the air. Most clinical staff truly want to help you. Sometimes, setting reasonable expectations for both you and the nurse may help. Communication is critical, so be sure to share your concerns with the IVF staff and work with them to get the best result for everyone.

Dealing with the loss of control, or not being the best in the room

There you are in the waiting room, listening to the person ahead of you brag about how well her cycle is going, how she's got 20 beautiful follicles, how good her partner is at giving shots, how she loves the nurses so much she's making them each a ceramic something to say thank-you, how great her veins are, and how happy she is to be alive. You look at your poor black and blue arms and think about how you have only seven follicles on ultrasound, how your partner seems to hit a nerve every other day, how much you hate all the nurses, and how much you hate this whole process.

In some centers, the waiting room is like group therapy in a psychiatrist's office: All the patients pull their chairs together while waiting for their ultrasound appointments and talk about IVF and life in general. This kind of place can provide you with new friends who know exactly what you're going through, but it can also turn into a sort of golf course with chairs — she got pregnant on the first try, she has the most follicles, she's doing better than she did last cycle, she's having twins, she's having triplets.

REMEMBER

Stay out of the comparison contests, if you can. Everyone responds differently to medications, and in the end, the person with three follicles may get pregnant, and the person with twenty follicles may not. Remember that the only thing that matters is you achieving a successful pregnancy.

TIP

If talking to other people about your problems makes you feel worse, don't join in. Bring a book and headphones and put an unapproachable expression on your face. Arrive as close to the time of your appointment as you can, get engrossed in the TV, or hide in the bathroom!

On the other hand, if you can listen to other women's tales and not compare yourself to them, the waiting room can be a great source of camaraderie and a place to make lasting friendships.

Why feeling blue is normal

REMEMBER

We can't stress enough that mood swings are normal when undergoing IVF due to the increased levels of stress and the hormonal manipulation. You may also experience a letdown feeling when doing an IVF cycle. You've planned for it and fantasized about how things would go, and now it's almost over. It's like Christmas: Sometimes the anticipation surpasses the reality. When you're almost ready for egg retrieval, you can't change things. It's too late to say, "We should have waited another month" or "I should have taken more meds, less meds, or different meds."

Taking a Shot in the Dark: Time for hCG

After 10–12 days of stimulation, there will come a time when the clinical staff will call with: "It's time for hCG!" If you've read your protocol, you know what hCG (human chorionic gonadotropin) is; if you haven't, here's a refresher course.

Understanding the purpose of hCG

hCG is a crucial part of your IVF cycle. It is given 32 to 36 hours before your egg retrieval; its job is to mature your eggs and prepare them to be fertilized. This is called the trigger. Recently antagonist cycles have been developed that use an agonist (Lupron) for the trigger. Using the trigger allows the retrieval to be at the precise interval between the trigger and the retrieval so that the eggs are at the proper point in their maturation. That's why the timing of your hCG is very important.

Setting the alarm: Timing is everything with hCG!

The hCG instructions include a specific time to take your injection, and following the directions is absolutely critical because timing really is everything. Your injection may be scheduled for midnight, or even a few hours later, if your center has a lot of egg retrievals to do on one day.

TIP

If your injection is scheduled for, say, 2 a.m., you can mix the medication ahead of time and put it on your bedside table; then set your alarm for the time you need to take the hCG. Giving the injection at an odd hour is easier if you don't need to fumble around mixing medications when you're half asleep. Just be careful to not accidentally push the plunger as you get it ready for later.

TIP

Just a reminder of the "'fess up" talk noted earlier. If, due to some act of God, you missed your scheduled hCG injection time (because that is really the only excuse, right?), *call your clinic!* Trying to hide this mishap will definitely change the outcome of your IVF cycle. More importantly, we are trained to try and fix it and often (not always) can. So, stop screaming at your alarm clock or partner, don't cry so that we can't understand you on the phone — just call and explain what happened.

Heading to the Big Dance: The Egg Retrieval

Almost before you know it, it's time for your egg retrieval. All kinds of emotions are probably churning around inside you and your partner. This is the culmination of several weeks of injections, emotions, and worries. It's your big day! How do you feel?

TIP

If you know ahead of time about an event that may conflict with your egg retrieval, tell your doctor about it *before* you start taking your stimulating hormones. Sometimes an egg retrieval can be held off for a few days if you take Lupron or birth control a few extra days before starting your stimulating medications. While minor adjustments to the timing of IVF can be done, why torture yourself? Isn't IVF stressful enough? Plan ahead for major life events. After you start stimulating medications, influencing the day of your retrieval is harder. The course of the FSH stimulation is set by the ovary and there is very little that can be done to alter this.

Looking at retrieval schedules

Some IVF centers do egg retrievals every day of the week. Others do retrievals only Monday through Friday and start their patients' medications all at the same time to avoid the weekends. Still others cycle patients through in batches, doing retrievals only every other month or a few months of the year. You probably won't have much say in what day or what time your retrieval is done.

Signing here . . . and here . . . and here . . .

Most centers have you sign consent forms ahead of time for your egg retrieval, and this process can take time as there is usually more than one informed consent document. Usually, a nurse reviews the consent forms with you after the doctor has explained your treatment plan. This may be done in a separate consult at the clinic, or you may be asked to read everything at home (or view webinars) and sign them electronically. No matter which method is used, the goal is to have you understand the IVF process and your specific treatment and to let the clinic know your choices and permission for certain procedures.

REMEMBER

If you decide to freeze your embryos, you will be asked to make decisions about the future disposition of these embryos. This will include considering what to do if you die, your partner dies, both of you die, or you get a divorce (or dissolve your relationship). Your choices will include letting your partner pursue a pregnancy, donating the embryos to someone else (known or unknown) to attempt a pregnancy, donating them to research (as allowed by law), or discarding them.

These are complex decisions and should be made thoughtfully, so don't rush just to get the paperwork done.

TIP

Some patients may defer decisions (especially about cryopreservation and future disposition of frozen gametes or embryos) until they "see" the results of the egg retrieval or fertilization. This means you may be making decisions on the day of the egg retrieval — maybe not the best idea. Keep in mind that your anxiety level will be through the roof, and the chances that you'll be able to read and comprehend 18 pages of legalese the morning of your retrieval are slim. Further, you may not remember to "fill in the blanks" about disposition and then the clinic won't have a clue what you really wanted to do. Since the outcome of the IVF cycle cannot be known in advance, there may arise rare occasions where decisions need to be made after the retrieval. Having thought about the possibilities ahead of time may make these later decisions more informed. Some centers let you make changes in the consent forms as long as they know what the changes are ahead of time and can have a lawyer review your changes. Here are the most common concerns that people have with IVF consent forms:

>> Having pictures taken of themselves, their eggs, sperm, or embryos, for use in any type of publication. Many people have no objection to this, but some do.

>> Allowing medical, nursing, or other students in the room to watch the procedure.

>> Using any sperm, eggs, embryos, or tissue for research. "Tissue" can mean fluid from follicles, endometrial tissue, or anything else removed at the time of retrieval or transfer.

>> Freezing of any embryos not transferred on a fresh transfer. Some people have religious objections to embryo freezing, and they want to inseminate only a few eggs, so that they can use up all their embryos and not have any left to freeze. Discuss this step ahead of time with embryology to make sure that everyone understands exactly what will be done.

TIP

If you have objections to anything in the consent forms, address them before the morning of your egg retrieval. If your clinic has a problem with your requests, it could delay or cancel your retrieval.

Meeting the retrieval team

A whole new group of unfamiliar people will be with you for the egg retrieval. During the egg retrieval, a nurse or a medical assistant may be in the room helping the doctor. An ultrasonographer may be present, and the embryologist will be nearby. The person in whom you may be most interested as you arrive in the IVF area (which you probably have never seen before) is the person who will give you the anesthetic medication for your retrieval. This can be an anesthesiologist (another doctor) or, more likely, a nurse anesthetist. Either one is fully trained to provide the type of anesthesia that your clinic uses for egg retrievals. While some clinics have staff anesthetists, more often these caregivers are contracted to provide anesthesia services. Either way, they are there to fully concentrate on one thing during the procedure — keeping you safe! Often you will "meet" them before your procedure during a phone call where they ask about your medical history, or directly before you go into the procedure room.

Previewing what happens in an egg retrieval

Different centers do things different ways, but in most centers, you're taken to the IVF suite, a part of the building you've never seen before and had no idea existed. You'll change into a gown, hat, and shoe covers because the IVF suite is a sterile area where an attempt is made to keep outside germs from entering.

An intravenous (IV) infusion is started. The purpose of the IV is mainly to have access for giving you medication, but it's also there in case any complications require you to be given large amounts of fluid quickly. If you know that certain of your veins are better than others for the IV, don't be shy about informing the person starting your IV!

In some centers, an embryologist may come in to see you before the procedure starts to ask you to verify your name, Social Security number, and information about your partner. The purpose of checking this information is to prevent any type of mix-up with eggs, sperm, or embryos.

The doctor generally comes in the room at the last minute, introduces herself, if you don't already know the physician, and instructs the person giving you medications to start giving them. Usually after you are asleep, the doctor inserts a speculum and washes the vagina and cervix thoroughly, trying to keep the area as clean as possible.

TECHNICAL STUFF

You won't remember the rest, so we explain what happens next. The doctor inserts the vaginal ultrasound probe into your vagina. On the top of the probe is a needle guide, an attachment that has a hollow, narrow, tube-like guide along which a long metal needle slides. The doctor locates your follicles on ultrasound with the probe and then punctures the back of the vagina with the needle, entering each follicle and sucking out the fluid. The follicular fluid is given to the embryologist, who examines it under a microscope and says, it is hoped, "Egg one, egg two," and so on. When the follicles are all emptied, you wake up and are taken to a nearby bed for a short time to recover. An egg retrieval usually takes about 30 to 40 minutes from start to finish, and you'll be asleep the whole time.

Sleeping on the job: Anesthesia's role in egg retrieval

IVF centers vary considerably in their methods of anesthesia for egg retrievals. Some centers do all their retrievals in a hospital operating suite, so a nurse anesthetist or an anesthesiologist (a doctor who specializes in giving anesthesia) gives your medications. Smaller centers may have only an assistant or the nurse giving medication under the guidance of your doctor.

Monitored anesthesia care (MAC) is a continuum of sedation and pain control that is used for surgical procedures. A lighter level of sedation is sometimes termed "conscious sedation" while the general term is MAC. Most patients are unconscious during the IVF procedure, and the level of sedation is determined by the anesthetist tailored to the patient's need. Commonly used medications include Versed, fentanyl, and propofol.

The degree to which you're awake during your procedure varies quite a bit between individuals, but almost all patients are unconscious. Your vital signs, including your heart rate, blood pressure, and respirations, are carefully monitored.

Certain medications, such as Versed, have amnesiac properties, which is a fancy way of saying that you won't remember what went on during the retrieval. This effect lasts for a short time after the procedure as well. Nearly every IVF patient wakes up after the procedure and asks, "How many eggs did I get?" at least three times before she's actually awake enough to remember the answer! You may not remember walking from the table to a recovery bed or chair, either, but you did!

Your Partner Is Busy Too

TIP

While you're doing your thing, your partner will be watching the movies most centers helpfully provide to make it easier for him to masturbate to produce a semen specimen. This can be a tricky issue for some men and downright impossible for others. If you think that your partner is going to suffer from performance anxiety on retrieval day, consider the following ways to take the pressure off:

>> You can have him freeze a specimen ahead of time. Most centers prefer to use fresh sperm, but if your partner knows a frozen backup is available, he may have an easier time in the producing room. And if he can't, the lab can use the frozen specimen; not as good as the fresh, but a whole lot better than nothing!

>> He can go to a nearby hotel or home if you live close enough — within 60 minutes away — and produce there.

>> You can help him produce. You may feel uncomfortable going in with him, but believe us, people do it all the time. But andrologists enforce two rules: no saliva and no lubricants. Either one can mess up the semen specimen. Make sure the specimen goes directly from the penis into the cup to maintain sterility as much as possible; no collecting it in your hand or elsewhere!

After the Dance: Do's and Don'ts for a Happy Recovery

There are as many post-retrieval experiences as there are patients undergoing a retrieval. However, there are some commonly experienced feelings. Most people will have mild to moderate pain. Some will have significant pain, which usually responds to IV pain medication. By the time a person is ready to leave the IVF center, the pain should be manageable.

Most people will also feel full, bloated, and somewhat uncomfortable for a few days after the retrieval. When pain is an issue, it is important to take the pain medication before the pain gets really bad. Some people will feel better and then in a few days they feel bloated and uncomfortable. These may be signs of OHSS and should be relayed to the IVF center.

Because the ovaries are making progesterone, the temperature will be slightly elevated. But any temperature greater than 101 degrees Fahrenheit taken twice a few hours apart, may signal an infection, especially if there is also increasing pelvic pain. The center needs to be contacted immediately.

Fainting is uncommon, and either call 911 or the notify the center immediately.

REMEMBER

The bottom line: If something seems wrong, contact the center immediately. If something seems really wrong, go to the nearest ER. Serious complications after a retrieval are uncommon but can be quite serious, even life threatening. Better to be safe than sorry.

Answering Common Post-IVF Questions

After a retrieval, almost everybody asks these questions:

>> **Can I see my eggs before I go home?** You can't see your eggs because they can be seen only under a microscope, and no embryologist in the world is

going to let a patient still lurching around in an anesthesia daze mess around with his extremely expensive microscope or those precious eggs!

>> **Why can't my partner come back to the retrieval room?** In some centers, partners are allowed to be present at the egg retrieval. Other centers don't allow anyone else to be in the room for the retrieval. Usually, the rooms are too small to allow extra people, and no one wants partners feeling woozy in the retrieval room and knocking over the ultrasound equipment if they fall. More importantly, these are akin to "operating rooms" (in other words, "clean" rooms), which may need to meet accreditation standards — and you would not have a partner in the room for your knee surgery!

>> **Do I have to have an IV?** Yes.

>> **Are you *sure* you won't mix up my eggs (or sperm or embryos) with someone else's?** Yes.

Centers are anxious to reassure patients on this topic, since all centers are very aware of the recent cases in the news and are being extremely careful to avoid such an incidence.

Most centers label all dishes, collection cups, and so on with the patient's name, date of birth, patient number, and sometimes a color code. Egg retrievals and embryo transfers are done one at a time — never two at the same time. Eggs and embryos go from labeled container to labeled container. And catheters used for embryo transfer are never reused, so someone else's embryo won't be stuck in your catheter! Today some centers use an electronic bar-coding system as well.

Post-Retrieval Pills and Potions

You may think that you're all done with medication after your egg retrieval, but you'll receive a sheet full of instructions about everything you need to take starting the day of your retrieval. Here's what you'll probably be given:

>> **Antibiotics:** An egg retrieval is surgery that goes through a "dirty" area: your vagina. Yes, your vagina is considered a dirty area no matter how personally dainty and clean you are, which simply means that in medical terms, the area is not sterile. (By the way, so is your mouth; medically "dirty" simply means that it is not sterile.) So your doctor will probably give you antibiotics for several days, starting on or before the day of your retrieval. Make sure that you mention any allergies or sensitivities.

TIP

If you're prone to yeast infections, you can take an over-the-counter pill called acidophilus, which maintains the balance of good and bad bacteria in your vagina. When the good bacteria are killed off with the bad ones, you get an overgrowth of yeast, which causes itching and a white cheesy discharge.

» **Steroids:** These may seem like an odd addition to your pill arsenal, but steroids may be given to protect your embryo from attack by white blood cells after transfer. Steroids decrease the number of white blood cells in your blood. The dose given is very low and usually for just a few days. Their use is controversial, and most centers don't use them.

» **Progesterone:** When it comes to progesterone supplements, you may be given pills, gels, suppositories, or — can you stand it? — injections. Some centers give progesterone injections to everyone because injections are the best absorbed. But progesterone injections do have a downside:

- **They hurt.** The needle used for progesterone needs to be at least a 22-gauge (relatively thick) variety because the progesterone is very thick, or viscous, and won't flow through a smaller needle. The progesterone is mixed in sesame or peanut oil, and a fair number of women have allergic reactions to the oils.

- **They're hard to find.** Commercially made progesterone in oil is sometimes hard to find. Some small compounding pharmacies make their own, as do some of the large mail-order pharmacies that specialize in fertility medications.

- **Insurance doesn't always cover the cost.** Some insurance companies don't feel that progesterone injections are medically necessary. Costs are reasonable — about $45 a bottle — but can add up if you're using a bottle every five days for several months.

On the other hand, some centers use vaginal suppositories. The downside aspects of these are

- **They're messy.** The suppositories leak, making it necessary to wear a pad.

- **They can cause yeast infections.** Because they keep you continually wet, you're more likely to develop a yeast infection or rash, which can be more than a little annoying.

Other progesterone options are the following:

- **Crinone:** This progesterone gel is manufactured by Serono, a drug company that makes many fertility medications. Crinone causes less leakage and irritation than vaginal suppositories. It comes in an applicator that is inserted vaginally. Crinone is more expensive than vaginal suppositories.

- **Endometrin:** This is a vaginal suppository containing progesterone made by Ferring, another drug company that makes many fertility medications. The choice between Crinone or Endometrin is arbitrary.

- **Prometrium capsules, or compounded capsules:** These are pills, which means that if you take them orally, they pass through your liver after being digested in the stomach. The main disadvantage is that the way they're metabolized causes drowsiness, which can be severe. Some women also complain about dizziness or nausea. The amount of progesterone you get this way is quite small. For this reason, most centers that use these advise patients to take the pills vaginally. The progesterone actually absorbs better than after swallowing them, and they're somewhat less messy than suppositories.

Other progesterone options are the following:

- **Crinone:** This progesterone gel is manufactured by Serono, a drug company that makes many fertility medications. Crinone causes less leakage and irritation than vaginal suppositories. It comes in an applicator that is inserted vaginally. Crinone is more expensive than vaginal suppositories.

- **Endometrin:** This is a vaginal suppository containing progesterone made by Ferring, another drug company that makes many fertility medications. The choice between Crinone or Endometrin is arbitrary.

- **Prometrium capsules, or compounded capsules:** These are pills, which means that if you take them orally, they pass through your liver after being digested in the stomach. The main disadvantage is that the way they're metabolized causes drowsiness, which can be severe. Some women also complain about dizziness or nausea. The amount of progesterone you get this way is quite small. For this reason, most centers that use these advise patients to take the pills vaginally. The progesterone actually absorbs better than after swallowing them, and they're somewhat less messy than suppositories.

The Waiting Game: Knowing What's Next

Before you leave the clinic after your egg retrieval, you will most likely find out how many eggs you have and be given a whole list of instructions on what to do next. Remember that the number of eggs resulting in an embryo is less than the number retrieved. Most clinics will tell you to take it easy at home and use the prescription pain medications as directed. Here are some other tips for the next few days:

» "Take it easy" means you should not be on the treadmill today! While we no longer expect bedrest (please don't do that!), many patients feel best if they take a short nap after the procedure and then treat themselves to an easy day at home in front of the TV or with a book.

» There are no points for "handling pain." This is not the time to be a hero, so take the recommended pain medication. Lisa always recommends taking the pain medication as soon as you get home and at least once more before you go to bed. For those who have had lots of eggs retrieved (more puncture sites!) taking pain medication every six hours for the first day after your retrieval is a good idea. Taking pain medication as prescribed after any procedure actually helps you recover faster!

» There may be vaginal spotting or bleeding. This is normal and should resolve within a few hours. Use a pad/pantiliner (not a tampon), and be sure to report any large amounts of bleeding to your clinic.

» Most patients can go back to their normal daily activities the next day.

Chapter **17**

The Care and Feeding of an Embryo: Amazing Teamwork in the Lab

The medical advances that enable IVF (in vitro fertilization) clinics to fertilize eggs and grow embryos in a lab are not only a science but also an art. The embryology team is skilled in working with the most precious of all biologic material: the eggs, sperm, and embryos that have the potential to become your child.

After you've completed the stimulation part of the IVF cycle and gone through an egg retrieval, everything is in the hands of the members of the embryology team. They're the ones who check your eggs, ready the sperm for fertilization, and keep those embryos growing until the day of transfer. They're often the gatekeepers of all news — good and bad — and you want to know everything they're doing.

In this chapter, we tell you what goes on in the lab, what the embryologists want to see, and what they *don't* want to see in eggs, sperm, and embryos. We talk about what you can find out from genetic testing on your embryos and how to understand genetic testing results. We also explain the transfer process and give some insight into how many embryos you may want to transfer.

Recognizing a Good Egg When You See One

Before you go home after retrieval (see Chapter 16), embryology will look at your eggs and may let you know whether they're mature, postmature, or immature. Mature eggs are needed for fertilization to occur, but immature eggs will often mature within 24 hours after retrieval. An egg retrieval often yields eggs that are both mature and immature, especially if you made a lot of follicles. If your eggs are postmature, they may not fertilize. However, the ability to judge eggs right after retrieval is somewhat limited by the fact that eggs are surrounded by a layer of cumulus cells, which protect the egg during ovulation but limit the ability of the embryologist to see details about the egg. They may not be able to tell you much about the eggs until the next day, when the sperm have dispersed the cumulus layer.

TECHNICAL STUFF

A mature egg is surrounded by a fluffy cumulus layer that allows the embryologist to see through it and identify the outline of the egg. In contrast, immature eggs have a tight, dense cumulus that has not yet expanded, which makes it very difficult to see the inner details of the egg. An immature egg still contains 46 chromosomes because the immature egg has not yet thrown off half of them, a step that's necessary before fertilization can take place.

When hCG or Lupron is given at the end of the IVF stimulation (or during the LH surge in a natural cycle), the egg, still in the follicle for 36 hours before being collected during an egg retrieval procedure, undergoes maturation. It separates its chromosomes in a process called *meiosis* and puts 23 of them into a small cell fragment called a polar body. This is what makes an egg "mature," meaning fertilizable. An immature egg has not yet successfully put out its polar body but may do so during the next day or so in the laboratory, becoming fertilizable at that point.

Embryologists use the term *postmature eggs* to describe those that are mature but may be dark and grainy looking. They tend not to fertilize and are sometimes associated with stimulations that go on too long; the embryologists say they are "overcooked." But this may not be the real reason the eggs don't fertilize, and postmature eggs may just be eggs that weren't meant to be embryos.

Prepping Sperm to Meet the Egg

If we have eggs, we will need sperm to create embryos! So, while you were having your eggs retrieved, your partner was probably collecting a sperm sample. Or, perhaps you are using frozen sperm from your partner or a sperm donor. Regardless of the method or source, the laboratory will be working with that specimen to get it ready to meet its partner. First comes identifying the appropriate specimen, and then the team takes it through a series of "washings" in special media to remove all the seminal fluid and isolate the sperm (pretty much like it's done for an intrauterine insemination). As the eggs are prepped, the sperm specimen is kept in an incubator until it's time to either inseminate the eggs by conventional methods or by going a little bit more high tech.

Conventional sperm insemination

If your partner's sperm is normal and your eggs are going to be fertilized in the lab with normal insemination, the next steps are as follows:

1. **The sperm are washed, and the egg is separated from the follicular fluid.**

    It still has its cumulus, which helps to activate the sperm.

2. **For standard IVF, your eggs (up to six to eight per dish) and sperm are placed a in dish that has wells so that each egg, or at most a couple, have its own chamber.**

    This step used to take place in a *petri dish,* a flat-bottomed round glass or plastic dish, which was labeled with your name, lab number, the date, and the number of eggs in the dish. This is so passé today.

3. **The dish is placed in an incubator so the eggs and sperm can be kept at body temperature. They're kept in a nutrient solution (culture medium), which provides conditions as similar as possible to those in the body.**

    Different labs use different culture media, and this is one way that labs differ from one another. However, today most labs purchase their media from a limited number of companies and there are only a few different types of media, so the media is standardized across the industry.

4. **Conventionally inseminated eggs are left alone for 16 to 20 hours.**

5. **The day after the retrieval, embryology takes the dish out of the incubator, strips off the cumulus (which has by now been greatly loosened by the action of the sperm), and checks the eggs.**

    What they hope to find is two pronuclear (2PN) embryos, or embryos that have two visible circles lined up next to each other (see Figure 17-1). These embryos contain the genetic material from each parent.

High-tech sperm injection

Since the advent of *intracytoplasmic sperm injection* (ICSI, discussed later in this chapter) the use of conventional insemination has decreased significantly. A report by the CDC states that from 1996 to 2012, the use of ICSI for male factor infertility rose from 76 percent to 93 percent and for couples without male factor from 15 percent to 66 percent. Using ICSI for male factor increases the chance that the egg will fertilize. Some men with male factor have sperm that can't penetrate the shell of the egg, and ICSI bypasses this problem. So, the use of ICSI for male factor makes sense. For couples with no male factor there is less of a need to do ICSI. The problem is that there is no test that accurately identifies the man with a normal semen analysis where his sperm can't fertilize the egg. The couple undergoes the entire IVF process, places the sperm and eggs together, and the next day finds that none of the eggs fertilized. This is not common but extremely disappointing when it occurs. For that reason, many IVF programs have significantly increased the use of ICSI.

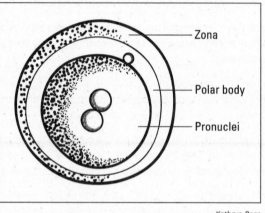

FIGURE 17-1: A 2PN (pronuclear) embryo.

— Zona

— Polar body

— Pronuclei

Kathryn Born

If you're planning to freeze some or all of your embryos for use at another time, your clinic may freeze them at the 2PN stage. Some centers grow all your embryos out to blastocyst stage and freeze only those that make it to blastocyst.

HAVING ATRETIC EGGS

Atretic eggs are dead; they're incapable of being fertilized. What would cause eggs to "die?" Some atretic eggs are postmature; they've been retrieved after their "peak freshness date," so to speak. This can happen when you have many eggs maturing at different rates; allowing time for smaller follicles to "catch up" may mean that a few of the larger eggs may become atretic. Some eggs are just poor-quality eggs and appear atretic.

Looking at What Can Go Wrong When Egg Meets Sperm

Good fertilization depends on the quality of the sperm and egg. At most centers, the fertilization rate is about 90 percent of the mature eggs. However, since the embryologists inseminate all the eggs, the overall fertilization rate that you should expect is closer to 60 percent. This reflects the fact that some eggs were not fertilizable. Why do they inseminate all the eggs? For one thing, judging maturity is not a perfect process, and even if an egg is immature at the time of insemination, it may still mature overnight and fertilize then. When embryologists look at the other 40 percent of the eggs, they may see things they'd rather not. For example, they may see the following:

>> Your embryos may be *polyploid,* meaning that they contain more than two pronuclei. This can occur when more than one sperm has entered the egg (polyspermy) or when the egg doesn't throw off the second polar body (which should occur at the time of fertilization). These embryos are never normal, because they contain too many chromosomes. Since each pronucleus contains 23 chromosomes, a triploid embryo (3 pronuclei) contains 69 chromosomes. Such an embryo will not grow into a baby and is not transferred.

>> The egg may still be immature. In this case, it may still be left in culture, even placed with sperm, with the hope that it will mature and fertilize later.

>> The egg may be mature yet show no signs of fertilization. In this case, the egg might be re-inseminated (by putting in some fresh sperm, hoping that the egg was immature when it started, has recently matured, and will now be able to be fertilized). Alternately, the embryologists may decide to fertilize the egg by using intracytoplasmic sperm injection (ICSI). Whereas fertilization can be achieved by this method, embryos resulting from "second day ICSI" have a lower chance of implanting, and some clinics feel that it is not worth the effort (or the cost!).

The High-Tech Meet-and-Greet: Doing ICSI

ICSI involves taking a sperm and injecting it into an egg. ICSI was developed to treat male factor infertility. Prior to ICSI, all eggs were fertilized by placing the sperm and eggs in a petri dish and hoping the egg would fertilize. Fertilization is a biochemical process, not a physical process. The sperm does not fight its way into the egg. There are proteins on the surface of the shell of the egg and on the egg that attach to proteins on the sperm. The initial attachment causes the sperm to release other proteins that digest a path through the shell. The proteins on the surface of the egg attach to the sperm, and the egg literally brings the sperm into the egg.

Since there are two ways to fertilize an egg, how do you choose which one to use? Information on the medical history of the man and his semen analysis are used to help decide if ICSI is needed. For example, the sperm from a man who has fathered any pregnancy, even if it was a miscarriage, and has a normal semen analysis most likely have the ability to fertilize an egg when they are placed in a petri dish — so ICSI is not required. However, sperm from a man who has never fathered a pregnancy of any kind and whose semen analysis is very abnormal, have a high probability of not being able to fertilize an egg. Here, ICSI is indicated. This leaves the gray zone. Many clinicians feel that ICSI is safe and will recommend ICSI for all patients to reduce the risk that the eggs will not fertilize (otherwise, a woman will go through the process of stimulation and retrieval for nothing).

If you and your doctor choose to do ICSI, after the eggs are retrieved, the embryologist removes the cumulus and the coronal layers from the egg, washes the sperm in a special solution, and then sits down at the microscope for a most delicate task. ICSI is done under a high-powered microscope and involves holding the egg steady with one pipette, while another is used to inject the sperm into its mid-section.

This task can be time consuming, and if moving, active sperm aren't available, the embryologist tries to pick out sperm for fertilization that are at least "twitching." Sperm obtained during a sperm aspiration (see Chapter 11 for more about sperm aspirations) are particularly notorious for not moving, and the embryologists sometimes put in extra chemicals to get them to twitch so that they can pick out the most viable ones!

TECHNICAL STUFF

ICSI is done with a very fine-gauge needle. The sperm is sucked into the needle, your egg is stabilized, and the needle point is slowly inserted into the egg. The process afterward is the same as conventional insemination. The ICSI eggs are left overnight and checked in the morning for fertilization. If the eggs haven't fertilized, ICSI can't be redone.

REMEMBER

Some studies have suggested that ICSI embryos may have a higher than normal rate of *aneuploidy,* or abnormal number of chromosomes. This higher rate may occur because some men with severe male factor have chromosomal abnormalities that can be transmitted to the offspring. Other factors that cause the man to have male factor infertility may also cause problems with his offspring and yet not be related to the ICSI procedure itself. For the most part, ICSI is safe and for many men with male factor it is necessary. However, as with any intervention, judicious use of ICSI can limit any hidden risks.

Answering the Call About the Embryos

An embryologist or clinical staff person usually calls the morning after your egg retrieval to let you know how many embryos you have and to discuss how many you are thinking you will want to transfer (the final decision will most likely have to be made on the day of transfer, when you will have a better idea of how they're growing). Freezing extra embryos has become very successful, in many cases more successful than transferring fresh embryos. Many centers prefer to culture all fertilized eggs for five or six days and only freeze those that survive. This reduces the number of nonviable embryos that are cryopreserved. Most physicians feel that today's improved culture conditions allow culturing the embryos for five days without compromising their ability to result in the birth of a child.

What "day" is it for the embryo?

You keep hearing the phrase "day-1, day-3, and so on" attached to your embryos, and you know it's not like the camel's question in the TV commercial. So why is the "day" so important? In a nutshell, the embryo day tells us what stage of development the embryo is (or should be) at. Day 1 is the first day after fertilization, day 2, the second day, and so on.

Embryologists refer to embryos as cleaving embryos or day 3 or day 5 embryos. On the day after the egg is fertilized, a normal embryo will have two circles, which are called pronuclei, and thus the embryo is called a 2 PN embryo.

Once fertilized, the embryo divides, and this is called a *cleavage stage embryo*. A two-cell, four-cell, or eight-cell embryo is a cleavage stage embryo. The four- to eight-cell embryo occurs three days after the egg is fertilized and thus is called a day 3 embryo. On day 4, the cells join and form a mass of cells, which is called a day 4 embryo or a *morula*. On day 5, the embryo forms a collection of fluid within itself, and since any fluid-filled space in the body is a cyst and the individual cells are called *blastomeres*, these embryos are called day 5 or 6 embryos or *blastocyst* embryos. As the blastocyst embryo develops, the fluid-filled space enlarges, and these are called expanded blastocyst embryos. Finally, sometime on day 5 or later, the embryo creates a hole in the shell and escapes from the shell. Just like a chicken egg, these are called hatching blastocyst embryos.

REMEMBER

Normal embryos follow a normal pattern of development, so any variation raises the chance that the embryo is not normal. For example, a morula embryo on day 6 will probably not be normal.

Understanding when embryos are checked

Everyone would like to know what the embryos are doing and, traditionally, the embryos were assessed daily. It turns out that embryos don't like that. So now it is common to put the embryos in an incubator, many times in their own tiny incubator, leave them alone, and only check them on day 5. Frustrating for those of us who want to know, but it makes for happy embryos — and we all want happy embryos. So don't be surprised if you do not hear about your embryos every day. Your center will tell you when they usually check and report on developing embryos.

Some centers still check the embryos on day 3. The embryologist looks at the embryo to see whether all of the cells look normal. Figure 17-2 shows a four-cell embryo. Some cells may stop growing, and many start to fall apart. This is called *fragmentation*, and the embryologist will try to estimate how much of the embryo has fragmented. Although a funny-looking embryo doesn't create a funny-looking kid, most embryologists do feel that an embryo with less fragmentation and more even-looking cells has a better chance of implanting. If you do get pregnant from fragmented embryos, the fragmentation does *not* mean that your baby will be abnormal in any way.

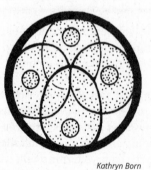

FIGURE 17-2:
A four-cell embryo.

Kathryn Born

Some centers remove the fragmented pieces before the embryo is transferred if the embryo has a significant amount of fragmentation. (See Figure 17-3 for a picture of an embryo with fragmentation.)

One study suggested that the size and location of the fragments was also important; removing large fragments improved pregnancy rates more than removing small or scattered fragments. However, fragment removal is one of those controversial areas of embryology; if the lab with which you're working doesn't do fragment removal, this doesn't mean they're not up to date. This is why embryology is not just science but also an art. Things that work in one lab may not work in another and may be felt to be unnecessary.

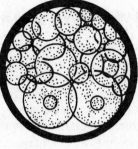

FIGURE 17-3:
An embryo
with a lot of
fragmentation.

Kathryn Born

Grading an embryo

On the day after the egg retrieval (day 1 of the embryo), an embryologist will review the status of your embryos. Over the years, considerable emphasis was placed on the quality of an embryo and the chance that that embryo would result in a successful pregnancy. Somehow, it made sense that an embryo that "looked good" under the light microscope would have a better chance of creating a pregnancy. And to a large extent, that is true. But the use of extended culture to five or six days and the introduction of preimplantation genetic screening for chromosomes numbers has altered the thinking about what it means when an embryo has a good score. Also, the use of timed cinematography has been applied to determine whether the embryo with the highest chance of success follows a certain timeline. Finally, considerable research is evaluating the metabolic status of the embryo as a possible help in finding the best embryo to transfer.

A current system for scoring blastocyst embryos is the Gardner scoring system. The system is based upon the anatomy of a blastocyst embryo, which has an outer shell of cells, an inner cell mass, and a fluid-filled cavity (hence the name blastocyst, where a cyst is any fluid-filled cavity). The numbers 1–6 are used to describe the cavity and the letters A, B, C are used to describe how many cells the outer layer and the inner cell mas have. Some centers have abandoned this system and just grade the embryo as Good, Fair, or Poor.

REMEMBER

A major reason embryos fail is that they do not have the correct number of chromosomes; the question is how accurately the appearance of an embryo reflects the chromosome number. The reality is — not much. Many studies have failed to find a significant correlation between the embryo scoring system and the number of chromosomes. Okay, fine. Now what are you supposed to do — test every embryo? That's probably overdoing it, so on a day-by-day basis using embryo scoring systems continues to provide advice about which embryos to transfer. Just be aware of the fact that a "beautiful" embryo may not be the "best" embryo.

Why are there fewer embryos than eggs?

You get the call about your embryos and there are only six — wait, wait, wait — you had ten eggs. What happened? Most people are surprised at how inefficient reproduction is considering there are almost always more eggs than embryos. Common sense would suggest that one egg = one embryo. However, even for women who have high-quality eggs (such as oocyte donors who are typically young and have no fertility issues) there is a large drop-off after fertilization between the number of oocytes and the number of embryos. When embryos are created from donor eggs, only 60–70 percent form blastocyst embryos, and of these as many as 30 percent are aneuploid. Eggs from older women have even fewer normal embryos, and for some, there will never be normal embryos. Since we expect fewer embryos than eggs in almost every case, you did great to get six embryos!

Testing That Embryo: Checking Genetics Before the Transfer

The word *genetic* is applied to a number of differing issues, and with today's technology, provides you with a number of options for finding out what is going on inside your embryos. Knowing about the number and quality of an embryo's chromosomes can help your doctor understand your fertility problem and give you a better idea of which embryos may lead to a live birth.

Considering your preimplantation testing options

Genetic disease refers to disease that is caused by errors in the genes and is passed from generation to generation. Advances in isolating and understanding genes now allow an embryo to be tested for abnormalities long before it is transferred back to a woman's uterus to try to establish a pregnancy. This is called *preimplantation genetic testing* (PGT). Today, there are several methods of testing that can give you very different, and more specific, information about your embryo. The choice of method often depends upon whether a specific abnormality is known, what information you want, and how much the procedure costs.

Checking chromosomes only: PGT-A

PGT-A, formerly called PGS, tests the embryo to count the number of chromosomes in the embryo. An embryo with an incorrect number of chromosomes is called an *aneuploid* embryo (which is the "A" in PGT-A) and is the leading reason why embryos fail to result in the birth of child. PGT-A is used to select out embryos that have too few chromosomes (like Turner syndrome) or too many chromosomes (such as Down syndrome). As chromosomes are being identified, this test is also used to determine the sex of the embryo and is helpful for patients who want to choose the sex of the embryo to be transferred. An embryo with the correct number of chromosomes is called a *euploid* embryo. Some embryos have some cells that have the correct number of chromosomes and other cells that have an incorrect number of chromosomes; these are called *mosaic* embryos.

Checking known defective genes: PGT-M

PGT-M, formerly called PGD, tests embryos to determine whether they have a genetic disease caused by mutations in a single (mono) gene, or, in other words, if there is a monogenic defect (the "M" in PGT-M). Some patients know that certain diseases such aa cystic fibrosis or Huntington's disease run in their families. There are literally hundreds of diseases caused by single gene defects, which may result in a child with an inherited disease because one or both parents have the gene defect, or the gene defect occurs for the first time *(de novo)*. The use of next-gen sequencing in PGT-M allows for the rapid diagnosis of gene defects so that using embryos that carry the defect can be avoided.

Checking structural defects: PGT-SR

PGT-SR, formerly called PGD, tests the embryo to determine whether the chromosomes have structural abnormalities — in other words, the chromosomes do not line up the way they are supposed to. The misalignment can be rearrangements, or the addition or subtraction of a chromosome. PGT-SR is indicated for patients who have balanced structural chromosome rearrangements (called balanced translocations or inversions) and are at risk for creating embryos with abnormal chromosome structures or numbers.

If you carry a genetic disease or sex-linked disease, are over age 35, or have a history of repeated miscarriage, you may want to check your embryo's genetic status before transferring. Pre-implantation genetic testing makes it possible to check an embryo for some common chromosomal abnormalities and can also determine whether the embryo will be a boy or girl. The procedure doesn't come cheap, however; centers charge around $5,000 (and up!) for PGD. The cost includes the laboratory charge for performing the test and the charges that the genetics lab charges for their testing, and these may or may not be covered by insurance. The charges may also include a fee for freezing the embryos because currently used testing blastocyst embryos requires freezing the embryos. Most laboratories base their charges on testing a set number of embryos (frequently eight) and then a per-embryo fee for any testing done on more than eight embryos. Finally, some women who produce a limited number of embryos may choose to batch by doing multiple egg retrievals where the fees are based upon eight embryos. For example, a woman may only have three embryos that survive to the blastocyst stage. She may choose to do another stimulation and retrieval to obtain more embryos and then have them all tested at the same time.

How is PGT (any kind) done?

Preimplantation genetic testing has undergone a major change from when it was first introduced into IVF. Originally, PGD was done by removing a cell, called a blastomere, from an eight-celled embryo, and then testing that one cell for either the number of chromosomes or for a specific genetic defect (like sickle cell anemia) or a genetic quality (like an HLA tissue match). The testing was done by a process called FISH and could only test for a limited number of chromosomes, which meant that many abnormalities were undiagnosed. Furthermore, removing one cell from an eight-cell embryo removes 12.5 percent of the mass of the embryo — probably not a good idea. Advances in the understanding of the biology of the embryo permitted embryos to be cultured for five or six days, where they became blastocyst embryos with over 130 cells. Furthermore, at the blastocyst stage the embryo is composed of an outer layer of cells that become the placenta and an inner cell mass that becomes the embryo. At the same time, genetic testing advanced significantly so that single errors in the genetic code could be detected using "next-generation" sequencing. Today, PGT is done by making a small hole in the shell of the embryo using a laser on day 4. The embryo starts to hatch through this hole so that on day 5, the embryologist can easily slice off a few cells for diagnosis — usually four to six. Thus, the embryo is at a later stage of development so that those embryos that are so abnormal that they don't reach the blast stage are not assayed. The assays are more accurate and test for all chromosomes. Finally, far less mass of the embryo is removed.

Does PGT improve my pregnancy chances?

On balance, advances in preimplantation genetic testing have added another valuable weapon to its arsenal for resolving fertility issues by helping us choose good embryos. Some IVF centers are reporting pregnancy rates of 50–70 percent per embryo. A far cry from the early rates of 5 percent. PGT can specifically test for the following, among others:

>> Common trisomies (meaning an extra copy of the gene is present), such as Trisomy 13, 18, and 21 (Down syndrome)

>> Single gene inherited genetic disease, such as cystic fibrosis, sickle cell anemia, and Huntington's disease

>> Anomalies of the X and Y chromosomes, such as Klinefelter (male child has 47 chromosomes, including XXY) and Turner (female with only 45 chromosomes; only one X is present) syndrome

>> Gender-linked disorders, such as hemophilia

REMEMBER

PGT does not increase the pregnancy rate per retrieval. Whenever a rate is used it is important to remember that a rate is one number divided by another. Consider, as an example, a retrieval results in ten eggs, and after adding sperm, three eggs create embryos that are normal or euploid. (Remember, it is unusual to get ten normal embryos from ten eggs, as some eggs will not fertilize, and some embryos may not be normal and will not survive.) So three out of ten eggs make normal embryos or a 30 percent rate. Suppose on day 3 only seven embryos survive to the eight-cell stage. The three normal embryos still remain, but now the rate of normal embryo formation is 3/7 or 42 percent. Now suppose only five embryos make it to day 5. The three normal ones are still there, but the normal blast formation *rate* is 60 percent. That sounds like the chance of having a normal embryo from the retrieval has increased, but in reality, the normal have been there all along. PGT-A information reduces the miscarriage rate and allows for single embryo transfers. It also gives information that can be used to assess a woman's ability to produce euploid embryos.

Choosing an embryo to transfer

Now that the embryos have been tested, catalogued, and are literally "on ice" waiting for the next step, how do you know which embryo should be transferred? If all the embryos come back labeled "normal" or *euploid*, the decision is fairly easy, and the discussion involves how many rather than which one. However, many PGT reports come back with a variety of labels. So how do you know what to do?

Understanding the PGT results

Reports from the genetic testing agencies are becoming very detailed and — for those who don't have a PhD in genetics — confusing. The easiest way to interpret these is to look at the column to the far right on most reports and see whether it says normal or abnormal. Usually the column to the left of this has a detailed structural description when the chromosomes are abnormal. But the best bet is to look at the body of the report, where there is usually a very detailed but understandable description of any abnormality (most physicians rely on this section of the report to help them understand any abnormality). If all of that fails, as it often will, there are genetic counselors at most of the testing laboratories who can help you understand what the results mean.

Making decisions about "mosaic" embryos

Of course, with any new technology, along with improved benefits comes a new set of problems. For example, testing four to six cells at a position away from the inner cell mass and not testing the inner cell mass raises the question about how accurately those cells that were tested reflect the true status of the inner cell mass, which forms the baby. It has also become apparent that not all cells in some embryos are alike. Some may have a normal number of chromosomes, but others may have an abnormal number of chromosomes. These embryos are called *mosaics*, and if the embryo is a mosaic, it raises the question about transferring an embryo that is *partially* abnormal. An embryo with a small percentage of abnormal cells can develop into a normal child. Those with a higher percent of abnormal cells usually do not result in a live birth because the embryo either doesn't implant or results in an early miscarriage. So, most tests now report the percentage of mosaicism, but this still creates a dilemma as there is still too little data to indicate much mosaicism is too much. The best solution for this dilemma is currently an area of considerable inquiry. Some patients choose to discard mosaic embryos, others choose to transfer them and take a chance on a normal child, and still others are keeping these embryos frozen until there is more information. Careful discussion between a patient and the physician is needed to make an informed decision about this problem.

What happens to the "abnormal" embryos?

Abnormal embryos can occur before genetic testing is done and are assessed by how the embryos appear under the light microscope. Very abnormal appearing embryos are nonviable, will not continue to develop or result in the birth of a child, and are disposed of in the laboratory. But an embryo may have major genetic abnormalities and appear perfectly normal under the light microscope. If these embryos are tested by PGT and are then found to be genetically abnormal, they are also discarded. However, low-level mosaic embryos may be kept, and possibly even transferred. As the "rules" on what is an abnormal embryo are changing, we may see more technically "abnormal" mosaic embryos retained (frozen for later use) while grossly abnormal or genetically defective embryos continue to be discarded.

Hatching Embryos — Come on Out of There!

Around 1994, embryologists came out with a new technique called *assisted hatching* (AH) to help human embryos implant in the uterus. The majority of IVF centers do hatching on at least some of their embryos.

Hatching was originally done only on embryos whose zona was thicker than normal or on embryos from women over age 37, whose embryos may have a harder time breaking out of the shell. Now, some centers do assisted hatching on almost all of their embryos, others still do AH only on certain patients, and some use it on frozen-thawed embryos. The use of zona drilling has come under criticism, and fewer cycles are having zona drilling.

Over time, there has been a change from transferring day 3 embryos to extending the culture period, creating day 5 or day 6 blastocyst embryos. These embryos can thin the zona as a part of their normal development, so AH on a blastocyst embryo is unnecessary. However, if the embryologists look at the embryo and feel that AH would help, they will frequently perform AH anyway. Where preimplantation genetic testing is being done, hatching is necessary to get the cells needed for the genetic tests.

Looking at the Embryos' Next Home: Your Uterine Lining

Embryos will implant only if the uterus is ready for implantation. Proper conditions for implantation are both anatomic and physiologic and way too complex to be tested. However, there seems to be a correlation between the physical pattern of the uterine lining (endometrium) and its appearance on ultrasound. This is particularly true for frozen embryo transfer cycles. Many centers use ultrasound to look at the uterine lining thickness and appearance, called the *pattern*, to decide whether your embryos have a good chance of implanting after transfer. Your lining may be described as triple lined, also called *tri-laminar* (TL) and describes the lining most clinics like to see before embryo transfer.

REMEMBER

Clinics vary on the importance of lining patterns, and your clinic may not even check the pattern or may have a different method for evaluating lining readiness. Some centers measure the estrogen level as an additional marker for the chance for an embryo to implant. Other centers do a mock cycle and perform an endometrial biopsy to see whether the biochemical profile is what it should be for the highest chance of implantation (*endometrial receptivity assays*). Most centers, however, do check the lining thickness before transfer; anything over 6 millimeters thick is considered adequate, although pregnancies do occur with thinner linings. Your center's emphasis on the importance of the lining thickness or pattern may vary.

Undergoing the Embryo Transfer

Well, here we are. Another hurdle passed — you have embryos, they've been deemed "good," and you are all signed up for your embryo transfer. The clinic staff have given you lots of information on your medications (oh yeah — that progesterone was started!), and now you are ready for the next step in trying to get pregnant. This will be one of the easiest procedures you undergo in the IVF process, but it still has a few things to consider, like how many embryos to put back, what the transfer day is like, and what happens afterwards.

Knowing what to expect: How many embryos to transfer?

A few years ago, IVF centers became alarmed at the large number of higher-order multiples (triplets or more) their patients were delivering, and they started looking for ways to transfer fewer embryos and still maintain the all-important high pregnancy rates.

The topic of how many embryos to transfer has taken center stage with two forces at work. First, ASRM has published guidelines concerning how many embryos to transfer. (You can find them online at www.fertstert.org/article/S0015-0282(17)30227-3/abstract.) The actual decision is made in consultation with the embryologist and the physician since each cycle is different and using standard guidelines may not reflect the situation for a given couple.

The problem is that a majority of failed IVF cycles where embryos were transferred is due to the embryo having the wrong number of chromosomes. Looking at an embryo under the light microscope can identify those embryos that are abnormal and not viable. But an embryo may look perfectly fine and yet have a very abnormal number of chromosomes. Even when donor eggs are used, up to 30 percent of the embryos that look fine may have the wrong number of chromosomes. Therefore, transferring more than one embryo increases the chance that a normal embryo will be transferred.

In the early days of IVF, the chance that an embryo would implant (implantation rate) was as low as 5 percent. Advances in technology have now resulted in implantation rates in young patients as high as 30–35 percent. As women age, more and more of the remaining eggs are damaged and create embryos with the wrong number of chromosomes.

Looking at issues such as poor-quality embryos, multiple failed IVF cycles, or patients of advanced maternal age, the ASRM guidelines suggest transferring only one embryo when the conditions are ideal but not more than three even under unfavorable conditions. However, the increasing use of PGT-A has modified the issue of how many embryos to transfer. The ASRM guidelines are based upon the chance that the embryo will have the wrong number of chromosomes. If the embryo is tested and found to have the correct number of chromosomes, then the argument for transferring more than one embryo fades away.

Where the embryos have been tested and have the correct number of chromosomes, only a single embryo needs to be transferred. This strategy reduces the chance for twins to the lowest possible rate. The reason this is important is that while the concept of twins seems exciting to many couples, the fact is that twins have increased risks for almost all common risk factors in pregnancy. Most important is the risk of prematurity where the children are born very early and survive but are left with a lifetime of disability.

REMEMBER

Choosing how many embryos to transfer remains a difficult decision. But discussion among the patient, the embryologist, and the physician helps make a decision that when things don't turn out as planned still seems like the best decision viewed in hindsight.

What's a good transfer day? Day 3? Day 5? Any other?

Most IVF centers are doing day 5 transfers, but that is up to the center and the patient. There are pros and cons for each day. Sometimes the clinic may want to see if the embryos get to the blastocyst stage, and in other cases physicians are waiting for PGT results (which takes time). The reality is that there is no strong evidence to choose one day over the other.

Describing the "oh-so-much-easier" procedure

The embryo transfer process has been made quick and easy — especially the prep! Most centers let you eat and drink normally, and your medications generally stay the same — no middle-of-the night shots and no anesthesia! When you arrive for your embryo transfer, you'll be taken to the IVF suite.

When you get to the transfer room, you'll be instructed to lie on an exam table that can be tilted. The worst part of the transfer in most clinics is that you're lying there with a full bladder. Embryo transfers are done using ultrasound guidance. Most of these are done with abdominal ultrasound and require the bladder to be full. You will be instructed to drink about 32 ounces of fluid before your transfer time, so that you feel like you "gotta go *now*." A full bladder, uncomfortable as it is, makes it easier to see your uterus under abdominal ultrasound guidance. Your bladder, lying right over the uterus, pushes your uterus back when it's full; this also straightens the path into the uterus, making the transfer easier. Most embryo transfers are done under ultrasound guidance rather than blindly placing them through the cervix. In some cases, especially for patients who are obese or have a retroverted uterus, the physician may use vaginal ultrasound for the embryo transfer because abdominal ultrasound may not allow them to see the uterus as well.

An embryologist or your doctor may come in to speak with you before the transfer. That person will tell you how your embryos look today, may show or give you pictures, will verify your identity, and will confirm the number of embryos to transfer. You'll most likely receive something to sign that says that you agree to transfer X number of embryos, that you understand the risks of multiple birth, that you realize there's no guarantee of success, and that you are who you say you are.

The actual embryo transfer is a relatively simple vaginal procedure. You will be awake as an abdominal ultrasound probe is placed on your abdomen and your doctor places a speculum and slides a tiny introducer catheter through your cervix. The embryo(s) are "loaded" with a small amount of fluid into another catheter, which your doctor slips through the first catheter. The embryo(s) and fluid are then released into your uterus near its top. In case you are wondering, the ultrasound pictures do not show the embryos being inserted, as they are microscopic. Instead, your doctor is looking at the tip of the catheter for the best placement and the fluid being released. Ideally, the whole procedure takes about fifteen minutes, although you may lie in the transfer room for a few minutes longer until the clinic staff get you up, give you directions, and send you home!

Clinics vary widely in their bed rest requirements, and they may keep you anywhere from no time at all to up to a few hours. Recent research has suggested that less is better, and now many clinics have you rest on the transfer table for only a few minutes, after which you are free to do anything you want. This makes a certain amount of sense when you consider that women conceiving naturally never know when the embryo has entered the uterus and is about to implant. So medically, activity levels after transfer don't matter. The real question is what your mind will do if you do something or don't do something (rest for a day or two) if you don't get pregnant. Did lifting those heavy groceries from the car keep you from getting pregnant? No — but who cares if that's the guilt trip your mind is playing on you? So, in general: If you are considering doing something and you have any question about whether it might keep you from getting pregnant, don't do it — the life of guilt is not worth the price.

TIP

Embryos are placed directly into your uterus; emptying your bladder or bowels isn't going to dislodge them! Neither will coughing or sneezing. Any fluid discharge you may experience after the transfer is usually the fluid used to clean your cervix that may have pooled in the vagina. However, it's easy to get constipated during this time because you're usually taking progesterone and may have reduced activity. This will make you uncomfortable, never mind more worried about straining! It's best to take a gentle stool softener, like milk of magnesia (which doesn't absorb from the bowel) or add extra fiber in your diet.

"Fresh" transfer prep

If you're not doing any PGT on your embryos, you're not in danger of OHSS, and you don't have any other reason to freeze your embryos, you will probably have an embryo transfer within the week after your egg retrieval. As discussed earlier, you and your doctor will decide which day will be optimal for your transfer. Regardless of the day, these are generally known as "fresh" transfers — basically because the embryos were never frozen. In order to get you ready for a fresh transfer, you most likely had instructions to add certain medications (such as progesterone) to your IVF cycle med routine.

Choosing the "frozen" path to a transfer

The use of frozen embryo transfer has increased dramatically in the last few years. Driving this increase is the increased use of PGT-A, the reduced risk for OHSS (ovarian hyperstimulation syndrome, discussed in detail in Chapter 14) in PCOS patients, and the discovery that frozen embryo cycles have a higher chance of success under certain circumstance.

The process of embryo transfer is considerably different when comparing fresh verses frozen transfer. When doing a fresh transfer, the stimulation part of the cycle has prepared the lining of the uterus to accept the embryo. Furthermore, the ovary will produce progesterone after the retrieval even though most evidence suggests supplementing that with progesterone after the retrieval.

When the transfer is done using frozen embryos, there are two major ways to do this:

>> One way is to just monitor a natural cycle and transfer the embryo on the day it would normally be in the uterus. This has the advantage of simplicity. Many centers use this method with no compromise in pregnancy rates.

>> However, many centers prefer to artificially prepare the lining of the uterus and control exactly when to transfer the embryo based upon the age of the embryo and the time from the initiation of progesterone, which sets the "implantation window."

Each center has their own protocol for doing this so that they can maximize their success rates. Since there is no "best" way, the method that gives the center their highest chance of success is the appropriate method for that center.

Post Transfer Tips and Boosts

For the most part, it's all up to the embryo after the transfer! The best thing you can do to enhance implantation is to stay on your medications and follow your clinic's directions. After you're safely home, you may or may not be given restricted activity for a period of time, depending on your clinic's policies. Studies vary on the impact of activity after an embryo transfer, but most debunk the "don't move" myth. Try not to compare what you're doing to what anyone else is doing, because different centers have different policies. If you don't follow your center's policies, you're bound to feel guilty if you don't get pregnant, so follow your instruction sheet.

If your center restricts activity after the transfer, you'll be lying around on the bed or couch, getting up only to use the bathroom and eat meals. After your strict rest period is over, many centers still ask you not to lift anything heavy (over 15 pounds is typical), not to do any strenuous exercise, and not to have sex.

Sex may be restricted because it may cause uterine contractions, especially if you have an orgasm, so if your clinic ascribes to the no-sex rule, then the no-sex rule applies to *any* activity that could cause an orgasm, not just intercourse. So, follow this advice or find a clinic with no restrictions on sexual activity. Again, applying what happens to women conceiving naturally, sexual restrictions do not apply, and yet here we are.

TIP

Heavy lifting is another unsubstantiated (some say ridiculous) common prohibition that can cause needless concern. Women evolved to be able to be fully functioning during all phases of conceiving and childbearing. Just because you needed to use IVF does not put you into a fragile, handle-with-care class.

REMEMBER

If your IVF cycle resulted in increased ovarian response and a large number of embryos were retrieved, then exercise restrictions make sense until your ovaries have returned to their normal size. But for frozen embryo transfers, exercise restrictions are an unsubstantiated concern. Use common sense about working out and all physical activity, including whatever else you do to decrease stress and increase endorphins. Lisa has a rule of thumb with all post-transfer activity — if it is something that you will always regret doing if you end up "not pregnant" after this cycle, don't do it! The possibility of future guilt over that closet you cleaned out or the water skiing you did (it *is* just a little water skiing) is just not worth it.

Chapter **18**

Keeping Your Head in the Game: Successfully Waiting after an IVF Cycle

inishing up an in vitro fertilization (IVF) cycle brings a whole host of emotions. You're happy that the procedure itself was successful and that the shots are finished or at least greatly diminished. You're ecstatic about having your life back, without the frequent blood draws, ultrasounds, and phone calls. On the other hand, you may feel adrift when the intensity is over, and you've gone from constant monitoring to almost no contact with your clinic. Now it's time to wait for your pregnancy test. Because the test results won't be accurate for almost two weeks after your embryo transfer, this time period is often referred to by patients as "the two-week wait."

In this chapter, we review some of the do's and don'ts of the two-week wait and take a little peek into the future when you'll have an answer to the big question — am I pregnant or not? — and what you'll do in either case.

Not "Not Pregnant" — But Waiting for Proof

From a purely technical viewpoint, after the embryos are placed into your uterus, you're pregnant — in the loosest sense of the word, at least. Embryos don't float, though that's a common misperception. The embryos rapidly attach and begin to invade the uterine lining. None of this is perceptible to you because it is at the submicroscopic level.

This may be the first time in your infertility history where you can say without a doubt that you've formed an embryo and that it is where it needs to be to grow. You may have known that you made a follicle and been fairly sure that you got sperm where it needed to go at the right time, but you never knew for sure that the egg and sperm got together. Now you do.

Now comes the waiting period. The two-week wait is a time of "what ifs" and "if onlys" like no other time you've probably experienced. Because this is new territory for you, we give some ideas on how to make it through the two-week wait without driving yourself crazy.

Meds without monitoring and feeling a little left out by the clinic

After all of the monitoring, ultrasounds, blood draws, and so on, you would think that this would continue into the post-transfer period. You would be wrong. As illogical as it seems, once the stage is set, the players — the embryo and the uterus — do their part with very little ability to rewrite the script at this point.

The fact that the clinic is not hounding you daily doesn't mean that they don't care. They do, and if you could see how the members of the IVF team wait daily for the pregnancy test results and see the exaltation or rejection they feel with the positive and the negative test results, you would appreciate the fact that they care very much. Like you, the IVF team wishes they could do something to make the cycle a success, and frequently, like you, they feel the frustration of having to wait.

Keeping busy: do's and don'ts

REMEMBER

Although you may be tempted to just relax and wait, unencumbered by other responsibilities, the truth is that sitting around waiting is hard work, a lot harder than keeping yourself busy with everyday tasks. Waiting for water to boil and staring at it is a quick recipe for instant irritation, and so is staying idle during these two weeks. More importantly, relaxing and waiting does not improve the outcome, nor does keeping busy. Which one works best for *you?*

TIP

Try to plan as many activities as you can manage (after your post-transfer rest period). If you work, consider it a blessing and immerse yourself in your responsibilities. Many women suggest reading a good book to get you through this time. Try to keep the book as far away from the topic of fertility as possible. Exercise is also a good way to keep busy, but keep it mild, like walking around the block. Many couples find that the two-week wait is a great time to take a vacation. What better way to distract yourself than with a little R&R? However, Dr R. isn't so sure a vacation at this time is a good idea if you will spend it worrying whether you are pregnant or not. Not knowing can drive you crazy, not to mention influence whether you can have that cocktail, go parasailing, and so on. You may want to wait until you have an answer and then decide on an appropriate trip — either to celebrate or regroup for the next step in your fertility journey.

If the tension does begin to run high, assemble your backup plan. What will you do next, pregnant or not? This type of planning often alleviates the fear and uncertainty that accompany the two-week wait.

Making your to-do or not-to-do list

Taking care of yourself during the roller coaster ride of trying to create a baby is crucial. For some women, this may mean a trip to the hairdresser, manicurist, gym, or all of the above. But you should consider a few limitations as you wait out these last few weeks before your pregnancy test.

Coloring your hair

For those whose follicle challenges begin at the top of their heads, hair coloring is more than just a luxury; it's a way of life. To color or not to color has been a long-time topic of discussion among the newly pregnant. According to the American College of Obstetricians and Gynecologists, hair coloring *is* safe during pregnancy. Based on this opinion, coloring your hair during the two-week wait is also presumed to be safe (unless, of course, your colorist turns your hair orange!). However, keep in mind that the two-week wait is only two weeks. If you're at all concerned, staying off the bottle (of color, that is) for the time being may be the best advice for you.

Manis and pedis

The greatest danger that we know of in manicures and pedicures is for those who give them. You may have noticed that many manicurists now wear masks to protect themselves from the fumes and toxins generated by the products. A simple polish-and-go won't hurt you during the two-week wait. Those with acrylic nails are advised to refrain from having this service during the two-week wait, and those who don't have acrylic nails but want them are better off waiting until after the two-week wait, and after the first trimester of pregnancy for that matter. If you already have acrylic nails, don't panic, but you may consider having them removed before your cycle.

Getting your exercise

REMEMBER

Exercise can be a great way to take your mind off your waiting and your worries during the two-week wait. Here are two basic rules to remember with exercise during this time:

>> Don't start up a brand-new routine during the two-week wait. In other words, if you're not a runner, don't become one now. Keep your exercise routine consistent with that in which you engaged before.

>> Keep your heart rate equal to or lower than 140 beats per minute. This rate is also recommended during pregnancy, so this is a good time to get used to keeping track of it. Most fitness stores sell inexpensive heart rate monitors, and certain exercise machines (such as particular brands of treadmills) have a built-in monitor that can read your heart rate when you grasp the metal sensors on the handlebar.

Keep in mind that moderation must become your middle name, in judgment and in exercise. Should you choose the two-week wait as the ideal time to scale Mount Everest? We think not. Nor do we recommend skydiving for novices (or even experts) during this time. Both activities, aside from being highly dangerous, also pose the added risk of high altitude, which may be hazardous for those unaccustomed to it. However, if you live in Denver, the mile-high city, you don't have to move.

The age-old recommendation surrounding pregnancy and then IVF was "take it easy." That concept has been challenged, and there is mounting evidence that this advice is unnecessary. Consider that women evolved in an incredibly harsh and physically/nutritionally challenged world. None of us could live more than a few days as did our early ancestors. So, evolution designed the body to handle these harsh conditions.

Also consider that the world of the early embryo and uterus is a microscopic world. It is *impossible* to physically damage an intrauterine embryo or pregnancy without severe damage to the mother. You could, it you really wanted to, alter some of your chemistry, but even here you would need to do significant damage before being able to influence the outcome of the IVF cycle.

There is an abundance of evidence that exercise does not reduce the chance for success with IVF, and some forms of exercise may actually be beneficial. There is a caveat to all of this. If you have had any form of ovarian stimulation (clomid, letrozole, FSH of IVF), then your ovaries are larger than they normally are. There have been reports that exercise during the time the ovaries are enlarged can result in the ovaries twisting and shutting off the blood supply to the ovaries (this is called *ovarian torsion*, which is an emergency situation that usually requires surgery to correct). The symptoms are sudden onset of severe pain on one side of the lower abdomen. If this happens, go immediately to an ER where they can do an ultrasound using color-flow Doppler to see if the ovaries are being perfused with blood. If diagnosed early, the ovary can be saved and, for the most part, the surgery will not influence the outcome of the pregnancy.

REMEMBER

The two-week wait calls for maintaining the status quo. Leave the new stuff for later.

Traveling — particularly out of the country

Travel during the wait time won't influence the outcome. But a little common sense seems in order (and you really need to read the section on Zika in Chapter 4).

First, if you are out of reach from your IVF clinic, they can't help you if you run into problems. Most developed countries have excellent reproductive services, but unless you are fluent in that country's language, you won't understand what they want to do — no matter how appropriate — and they won't understand your issues. Not uncommonly, an IVF clinic will get a frantic call from a patient in a foreign country because her medication got lost, broken, or she ran out, and now needs to get medication immediately. This is not always easy far away from home.

TIP

Traveling immediately after your IVF cycle is not a clear "no-no," but you have to ask yourself, *Is it really that necessary?* A trip three states away to a family wedding (where there is great medical care and you speak the language) weighs a whole lot differently than a romantic week in Bora Bora (where they speak French).

Having sex during the two-week wait

WARNING

Historical statement:*"For those going through the two-week wait after in vitro fertilization, sex is considered a no-no (at least by most doctors). You've had surgery (albeit minor), and the risk of infection may be greater, so hands (and other body parts) off during this time. Another concern is that female orgasm may cause a series of uterine contractions, which are not ideal in creating a hospitable environment for baby embryo. Read a good book instead."* PLEASE KEEP READING . . .

Let's take another long look at the preceding warning. Like many older recommendations, the concept of abstinence around IVF is losing its credibility. First, IVF is not really surgery — a hysterectomy is surgery; a delivery is surgery — but not IVF. IVF is more like a biopsy where a very thin needle is passed through the vaginal wall. Antibiotics are used to prevent infection, and the puncture site closes over very rapidly — often before you get home. Also, for a while, it was popular to place semen in the vagina at the time of ART because the thinking was that it actually helped in implantation. An article published in 2000 concluded that exposure to semen around the time of embryo transfer actually increased the implantation rate. Thus, for a frozen embryo transfer where there is no retrieval and no enlarged ovaries, intercourse may actually be helpful — certainly not harmful — and may actually be fun.

But what about after an IVF cycle where the ovaries are stimulated? Most women will experience discomfort if they have had a good stimulation because the ovaries are large and bouncing them around hurts. So again, use moderation and common sense — if it hurts, stop. And that includes pain to your psyche as well. Remember, pamper yourself during the two-week wait — doctor's orders!

TIP

Dr. R. isn't so sure that all the planning to relieve tension during the two-week wait is going to be helpful. All the planning in the world does very little to actually alleviate the tension of waiting for something this important. His suggestion: Admit your feelings and for two weeks let the world deal with it — you earned that right!

Sensing Every Little Twinge: The Truth about Pregnancy Symptoms

Of course, you're anxious. Of course, you're anxiously examining every twinge and cramp you have for some indication of whether you're pregnant. If you're taking progesterone, as you most likely are after an IVF cycle, the symptoms of pregnancy can easily be confused with symptoms of progesterone supplementation, because an increase in progesterone is associated with many common pregnancy symptoms. What might you experience, and which signs are good, bad, and meaningless? Here are some symptoms you may experience and what they mean:

>> **Sore breasts:** Tender breasts are almost a universal sign of pregnancy, with or without feelings of heaviness or tingling in the nipples. Unfortunately, sore breasts are caused by increased progesterone and estrogen, so sore breasts may be caused by the ovarian stimulation you underwent or your suppositories rather than by a growing embryo.

>> **Spotting:** This symptom is very common in very early pregnancy, whether or not you've undergone fertility treatment. If you're taking progesterone suppositories, irritation from the suppositories can also cause some spotting.

>> **Cramping:** This discomfort is typical in the two-week wait and may be caused by the enlarged ovaries if you've done a medicated cycle (taken ovarian stimulating medications, as discussed in Chapter 14).

>> **Fatigue:** This symptom is often related to higher-than-normal levels of hCG (human chorionic gonadotropin, the injection given 36 or so hours before an egg retrieval) and progesterone, both of which can be from the growing embryo or from your hCG trigger shot. Progesterone pills are particularly noted for causing extreme fatigue. Plus you're probably emotionally exhausted from the IVF cycle! This is a perfectly good time to get extra rest.

>> **Nausea:** This symptom is fairly common with progesterone, especially in pill form, and also with high levels of hCG. Higher-than-normal levels of estrogen can also cause nausea.

So how can you tell whether you're pregnant in the two-week wait? Unfortunately, you really can't. Lisa can name dozens of patients who swore they were not pregnant — even one who had a full period. Continue taking your meds even if you're *sure* you're not pregnant, because you might be wrong!

WARNING

Never, never, never (did we say "never"?) stop taking your meds until directed to by your fertility clinic.

Checking on Your Own: Home Pregnancy Test Traps

Most women find the temptation of a home pregnancy test (HPT) impossible to resist. Those little packaged sticks promise immediate results and an answer to the question "Am I pregnant or not?" Before you go out and buy up your druggist's supply of home pregnancy tests, consider the following:

>> Many home pregnancy tests require a minimum amount of hCG in your system in order to register a positive. Early pregnancy may not result in a high enough number to register, even if you are pregnant.

>> You were most likely given an hCG shot to trigger ovulation before your IVF retrieval. That shot of 10,000 units of hCG doesn't leave your system overnight. Furthermore, it's the same hormone (the pregnancy hormone) measured in

home pregnancy tests. For some women, the traces of the hCG shot can take 10 to 15 days to disappear. Your HPT doesn't know that though! This can result in a false positive and a big letdown when the moment of truth arrives.

>> Home pregnancy tests (HPTs) are, first and foremost, over-the-counter devices. They do not replace a *beta hCG* — a blood test that measures the level of hCG. Don't expect the same accuracy or reliability from drugstore pregnancy tests. (See Chapter 6 for more info on HPTs.)

WARNING

Many women get on the HPT roller coaster, allowing their emotions to rise and fall with each subsequent pee stick. It isn't worth it. Wait for the real thing, as hard as the waiting may be. You have no reason to subject yourself to a test that could very well yield incorrect results.

Coauthor Jackie spent *far* too much time and money "testing" with HPTs. When she didn't see a visible line, she would hold the stick up to a variety of stronger lights to see if a "shadow" existed. Imagine her disappointment (*long* after the fact!) when Lisa shared with her that the line she was seeing (in shadow form, no less) was the one "built-in" to be activated by hCG, if present. All that money spent then (HPTs are *not* cheap!) could have bought a whole lot of Starbucks today!

Waiting for the News

It's beta day — the day your blood tests reveal whether you're pregnant or not.

Waiting for the phone to ring is almost always unpleasant, but modern technology has given us answering machines and voicemail so that you don't have to sit by the phone! Take advantage of this technology.

Deciding how and where you want the news

If you choose not to be home when the phone rings, alert the nurse or doctor who will be calling you with your results. Do you want that information left on your answering machine? Is there a chance that your little sister, mother, or cleaning person might hear the results instead, and perhaps forget to tell you? Work out these details ahead of time and communicate them to those who'll be delivering your results.

Planning to receive this call at work may not be the best idea, unless you have a private area and/or supportive people around you. If you don't want to be called at work, make this fact very clear to the nurses and/or doctor as well. Some choose to have their partners receive the news. If you feel that hearing the news from someone close to you would be easier, consider this option and put it into action. You can't control the news you'll hear, but you can control the way you hear it.

Understanding what the test results really mean

So, you got the call or the email or the text and the news is your beta hCG is "X." Is that a positive or a negative? Are you pregnant? Are you not pregnant? What does that number mean? False positives are rare in pregnancy tests. You're most likely to get a false positive result on either a home pregnancy test or a beta sub-unit if it's been less than two weeks since you took hCG. Some doctors give hCG "boosters" during the two-week wait because it helps the corpus luteum, the remnant of your follicle that produced an egg, put out more progesterone.

Although anything over 5 IU is a positive test, the chances of a pregnancy with such a low starting level succeeding are less than if the beta were higher. However, sometimes a pregnancy may implant a few days later than normal, giving an initial low positive. These pregnancies may pick up steam quickly, and the beta will start rising appropriately.

TECHNICAL STUFF

A beta that is positive for only a few days may be called a biochemical pregnancy by your doctor. A *biochemical pregnancy* is one in which the embryo starts to implant but fails to grow normally, so that a low level of hCG may be picked up for a short time. The beta in these cases may be negative a few days later if you repeat the test. (See Chapter 13 for more about biochemical pregnancies.)

TIP

Most clinics urge cautious optimism if the first beta level is lower than they would like to see it. Don't broadcast the news to anyone except those closest to you if your initial beta isn't very high.

REMEMBER

It's not unusual for beta hCG results to be low after a frozen embryo transfer, so don't despair on the first result and — can we repeat it often enough? — do not stop any of your medications on your own!

Responding to Good News: OMG!

After you get the call from your center that your test was positive, your initial elation may quickly change to worry: Will everything go well? Are your numbers too high or too low? Should you tell anyone yet? After almost constant contact with your clinic for weeks or months, it can be scary to think that you'll soon be leaving the people you've come to know and trust.

Don't panic. Most clinics continue to see you for a few weeks after your first positive test to make sure that your pregnancy is going well.

Cautiously pregnant and continuing tests

Some centers continue to check your beta and your progesterone levels for several weeks to make sure that your pregnancy is a good one. Because you may not be able to see an obstetrician for a few weeks, this monitoring ensures that if you have an ectopic pregnancy, you'll be diagnosed promptly, to avoid life-threatening complications. On the other hand, doing frequent monitoring will not affect the outcome so frequent monitoring is not necessary.

Your clinic usually wants to see your beta double every two to three days for the first few weeks. The following numbers are typical milestones based on a day 3 embryo transfer (three days after the egg retrieval). If you transferred blastocysts on day 5, subtract two days. Obviously, there are many exceptions to the "rules" here. This list gives only the averages.

>> **9 days post-transfer:** Average bHCG 48; range 17–119

>> **10 days post-transfer:** Average bHCG 59; range 17–147

>> **11 days post-transfer:** Average bHCG 95; range 17–223

>> **12 days post-transfer:** Average bHCG 132; range 17–429

>> **13 days post-transfer:** Average bHCG 292; range 70–758

>> **16 days post-transfer:** Average bHCG 1,061; range 324–4,130; yolk sac may be visible

>> **By the sixth week of pregnancy:** Average bHCG 17,000; heartbeat seen by end of sixth week

>> **End of sixth week:** Average bHCG 30,000; embryo seen

If your beta isn't rising appropriately, no one can do much but wait to see what happens. Some clinics monitor your progesterone levels and add more progesterone if your numbers are a little low, but adding progesterone won't save a bad pregnancy, especially if the pregnancy is genetically abnormal. Normal progesterone levels in early pregnancies are 12–20 ng/ml in weeks 5–6 and tend to rise linearly throughout the first trimester. A progesterone level of <12 ng/ml suggests an abnormal pregnancy, and the miscarriage rate can be as high as 70 percent.

The use of vaginal progesterone preparations in frozen embryo transfer cycles makes these numbers meaningless.

A beta that starts out high and rises very quickly may mean a twin or triplet pregnancy.

So, what is the real story of how rapidly the early beta level should rise? The standard rule of thumb is a doubling every 48 hours, but that actually is incorrect. So, if the beta does double or more, then that is reassuring. What if it only rises 95 percent, or 75 percent, or — horror of horrors — 60 percent? Actually, these are all normal. The expected rise depends in large part upon what the starting value was. If the starting value was <1,500 then anything above a 50 percent rise is considered normal. If the staring value of the beta was >3,000, then any rise above 33 percent is considered normal. Once the beta continues to rise, the next best thing to use to try to determine whether the pregnancy is normal is an ultrasound.

Expect ongoing monitoring

When will you get to see your baby on ultrasound? Some clinics schedule an ultrasound around six weeks, or two weeks after you've missed a period. Don't expect to see much at this point. The enthusiastic ultrasonographer may be able to point out the fetal pole and the yolk sac to you, but these features resemble a blob much more than a baby.

For historic reasons, obstetricians count the "gestational age" from the theoretical first day of the last menstrual period, assuming normal cycles and natural conception. During IVF, the day of egg retrieval is considered the day of ovulation, or 14 days after the last menstrual period. So, six weeks of gestational age means four weeks after ovulation, or exactly 28 days after egg retrieval during IVF. If today is the 31st day after egg retrieval, then your gestational age is six weeks plus three days.

At this point, you should know whether you have more than one baby, but keep in mind that many times one twin or triplet will disappear by the next ultrasound. Very early losses of one or more embryos are very common, so wait until 12 weeks or so before you tell all the neighbors you're having twins or triplets.

By six to seven weeks you should be able to see a heartbeat, which you may actually recognize on ultrasound as a little flicker, and the embryo will be visible. (What you are seeing is *fetal heart motion* (FHM): Early heart monitors that sound like a heartbeat are actually Doppler flow machines, which artificially make the sound of a heartbeat.) Some clinics spend time determining the actual rate of the FHM. For every 10 beats per minute (BPM) below 130, the risk of a miscarriage increases by about 25 percent. But what if the FMH is 140 and the next time it measures 132. Is that a risk for miscarriage? Not really — that amount of variation can be physiologic or technical. The point is that it is easier to just see if it is rapid or slow and follow the pregnancy with ultrasound. At this point, your baby will resemble a fish more than a human being. No one will be willing to guess if you're having a boy or girl for another seven or eight weeks. Remember that ultrasound guesses aren't always accurate, so don't decorate the nursery in pink or blue just yet!

WARNING

One of the most accurate ways of making sure that your baby is growing the way it should is to measure the crown-to-rump length. The embryo can first be measured around six weeks, when it's about 4 millimeters long and the heartbeat can first be visualized. Fetal growth in the first 12 weeks is fairly exact, and your baby's gestational age can be determined from the crown-to-rump length. (This is more important when women are not sure when they conceived, but during IVF it helps to reassure you that the pregnancy is growing according to schedule.) Here are what the measurements should be at different stages:

>> **Six weeks:** 4 millimeters

>> **Seven weeks:** 10 millimeters

>> **Eight weeks:** 16 millimeters

>> **Nine weeks:** 23 millimeters

>> **Ten weeks:** 31 millimeters

>> **Eleven weeks:** 41 millimeters

>> **Twelve weeks:** 54 millimeters

Graduating from your fertility clinic

Some fertility clinics monitor you through the first few weeks after you become pregnant; others wave goodbye with your first positive beta test. Most clinics don't want to keep you too long as a pregnant patient because they don't want to deal with pregnancy issues. Also, malpractice insurance for gynecologists and reproductive endocrinologists does not cover taking care of patients beyond the first trimester. But you may have a hard time getting an appointment with an obstetrician until you're ten weeks pregnant or so, leaving you in sort of a no man's land of medical care.

TIP

Establish yourself as a patient of an obstetrician even before you get pregnant. That way, if you have any problems in the first few weeks, such as spotting, cramping, or severe pain (as in a possible ectopic pregnancy), your obstetrician can take care of you, even if your clinic doesn't deal with these issues.

Knowing when high-risk monitoring may be necessary

Don't think of yourself as a high-risk pregnancy just because you did IVF to get pregnant. Most of the time, IVF doesn't increase the risk of complications in pregnancy. The complications come from whatever caused your infertility, such as your age, uterine shape, or other health issues.

Most doctors consider you high risk for the following reasons:

>> You're over age 35.

>> You have a uterine malformation that may make it hard for you to carry the pregnancy.

>> You have multiples (twins or higher).

>> You have a health history of cancer or a disease such as diabetes, lupus, or heart disease.

>> You have a history of incompetent cervix.

>> You have had several previous cesarean sections.

>> You're significantly overweight.

If you're a high-risk patient, you'll probably be seeing your obstetrician more often than once a month in the first trimester. You may be doing additional testing, such as chorionic villus sampling (CVS), to check for chromosomal abnormalities in the first three months.

Taking the Next Step if IVF Doesn't Work

Every day, a patient asks coauthor Lisa how she could *not* be pregnant. "But my embryos looked perfect. My lining looked great, and I did everything I was supposed to. How could it not work?" women say.

Unfortunately, some of the time the answer is "We don't know." Statistically speaking, if you have a 50 percent chance of getting pregnant, you have an equal 50 percent chance of not getting pregnant, but this isn't the answer a disappointed patient wants to hear. You want an answer, something you can fix in the future.

Grasping the importance of follow-up after bad news

A consult with your REI after a failed cycle may provide information about what may be done on a repeat cycle to improve the chance of conception. Even if there is no immediately identifiable problem, the chance of conceiving if you try IVF again can be calculated. It is important to paint a broad picture here and consider all facets of how you got to this point: age, length of infertility, diagnosis, and response to IVF. For some people, repeated IVF cycles can provide a very good chance of success, while for other people, repeated cycles of IVF will be unsuccessful.

TIP

As hard as it is to pick yourself up after a cycle disappointment, it is important to sit with your doctor and review what happened and re-group. Whether you want to try again or move forward with a different type of treatment, you owe it to yourself to make your next decision with all available information.

Some clinics will make you wait to see the doctor until you get a menses, so don't be surprised if they refuse to get you in the day after your negative pregnancy test. No, they are not trying to stall you. They actually want to make sure that they have all the details of your cycle together and you and your partner are in a better place to make new plans.

Figuring out what happened

What happened? One of several things happened if your pregnancy test was negative:

>> **The embryos may not have implanted at all.** The most common reason for embryos not implanting is that their development stopped prior to reaching the implantation stage. The older you are, the more likely this is to happen, but the cessation of embryo development is thought to be the most common cause of lack of pregnancy at any age, and in fact, even during natural conception.

>> **The embryos started to implant and then stopped.** Usually this happens because the embryos are abnormal chromosomally. The only way to tell whether embryos have the right chromosomes is to do pre-implantation genetic testing (PGT), a procedure in which one cell is removed from the embryo before implantation and its DNA is analyzed for abnormalities. This procedure is expensive, and not all centers do PGT (see Chapter 17 for more about PGT).

>> **There may have been a problem with the uterus.** There isn't any way to test the endometrium specifically during the actual cycle, because an endometrial biopsy would damage the lining and might actually prevent the implantation. Most centers merely measure the endometrial thickness with ultrasounds. It is also important to check the cavity to make sure there aren't any fibroids or polyps that might interfere with implantation. Other than these two tests, there isn't any other testing that has proven to be useful.

Questioning God and your doctor

An unsuccessful attempt at IVF can be devastating financially, physically, and emotionally. It opens up the floodgates for a host of worries and fears that can be overwhelming. For this reason, your best thinking probably doesn't come on the day of or the day after an unsuccessful attempt. You may need to put some time and space between the cycle and your next steps or you may need immediate answers. Remember that your hormone levels are probably off kilter as well. They'll eventually return to normal and probably your mood will, too, as the days pass.

As you prepare your list of questions for your doctor, try to be as specific as possible. "What went wrong?" may be a good question with which to start, but you're better off breaking this broad question down into more specific questions, such as the following:

>> Did I respond as expected?

>> How was my egg quality? This really comes down to: How was my embryo quality?

>> What particular stage in the process did you feel posed the most problems?

>> What did you learn about me and my situation through this process?

>> What would you recommend as a next step? Why?

REMEMBER

Remember that your doctor doesn't have all the answers that you may want. Fertility is a complex process under the best of circumstances. If doctors knew exactly why it all worked or didn't work, they would save you and themselves a lot of time. Unfortunately, medicine doesn't have all the answers for anything, including fertility.

TIP

Your doctor may be a great source of comfort but consider taking the "Why me?" question to a therapist, a religious person, or God. Use your doctor for the knowledge that the doctor does have and seek other avenues for the answers that your doctor doesn't have. Your doctor *does* care — likely, enough to want you to seek the best source for answering a question far more in the spiritual realm than the medical one.

Grieving your loss

Whether you are stoic or devastated, a negative pregnancy test for most fertility patients feels like a loss. And it is. Perhaps the best way to deal with the morass of emotions brought on by an unsuccessful cycle is by looking at the grief process. Elisabeth Kubler-Ross, the author of *On Death and Dying*, identified the five stages of grief following the death of a loved one: denial, anger, bargaining, depression, and acceptance. The death of a dream, even if it's only a temporary condition, is much the same. You can treat this disappointment as a loss, and some women even liken it to miscarriage. Consider the following stages and how they may apply:

» **Denial:** "Maybe the test results are wrong, and I really am pregnant," you may say. Denial is perhaps one of the most time-honored human traditions in dealing with painful situations. Although denial provides you with a brief respite from your pain, it isn't something that can successfully carry you out of your grief. Realizing that you're not pregnant (after your doctor has confirmed it), no matter how much you want to be, is the first step.

» **Anger:** "My doctor doesn't care" or "Somebody messed up" may be a typical response. Anger is also a perfectly natural and understandable response to grief. You may find that, as your emotions (and hormones) subside with time, your anger may not seem as urgent. Remember that physical force or verbal intimidation are never appropriate, no matter how angry you are. If you feel this way, you need some time to cool off and perhaps some professional help to do so.

» **Bargaining:** "If only I could be pregnant, I would never again (pick one) yell at my mother, slack off at work, speed, or engage in any other bad habits." Bargaining is similar to foxhole prayers, those pleas for help that come at desperate times. It's also a normal reaction to grief, albeit not a very useful one. Allow yourself time to move through this stage (as with all the stages that you experience). This too shall pass.

» **Depression:** "I'm not pregnant. I'll never have a baby. My life is worthless." Also known as "stinking thinking," depression can cast a cloud over your thoughts and feelings. This is another (normal) stage of grief that often doesn't let you take into account the positive realities in your life. If your depression lasts longer than two weeks, consider seeking professional help, whether from your doctor or a therapist. She or he may prescribe antidepressants to get you through this difficult time.

>> **Acceptance:** Remember that acceptance doesn't equate to agreement. You may accept your circumstances as they are today and yet continue to feel that the situation is unfair — and it is. Remember that you can change your circumstances now that you've passed through your period of mourning.

You may go through these stages of grief more than once. You may skip a stage or repeat it twice before you come to accept what has happened. Regardless, don't rush yourself. You'll get there when you get there, and not a moment sooner.

Taking time out for you and your partner

While you're grieving, your partner may be grieving as well. Your partner may be stuck in a particular stage of the process, such as denial or anger. Look for signs that they may need some additional help to work through their feelings.

Use your follow-up doctor's visit as a springboard to discuss your future plans with your partner. Remember that you're both playing on the same team. If your goals appear to be different at this point, give one another the space and time to consider both sides. If you need help arriving at a mutually agreeable decision, you may want to consider visiting a therapist or a religious adviser.

Keeping Embryos on Ice

If you have embryos frozen from a fresh cycle, you may be concerned that if you don't use them, you'll lose them. This thought may have you rushing into another cycle before you're emotionally ready or doing another cycle soon after you deliver Baby Number 1.

While there's nothing wrong with doing a frozen embryo transfer as soon as you're ready, you don't have to worry that your embryos will get freezer burn if left in the tank too long. Embryos have been successfully thawed and created perfectly normal children even after being frozen for years.

Some clinics are imposing time limits on keeping embryos frozen on-site because of limited storage capacity. Your clinic will tell you how long they'll store embryos at the time of freezing and what the costs for that storage will be. Today, many IVF centers are keeping frozen embryos on-site for shorter periods of time, so you may be asked to move your embryos to long-term storage facilities. No matter where your embryos will be stored, you will have to sign documents that allow the clinic to freeze and initially store your embryos (usually called an informed consent and disposition document). If your embryos go to long-term storage (don't worry about choosing one — your clinic will tell you), you will also have to set up an account with the long-term storage facility and sign a disposition of embryos contract. We explain a lot more about future use of your embryos in Chapter 22.

Regrouping and Future Planning

Knowing when to say when may come sooner for some infertility patients because of basic reasons: a lack of money, time, or opportunity. But even for those who've figured out ways to juggle limited resources a little bit longer, knowing when to say when still isn't easy. A good friend counseled coauthor Jackie one day when she felt she couldn't take the fertility treatments anymore.

"When do I give up?" Jackie cried to her over the phone.

"When you just can't walk another step," her friend replied firmly.

PERSONAL STORY

Jackie had moments and even days when she felt that she couldn't take one more blood test or one more ultrasound or answer one more phone call. During those times, the wonderful support of her online network, friends, and family helped her through. It often took what felt like a Herculean effort to do the next right thing when it came to fertility. Along the way, however, Jackie also "gave up" in little pieces. By her last cycle (the one that worked after three-and-a-half years), she had put away her extensive filing system in which she cataloged every test result. Instead of comparing her daily results to past results, she stuffed the files into the bottom of a cabinet and just looked at the day in front of her. Was she giving up or letting go? Perhaps a little bit of both. And although the cycle was successful, she realized that it was not *because* she let go. Letting go at the time was her only option in order to continue taking the necessary steps.

For many people, giving up and letting go are one and the same. For Jackie, both actions allowed her to take the responsibility and the results off herself, where they don't belong anyway. This attitude allowed her to continue without a death grip on every last detail, many of which are truly insignificant in the long run.

REMEMBER

Let go if you can, sooner rather than later. Doing so helps you maintain your spirit throughout the process, whether it is short or long. And, if this stop working, and you just can't walk another step, consider your other options.

Chapter **19**

Staying Afloat When You're Drowning in a Sea of Fertility Data

"Big Data" and "artificial intelligence (AI)" are among the latest buzzwords. Everyone is talking about how AI will solve all of our problems. There are more websites that tell you what to do than there are good-intentioned relatives. And yet, here you are — not pregnant and most likely confused. Don't worry; you are not alone. The world's experts can't agree and are just as confused as you are. If everything was so clearly predictable, there would be no need for experts, countless publications, and endless debate over oodles of data. However, making predictions can be much more accurate when you utilize all the information — *with* a clear head.

At the end of the day, decision making is a guess, and after arming yourself with as much information as tolerable, your instinct is probably as accurate for your life as that of any expert, AI prediction, or mother. Understanding what AI and the digital revolution are about can help you sort through a lot of useless information so that you are well armed to make the best decision possible.

WHAT IS "BIG DATA" AND WHERE DID IT COME FROM?

The digital revolution started between the 1950s and early 1979 when there was a shift away from the analog world to the digital world and the introduction of digital computers and information storage. The digital revolution coincides with what has been called the information age. The information age started after 1947 with the invention of transistor. During the 1050s and '60s the government and the military used transistors to invent the computer. The personal computer became popular in the 1980s. Apple introduced the Apple I in 1975, and IBM introduced the IBM PC in 1981. The world wide web was functional by 1992, and the internet was incorporated into business after 1996. The result was a trio of components working together that included increasing computing power, the ability to store reams of information digitally, and a fast means for communicating and transmitting data — the internet. This amazing combination gave us "Big Data."

Big Data is to a certain extent what the phrase implies — a large amount of data. But having a large amount of data is useless unless it can be used to provide information about a topic or help in making decisions. Consider this definition from a Google search: "extremely large data sets that may be analyzed computationally to reveal patterns, trends, and associations, especially relating to human behavior and interactions."

So, while Big Data implies the data, the term itself actually describes a process, referring to a large set of data that has been collected and stored. The data can be of many different types such as files, photos, emails, and data from the internet, to name a few. The data can be moved and used with great speed, and there has been some attempt to ensure that the data is accurate. Thus, Big Data is actually described by these four terms: volume, variety, velocity, and veracity. In simple terms, the amount of data, the type of date, the speed of the data, and the accuracy of the data.

Exploring the Link Between Information and the Care You Receive

The process of Big Data allows the use of a vast amount of data to create information. Data without meaning is useless. The New York phone directory digitalized and stored on the cloud is Big Data. Using a program that allows a person to search for a friend's address gives that data meaning. Without the program, the file is meaningless, and since it is stored in a language of 0s and 1s, it is nothing more than gibberish.

But along with the capability that Big Data provides, there have been rapid developments in the field of statistics that deals with analyzing the data so that it can be useful. For example, if the age of a woman, her weight, her AMH, and her problem are recorded in her electronic medical file, a physician can use a program that can help predict the ability of IVF to help her achieve a pregnancy. Given that information, said person can decide whether IVF is for her. The program creates a math formula that is developed from all patient information stored in the electronic medical record. The program tries to find patterns that help predict future events. So, if age has a negative impact upon a woman's fertility, using that can help predict a woman's potential to achieve a pregnancy based upon her age. For example, a 25-year-old using IVF with the diagnosis of severe male factor has a 40–45 percent chance of conceiving with one IVF cycle. But a 44-year-old using IVF for age-related infertility has only less than a 4 percent chance of having a pregnancy.

This is the essence of the hope for Big Data and the field of analytics — that the large amount of data can be used to help make predictions that will improve the accuracy of decision making. At the end of the day, making decisions is guesswork. Using Big Data and analytics tries to make the guess more accurate, but it is never precise. For example, in IVF the complication rate determined by the number of people who have hyperstimulation syndrome, bleeding, or infection is less than 0.8 percent. When the process of IVF is explained, usually in an IVF "consult," the explanation covers risks. The person trying to decide weighs the risk of these complications against the success of IVF. The risk rate seems quite low and acceptable given the success rate for IVF. Suppose that person decided to do IVF and developed a severe infection after the retrieval such that she required surgery and an extended hospital stay. Would she still have decided to do IVF given this as an outcome?

So, using Big Data can't guarantee an outcome, and hindsight is always better than decision making. But Big Data and analytics are powerful tools that a person can use to improve the outcome that person desires.

Knowing how medical decisions are made

The information age has provided everyone with massive amounts of information. How is this information used to make medical decisions? At its core, medicine strives to be a science and use the scientific method for decision making. The *scientific method* uses structure, measurement, and experiments to formulate hypotheses.

For example, a couple is considered infertile by ASRM if they have been trying to conceive for over a year and have been unsuccessful. How was this definition determined? Suppose you are tasked with defining infertility. First, define fertile. Most would agree that a woman who delivers a child is, at the moment of delivery, fertile. Maybe not in a year or so, but at that moment the birth is proof of fertility.

Ask 1,000 women who gave birth how long it took to conceive the pregnancy that resulted in the birth. Then apply math (simple addition and division) to determine how many were pregnant after three months. While the data vary, one estimate says that after three months, 65 percent of fertile women had achieved a pregnancy. After six months, 85 percent had achieved a pregnancy. But after a year, the chance of conceiving in any given month was quite low. So now draw a line and say that after one year, a couple can be considered infertile. Does that mean they will not conceive on their own? Not at all, but it does say there may be a problem, and knowledge about that problem may help them conceive.

The diagnosis of infertility has three groups: One group will conceive on their own at some point in the future, one group can conceive but will need help, and one group is sterile and will never conceive. The goal of using medical information for decision making is to help decide which group a couple falls into and what treatment, if any, may help achieve a pregnancy.

Sifting through medical studies: All data is not created equal

What information does the medical community rely upon? The medical community relies upon studies that are conducted under established guidelines. Not all studies provide the same level of information, and different types of studies are ranked by how reliable they are.

For example, the least reliable studies are called case studies. Here a researcher describes what happened in a particular case or maybe a few cases. This is the same type of information that can be gotten from friends telling their story or their "friend's" story, or from mom or her friends and their daughters. Fascinating stories . . . but not reliable when applied to a different couple. A higher level of reliability comes from what are called *observational studies,* which are recorded in a very defined fashion with results and outcomes for a large group of patients.

Formerly, the most reliable study was the randomized control study, where a very defined group of patients was randomized to either treatment or placebo and then compared for outcome. Currently, the highest level of reliability comes from combining the results of many studies into one evaluation, and these are called *systematic reviews* and *meta-analyses.*

The internet has allowed everyone access to medical literature. But can we rely on what we read? A person can use Google search or PubMed and find hundreds to thousands of articles on a topic. Given this access, it's become more important for people to realize the limitations of medical research. Currently, professional organizations are making efforts to ensure that research is conducted according to guidelines for properly conducted research.

The European Society for Human Reproduction and Embryology (ESHRE) formed a workshop group and published their report with the title "Protect us from poor-quality medical research" (Human Reproduction 2018 33:770). In the article, the authors state: "We recognize up front that perfectly reliable/credible and useful research is clearly an unattainable utopia. However, there are many ways in which the existing situation can be improved. It has been estimated that 85% of all research funding is actually wasted due to inappropriate research questions, faulty study design, flawed execution, irrelevant endpoints, poor reporting and/or non-publication" (Moher et al 2016). This is very distressing given the emphasis placed upon medical research.

One way to put this in perspective is to be extremely cautious of newly released results that show a marked improvement. Studies are published because they do show a difference. However, over time as more information is accumulated, those early positive results prove not to be an improvement at all. Also, it is tempting to apply the positive results of a study used for a very defined group of patients to other patents who may be in a different group where the treatment will not work. For example, the use of information from endometrial biopsies for patients with recurrent pregnancy loss may not be useful for patients doing IVF with recurrent implantation failure.

REMEMBER

Medical decisions are influenced by the person making the decision. A physician's training and experience influence how the physician interprets the literature. This influences how the information is presented to a patient. Rational decision making is a clever thought but never really attainable. People have unconscious biases that influence decision making. A common bias that everyone has is called *confirmation bias.* In other words, a person thinks something is true and then looks for information that confirms that bias. For example, a 47-year-old patient wants to have a child using her own eggs and cites a famous Hollywood star as having a child at age 47. True, but that Hollywood star most likely used donor oocytes. Or a 27-year-old patient has a friend who conceived using Clomid and now wants to use Clomid. Maybe that is fine, but what if the problem is that her partner has a very low sperm count? Treating *her* with Clomid will not help him get more sperm.

Stacking the deck: why diagnosis matters

The story of a patient going to her doctor asking for Clomid "because it worked for my friend" shows why knowing your diagnosis is critical. Since we don't know the patient's problem, how do we know whether Clomid will work? Medical literature is designed to answer questions about very specific problems. Knowing your diagnosis allows you (and your doctor) to apply the appropriate information so that you can use the most successful treatment. For example, Clomid is widely used for the treatment of infertility. Not uncommonly, a gynecologist will prescribe Clomid when a patient has been trying to conceive for over a year without success. Some patients will conceive using Clomid; many will not. The real questions are these: Did the Clomid make a difference? Or, did this couple conceive without any treatment? That is called the *treatment independent pregnancy rate*.

TECHNICAL STUFF

The treatment independent pregnancy rate is a very useful statistic because it sets the floor for expectations and helps direct appropriate treatment. But the rate is influenced by the diagnosis. For example, a young couple who have a fertility work-up that comes up "normal" may choose to forgo treatment for a little longer since their rate may be as high as 5–15 percent without treatment (in other words, if they keep trying, they have up to a 15 percent chance of conceiving). However, a 42-year-old patient with a low AMH may choose to move to IVF right away since her monthly treatment independent rate is less than 1 percent.

Knowing the treatment independent rate also allows for a more accurate assessment of treatment options and how long to use a particular treatment. Most fertility treatments work within the first three or four tries. After that, the treatment dependent rate approaches the treatment independent rate and suggests that further use of that treatment is not helping.

REMEMBER

Knowing your specific diagnosis allows for a much better prediction of how effective any fertility treatment will be for you. Consider a couple who are diagnosed with solely male factor infertility (the woman has no fertility issues). If they choose to use Clomid/IUI treatments, they will have an estimated overall success rate of 15–25 percent. If they choose IVF, their estimated overall success rate is up to 40 percent for a single cycle and over 85 percent for multiple cycles. What a difference! This type of data is *so* helpful and supports the need for muscling through all of that testing we talk about in Chapters 12 and 13 to find out your diagnosis.

Calling Dr. Google! Okay, the first place you went when you weren't getting pregnant was to the internet, right? 'Fess up — of course you did! Most of us do online searches when we have any medical questions (or any questions) so why would your question about getting pregnant be any different? Then why does your clinic tell you to stop going online?

Coauthor Dr. Rinehart says the real issue with the internet is not that you shouldn't consult it, but rather now much weight you should give to your search results. All physicians occasionally learn something new from a patient search. However, an emerging job for the medical staff is to help patients understand and appropriately apply information found on the internet. It is hard to keep up with the growing online journals that publish loosely reviewed articles, sometimes just because the author is willing to pay. Many publishers are rushing articles into print and online without verifying the data. So, it is exceedingly difficult for patients to truly understand what it all means. Most healthcare providers realize the influence of the internet and are prepared to help patients understand what they are reading. But remembering the commercial using the line, "It must be true if it's on the internet" highlights the Wild West nature of online information.

Choosing What's Best for You

Finding out your diagnosis, adding the power of Big Data, and having all the treatment options laid out for you by your clinic may leave you shell-shocked. All you wanted was for someone to tell you what to do so that you could have a baby. How on earth are you going to figure all of this out and choose the right path for you?

Figuring out your true conception goal

Medicine is hampered by well-intentioned people trying to help. Often that is interpreted as having to *do* something. Many times, not doing something is more helpful than repeatedly doing something that is not helping. In today's infertility world, we see this when IVF is done over and over again with no term pregnancy resulting. Doing the same thing over and over and expecting different results is one definition of insanity! Both patients and the healthcare team may focus on doing IVF because it is *something to do.*

If the goal is to do something — anything! — then doing more IVF achieves that goal.

However, rarely is the ultimate goal of IVF just to do IVF, nor should it be. Most people do IVF to have a child — which highlights the fact that most people utilizing infertility services are doing so to have a child. Having a child is the ultimate goal. But many people will not have a child using all of the available technology.

Even under the best of circumstances where people use up to six cycles of IVF, as many as 15 percent remain childless. Ultimately, the most overarching goal is to help resolve a person's or couple's fertility-related issues. That may mean helping people to deal with remaining childless, opening doors to third-party reproduction, or encouraging adoption. When making a plan, the most important question is how you would feel in ten years if the decision did not meet the ultimate goal.

PERSONAL STORY

Co-author Lisa remembers working with a couple (let's call them Sally and Ben) who were struggling with deciding on moving to IVF using donor eggs. Sally was 44 years old. They had done two IVF cycles, and none of the embryos were viable. As Lisa sat with them talking about options, she asked them what their goal was in pursuing fertility treatment. Did they want biological children, or did they want to be parents? She told them that if biology was the goal, the chances were almost nonexistent given Sally's age. But, if they wanted to be *parents*, there were many options to help them succeed. Turning the conversation into "What is your goal?" opened so many more doors and helped Sally and Ben make the decision that was right for them. (P.S. They used donor eggs and now are parents of a beautiful baby girl!)

Teaming up to decide what is best

Very few important and complex decisions are made in a vacuum. Starting a family and having children is one of life's most important decisions. Tom Brady did not become one of the most successful quarterbacks in the history of football by doing it alone. Coach Belicek and Brady assembled some of the most talented pro football players and then maximized their abilities.

That method can be applied to infertility. The team includes healthcare providers, psychosocial experts, financial advisers, family, and friends. Anyone who is willing to work hard for the positive promotion of solving the infertility problem can be a member. Anyone who is not a strong team player needs to be traded.

Knowing where to go for useful information

The internet is a valuable tool when placed in perspective. The American Society for Reproductive Medicine (ASRM) and the European Society for Human Reproduction and Embryology (ESHRE) are two societies established by the medical community. Both have patient information that has been reviewed by the societies.

Many websites are in essence advertisements for medical practices, and while they often have very useful information, it should probably be viewed from the perspective of infomercials. Know the difference! Other patient-organized websites also have very useful information, and chat groups and social media can be helpful. We talk more about this in Chapter 8.

Go one-on-one with your doctor

A critical aspect of a physician role in today's medicine is to provide patients with understandable, useful, honest information so that they can make an informed decision about their healthcare given their set of circumstances.

Physicians have their own bias and moral compass. Accepting that, a patient's interaction with a physician should always be patient focused. Further, in today's healthcare environment, much of the care is provided by the healthcare team and not solely by the physician. The most successful outcomes are achieved when the care is cooperative.

5

Exploring Alternative Routes to Conception

Consider the use of donor eggs, sperm, and/or embryo and whether it may make sense to consider gestational surrogacy.

Decide when "enough is enough" and discuss other options for having a family.

Take a trip to the future and look at new advances and concerns in fertility treatment.

Chapter **20**

Considering Third-Party Reproduction Options

The traditional family of Mom, Dad, and 2.7 children has changed considerably over the past few decades. In 2018, the average number of children per family was only 1.9. Families today may contain biological children; adopted children; children with single parents of either sex; gay parents; children born from donor eggs, sperm, or embryos from third parties; as well as children carried through pregnancy by their grandmother, their aunt, or a total stranger.

The legal and emotional issues involved with using eggs, sperm, or uteri from someone else can be tricky. In this chapter, we discuss how to decide whether third-party — or even fourth- or fifth-party! — reproduction is right for you, and how to proceed after you make your decision.

Deciding to Use Donor Eggs, Sperm, or Embryos

Deciding to use donor eggs, embryos, or sperm is a difficult decision that opens up a host of emotional and legal issues. Usually, you make this decision because you have to — because one or both of you has a fertility issue that can't be fixed. Or you make the decision because you're a same-sex couple or a single parent; obviously, you need some type of donor in these cases.

Why do I need to do this?

To achieve a pregnancy, three things need to work: eggs, sperm, and uterus. Therefore, one reason to use third-party reproduction is gonadal failure of either testes or ovaries. Severe problems with the ovaries may result from being born with ovarian failure or experiencing premature menopause (menopause before the age of 40), chemotherapy, radiation therapy to the ovaries, or surgery removing the ovaries, just to mention a few causes. Likewise for the male, there may be congenital testicular failure, no sperm (*azospermia*) as well as chemotherapy, radiation therapy to the gonads, traumatic injury to the genitals, or surgery. Either the man or woman may carry a serious genetic disease that they don't want to transmit to their children. The use of preimplantation diagnosis has reduced this category. Another reason is advanced maternal age to a point where no more normal eggs exist. Finally, third-party reproduction may be indicated for couples who have had very poor embryo formation after a number of IVF attempts.

Getting started down the third-party road

You never thought you'd be talking about having a baby through IVF, let alone using donor eggs or sperm, donor embryos, a gestational surrogate, or some combination of these. It is a more complicated path, but for many, it's the way to successful family-building. Now that you are here, there are a few practical steps you can take to make it work better:

>> **Recognize that this IVF cycle is going to take time** — more time than any cycle you may have gone through before. You have several preliminary steps to go through before anyone starts taking medication, such as deciding on the fresh or frozen route (or eggs), making your donor choice, and — if your plan calls for it — picking a gestational carrier. So sit back and take it one step at a time.

>> **It's going to cost more.** Very few insurance plans cover all the medical costs of third-party reproduction. You may be one of the lucky few, but you'll still have to bear the legal costs of most arrangements.

>> **You have less control.** Even though this is your baby — and everyone knows it is your baby — you will not have the same input you did before. Coauthor Lisa always says that her infertility patients are some of the most educated patients she's met, and with that knowledge comes a lot of input. When you are dealing with a "third party" in your baby making, you have to release some of the control, and that can be hard.

>> **You may find yourself with a new title.** Patients who are using (or receiving) donor eggs or donor embryos are termed "recipients," and those who are using a gestational host are named "intended parents." These terms help the staff identify who is doing what in the third-party IVF cycle.

REMEMBER

If you're moving to donor eggs or sperm because you have an unfixable problem, you need to come to terms with your loss before moving on. As an infertility nurse, Lisa saw couples move too quickly to donor eggs and sperm and then struggle with their feelings about being pregnant with a child not biologically their own. Donor eggs or sperm will always be available; don't jump in before you're sure that you're emotionally ready.

If you decide to use donor eggs or sperm, the child created will be related to *one* of you. Is this fact going to be a problem if you and your partner separate down the road? Is it something that one of you may fling in the other's face if the child has a serious health problem or ends up in trouble with the law? Will the fact that one of you can see family features in your child's face while the other can't become a source of friction? You need to consider these questions, as well as any others that cross your mind, before you make the leap.

TIP

When these questions keep rattling around in your brain without a clear answer, it may be time to consult a mental health specialist who works with fertility patients. Fertility counseling has become a subspecialty, and many clinics have counselors in their facilities. Others have lists of preferred counselors. Either way, when you can't find answers on your own, these specialists are a wonderful resource.

Protecting Yourselves When Considering a Donor for Anything

Before entering into any type of donor situation that we describe in this chapter, whether it involves eggs, embryos, or sperm, you need to do several things. In this section, we cover how to find and select the best donor for you, as well as getting the legal support you need to get through the third-party process successfully.

Asking key questions

>> **Thoroughly check out the donor's health history but realize that a clean slate is no guarantee against a host of other potential problems.** For starters, we can only test for those diseases that we're aware of today. New communicable diseases and new strains of old ones, not able to be tested for today, may be uncovered in the future.

>> **Be aware of the limitations of genetic tests.** While most centers test for the most common genetic diseases such as cystic fibrosis, spinal muscular atrophy, or sickle cell anemia, they may only test for the most frequently recognized mutations. While this covers the majority of cases, as many as 10–20 percent of rare mutations that are not tested for may remain. Certain populations, such as Native Americans, tend to carry more remote, albeit just as harmful, mutations of diseases such as cystic fibrosis. These would only be found via extensive screening, which would need to be done at your request and on your bankroll as well.

>> **If you're a known carrier of a genetic disease, be sure your donor is tested for these specific diseases.** Less common genetic illnesses, such as Tay-Sachs disease or Maple Syrup Urine Disease, are generally not tested for in the standard centers.

>> **Be aware of the testing differences between donor sperm and donor eggs.** While donor sperm are frozen and quarantined for six months after initial testing, donor eggs are a different egg altogether! Because eggs aren't quarantined after the initial infectious disease testing, there's a small chance that infectious disease could be transmitted to their recipient. While you may be able to rule out the likelihood of certain diseases by your donor's lifestyle, partnership, or health history, remember that you're going on her word and that of the clinic compiling her information.

TECHNICAL STUFF

In 2005, the Federal Drug Administration (FDA) weighed in (heavily!) on preventing the spread of infection in transplanted tissue. Now it may not seem like you are getting a "transplant" when you use donor gametes or embryos, but it is tissue being placed from one human to another, so technically it falls under the guidance of the FDA's Good Tissue Practices regulation. Under this law, fertility centers must follow very specific testing guidelines to ensure that you, your donor, and/or your surrogate are not currently carrying and have not been exposed to certain infectious disease. So, each of you will be tested at least twice before any procedures are carried out. In addition, donors are screened with a physical exam and a questionnaire to rule out any risky conditions or behaviors. This list keeps changing, and the clinic will let you know what needs to be done and when. Keep in mind that it is not negotiable (if everyone wants to follow the law) and, as mentioned previously, it takes time.

Researching companies that find donors

Third-party reproduction is a business, and as such, there are a number of companies around the world who provide gametes and embryos. While it may seem crass, gametes and embryos are things to buy, so *caveat emptor*. Many REI practices have their own programs. The upside of this is that they are a known entity. The downside is their limitation to the options and the potential bias to want to sell their product. Many larger cities have companies, called "agencies" (even though they are not licensed), which provide gametes and match them with potential parents. Today, you can find many matching companies online as well. As in buying any other very important product, comparison shopping, searching for references and background, and careful interviewing increase the chance that things will go as planned.

REMEMBER

You'll pay a lot for using a matching company — sometimes even a fee to see their donor list even before you agree to a match. Also, the donor screening processes vary from company to company. Most do not do complete medical screening on the donor, so that would still have to be done (at your expense).

Embryos are usually obtained from REI practices, but some organizations provide embryos as a way to prevent their destruction. Many foreign countries offer gametes and embryos cheaper than can be obtained in the U.S. *Cross-border reproduction* (traveling to a country outside your home country to have fertility treatment) is a booming business, but remember, if you follow this route, you are no longer covered under U.S. law.

Recruiting a family member or friend

Some parents-to-be choose a donor they know, perhaps a brother or close friend of the intended dad. In these cases, fresh sperm can be used. However, if the insemination is done by a doctor's office, the doctor should insist on having all infectious disease testing up-to-date.

TIP

Fresh sperm no longer have a higher pregnancy rate than frozen sperm. Prior to the AIDS epidemic, donor sperm was done using fresh specimens. The fact that a man could be infectious for HIV before the test turned positive forced an evaluation of frozen sperm. Amazingly, the number of sperm required to maximize the pregnancy rate was known for bulls but not for humans. Once this was discovered, attention was directed at making sure that once the specimen was thawed, there were enough live, motile sperm and — voilá — the pregnancy rates were the same regardless of whether the sperm were fresh or frozen. If you are using a known donor, keep in mind that the donor will need to be tested for infectious diseases. Most clinics still prefer that the sperm be frozen and quarantined, and in this case, there's a waiting period of six months before the sperm can be used. This gives the clinic time to retest for infectious diseases — many infectious diseases (like HIV) take up to six months to show up in the blood. Many centers won't use fresh sperm at all, but its use is within the new FDA guidelines.

With known-donor insemination, of course, the chance that the child will find out the truth about his conception is much higher, because more people are involved in the process. For some couples, the psychological issues of using a known donor may be too complicated for them to handle. However, couples who want a genetic match that's as close as possible and who can handle the psychological problems may find this method to be a good solution.

WARNING

Although such a topic may be difficult to discuss, some type of legal document should be drawn up to make it clear who the parent is if a pregnancy occurs, among other things. This document should also address such issues as how much say the donor will have in the child's upbringing, how much contact he'll have with the child, and whether he'll have legal rights to the child if anything happens to you. Finally, you need to consider if and when you will disclose to a child that he or she was born using donor eggs or sperm — and who donated. This is becoming an increasingly sensitive legal issue.

Of course, you may never experience any emotional or legal problems as a result of this donation. The donor may see your child as just another niece or nephew and never give it a second thought. You know your own family best, but covering the possibility of interference down the road is always a good idea.

What if your partner's *father* is interested in being your donor? This happens more often than you may think. He *is* a genetic link, but remember that grandparents in general can be too outspoken about your child's upbringing. (Why do you let that kid have so many cookies? Why do you let him scream like that?) Ask yourself whether his being the silent "parent" as well as the grandparent may cause problems in your relationship.

Getting the lawyer involved

Whether you are considering using donor eggs, sperm, or embryos — from a known or contracted donor — you are definitely going to need to ensure that your rights are protected. This means you need a lawyer on your side. This is a highly emotional decision, and you need someone objective to make sure that you understand what you are agreeing to and your financial obligations. Most attorneys familiar with reproductive law will be able to discuss all of these issues with you and help you make the best decision for you. Many clinics have referral lists to such attorneys, but if they don't, you can turn to a well-respected national organization for a referral in your area — the American Academy of Adoption and Assisted Reproductive Technology Attorneys (AAARTA) at www.aaarta.org.

REVIEWING FDA REGULATIONS

In 2005, the FDA (Food and Drug Administration) implemented stringent new rules regarding donation of oocytes and embryos. The new regulations mean that egg donors must 1) have a physical exam; 2) complete a detailed lifestyle questionnaire; and 3) be tested twice for a number of communicable diseases (this means blood tests): once within 30 days before the planned egg retrieval and second within 7 days before their eggs are retrieved. Couples who may want to donate their embryos in the future also need to complete testing within 30 days before egg retrieval.

In the meantime, keep these tips in mind:

>> **Put things in writing.** If you're using donor eggs, embryos, or sperm, your clinic's legal documents are only the beginning and may not be enough.

>> **Retain a competent lawyer to represent you**. Think ahead and consider things such as divorce. You may think that you and your partner will never separate, and it is hoped you won't, but it's always a possibility. You owe it to yourselves and your potential child to be prepared. Nobody needs an attorney until they do. Attorneys are like physicians in that they specialize in reproductive law. Your uncle Harry, who is a real estate attorney, is *not* the best choice.

>> **Consider discussing all your options with a mental health professional.** You will be faced with may future disposition decisions, as well as having to deal with the loss of your own gametes and the acceptance of nonbiologic gametes or embryos. A mental health professional can help you navigate these complex issues.

TIP

If you're using a gestational carrier or surrogate (see "Enlisting the Aid of a Surrogate," later in this chapter), make sure that everything is in writing. *Everything.* Legally controlling another person's actions is very difficult, so bring up just about any possibility you can think of. Having something in writing may save you from some heartbreak down the road.

REMEMBER

Some jurisdictions do not allow gestational surrogacy. This means that it is against the law in certain states. Check with a reproductive law attorney for more information in your area.

TIP

Co-author Lisa thinks it is important to include letting go of biology as one step in moving to third-party reproduction. While it sounds so easy to say, "Sure, let's get pregnant with donor sperm, eggs, or embryo," deciding to use someone else's gametes is easier said than done for some patients. If you have already accepted the possibility of adopting to build your family, you may be a step ahead. So, do some soul-searching and maybe get some help to work with any issues. ASRM has a list of people specially trained in reproductive support through their Mental Health Professional Group (MHPG).

Heading to the Bank — the Sperm or Egg "Cryo" Bank, That Is

Donor sperm has been used for artificial insemination for more than 100 years. About 50,000 children are born each year as a result of donor sperm insemination, also known as TDI (therapeutic donor insemination) or AID (artificial insemination — donor). Sperm banks are licensed by the state in which they're located, and they have stringent requirements for donors. Many sperm banks are certified by the American Association of Tissue Banks (AATB), which adds an additional level of safety by setting standards.

Picking donor sperm can be similar to buying a house; it sounds like fun until you have to really do it! Then the "what if I choose wrong" fears start to set in and the process becomes more nerve-wracking than fun.

Choosing the right biological donor for your future child is far more important than buying a house, but many of the same caveats apply. Don't be too heavily swayed by externals, don't let fear of the unknown keep you from making a decision at all, and don't agonize over your decision once you've made it! These next sections can help you understand the donor sperm process and help you choose the best man for the job.

Why fewer couples are using donor sperm

Use of donor sperm has decreased since 1992, when it became possible to inseminate an egg with a single, carefully selected "ideal" sperm (as ideal as existed in the male's sample, anyway) in a process known as *intracytoplasmic sperm injection,* or ICSI. (See Chapter 12 for more about ICSI.) Men whose sperm counts were very low or those with poor sperm motility, or movement, could now become biological parents — as long as they could afford to do in vitro insemination.

Many couples, however, can't afford or don't want to do IVF, so they use donor sperm. Also, those men who have no sperm at all, such as those with Sertoli cell only syndrome (see Chapter 12 for more on this syndrome), still depend on donor sperm to become parents.

Reviewing donor sperm requirements

In case you're thinking that sperm donation may be a way of making a little extra money, here's a list of requirements for donors from some of the most popular donor sperm centers with the most stringent requirements:

» **Health:** All donors should be in good general health and have no genetic diseases.

» **Height:** Most people request a donor between 5 feet 10 inches and 6 feet 2 inches.

» **Weight:** The donor's weight should be proportionate to his height.

» **Age:** The donor should be between the ages of 21 and 34 for oocyte donors and below 40 for sperm donors.

» **Sperm specs:** The donor must have 70 percent motile, or moving, sperm, 60 percent with normal appearance (morphology), and a sperm count of 70 million/milliliter. A donor must have better than average sperm because some will be lost in the freeze-and-thaw process.

Testing donors and taking precautions

Here are some common precautions taken to ensure you receive good sperm:

» **Infectious disease testing:** The donor is tested for all infectious diseases as well as certain genetic diseases, depending on his genetic background. He's also required to fill out a very detailed questionnaire about his background, his family background, his interests, and his likes and dislikes. He may be asked to submit a baby picture.

TECHNICAL STUFF

Some centers, concerned about donors bringing in a "ringer" to produce a specimen for them, have the donor's hands recorded on a three-dimensional biometric device. The donor then has to "sign in" and match the hand key before he's allowed to produce. Of course, this assures the bank that all the specimens for a given donor match up with his blood tests, and so on.

» **Use of frozen sperm:** Because the risk of disease transmission is too high, sperm banks no longer use fresh sperm (although some clinics may allow this under special circumstances). Instead, sperm are now frozen, and the donor is retested for infectious disease before the sperm are released for use — usually a waiting period of six months.

>> **Number of children a donor can father:** To avoid, it is hoped, unknowing incest between half-siblings years down the road, many countries and a few U.S. states have adopted laws to limit how many children a sperm donor can help create. Also, the American Society for Reproductive Medicine (ASRM) guidelines suggest that a donor be allowed to father no more than ten children. Sperm banks routinely follow up with questionnaires to centers using donor sperm to ask whether the donation resulted in a live birth. The ASRM recommends that oocyte donors should be limited to six or fewer donations. There are no national donor registries, so it's not always easy to know how many children have been born from a given donor.

Ordering sperm

You can choose between sperm that has not been washed and is therefore only ready for intracervical insemination (ICI ready) or sperm that's already been washed and is therefore ready for intrauterine insemination (IUI ready).

Some fertility centers prefer that the patients bring in ICI sperm, and then do the sperm washing themselves, because they feel that it gives them a better specimen; check with your center before ordering one or the other type. The technique for IUI, which places the sperm directly into the uterus, is more complicated, but most centers report a higher pregnancy rate with IUI than ICI. Pregnancy rates for women under 35 are about 10–20 percent per insemination; rates decrease for women over 40 to 5–10 percent per insemination. The overall chance for pregnancy after six inseminations for women under 40 is about 85 percent and for women over 40 progressively declines with the woman's age. For women 40–42, the overall chance of success after six cycles is between 40 and 60 percent.

Shopping at an Egg Bank

Purchasing frozen eggs from an egg bank is very similar to buying sperm from a sperm bank. Recent technologic advances have made frozen eggs just as good as fresh. This has resulted in a number of commercial egg banks that sell eggs in lots — frequently six eggs per lot. The process for purchasing and using frozen eggs is simpler than for fresh eggs. For frozen eggs, there is no donor being stimulated and having a retrieval — that has already been done. So, the advantage is that you know there are eggs. You don't know if the eggs will work, but that is also true of a fresh cycle. The recipient undergoes preparation of the uterus to accept the embryos created from the eggs. The way this is done is not standardized, but the general principle is to use estrogen to grow the lining and when appropriate add progesterone to change the lining and set the time when the embryo can implant. Centers vary in terms of the amount of control they want over the cycles, so some use the start of a period while others may use oral contraceptives and Lupron. The eggs are thawed, and sperm are added using ICSI. The embryos are cultured for three to five days, and then an embryo is transferred to the uterus by flushing it into the uterine cavity. Usually progesterone is added until a pregnancy has been established and verified by ultrasound.

Just like sperm donors, egg donors should be women in general good health with no genetic or infectious diseases. While many patients look for a donor to match their own physical characteristics, now is the time to consider "fixing" something about yourself that you want to change — for example, if you want to be taller, choose a tall donor! Other considerations include

>> **Age:** Donors should be of legal age in your state, most likely between the ages of 21 and 34.

>> **Previous pregnancy:** Proven fertility is very helpful, but not always required.

>> **Personal history:** There should not be any indicators of genetic or health risks such as illicit drug use or sexually transmitted disease.

REMEMBER

Gametes (sperm and eggs) and embryos can be frozen nearly indefinitely. They're kept in liquid nitrogen containers and shipped out when requested. The cost for a vial of donor sperm runs about $150 to $300, or more if you have specific requests, such as a Nobel Peace Prize winner. Most clinics suggest that you order at least three vials at a time. Currently, the cost for oocytes is approximately $12,000 for six oocytes.

Selecting a Donor for a "Fresh" Donor Egg Cycle

Unlike sperm donation, which has been around for decades, the use of donor eggs is a relatively newer phenomenon (the first baby conceived with a donor egg was born in 1984). It required the invention and perfection of in vitro fertilization (IVF) in order to become practical. (See Part IV for complete information about IVF.) Egg donation is a growing national trend, with approximately 30,000 babies born in the United States as a result.

The choice between using frozen oocytes and fresh oocytes is complicated. Fresh donor cycles usually produce more eggs. Many fresh donor oocytes cycles result in over 1 –20 oocytes. Since the pregnancy rates are comparable, issues of cost and future pregnancies arise. The cost of a cycle using frozen oocytes is cheaper than a fresh cycle because there is no donor IVF cycle. However, for couples having insurance benefits, the cost may be cheaper for fresh cycles because of the increase in the number of oocytes usually obtained.

For those who decide that fresh egg donation is the way to go, this section covers the basics of what you need to know.

Matching with a "fresh" egg donor

Perhaps you're wondering how you can obtain donor eggs (that are not frozen — because you can use a frozen egg bank as discussed earlier). You have several options:

>> **You can be matched with a paid IVF donor at your clinic.** These women donate all their eggs to one or possibly two recipients for a fee.

>> **Use a broker.** Commercial donor matching companies, or brokers, can also be found on the internet by entering "donor eggs" into a search engine. Using a broker is currently the most common form of egg donation because most clinics have given up recruiting their own donors. The advantage of brokers is that they provide more choice of donors; the disadvantage is that they add considerable cost.

>> **You can be matched with a fellow infertility patient at your clinic.** Some clinics are still offering egg-sharing programs. This involves a woman willing to share half her eggs with you in exchange for your paying her IVF costs. The availability of this type of donation varies widely from center to center, with some centers favoring this type of arrangement while others don't offer it at all.

>> **Find a willing friend or relative.** If you're fortunate enough to have a friend or relative who agrees to donate eggs to you, you'll both be screened through your clinic for infectious diseases, and then your cycles will be coordinated so that you can have a fresh embryo transfer. This is the second most common form of egg donation. The obvious advantage of using a relative is that she shares some fraction of your DNA. In the case of a sister donor, you share 50 percent of your DNA — and the child will have the same grandparents as if you were the genetic parent. Furthermore, because your husband contributes 50 percent of the genes and your sister the other 50 percent, you can think of the baby as 75 percent genetically "yours" as a couple.

Keeping the facts in mind

Although your reason for using egg donors is similar to that of using sperm donors, differences do exist. Keep the following in mind when thinking about using an egg donor:

>> Using donor eggs is more complicated than using donor sperm; IVF centers usually try to coordinate the menstrual cycles of the egg donor and recipient so that the recipient can transfer into her uterus fresh embryos that were created a few days before in the IVF lab. This transfer requires monitoring at an IVF center to make sure that the uterus is ready to receive the embryos.

>> Asking someone to be an egg donor is much more complicated than asking someone to be a sperm donor. Egg donation involves several weeks of injections, blood draws, ultrasounds, and, at some clinics, psychological testing. Plus, you'll need to explore the emotional and legal consequences, just as you would if you were using donor sperm. You'll also need a lawyer to draw up a detailed legal contract; you should do this even if you're using someone you know.

WARNING

>> One disadvantage of donor eggs is that, unlike donor sperm, you don't know what you're getting in advance. Because the egg donor is doing a stimulated IVF cycle while you're taking medication to be ready for embryo transfer, you won't know how many eggs you'll get or their quality until a few days before your transfer.

>> Although you may assume that a 22-year-old donor will make a good number of eggs in an IVF cycle, that doesn't always happen. Clinics usually have rules about what happens if your donor doesn't stimulate well, but chances are you'll still have to pay for the blood tests, medications, and ultrasound examinations that she had before the bad cycle was diagnosed.

Finding donor eggs

Most clinics are still doing traditional donor egg programs; seniority on the recipient list gets you first pick at the donor of your choice, all donors being paid the same. However, a search of the internet reveals a plethora of near-genius beauty queens ready to barter their eggs to the highest bidder.

If you really are looking for something very specific — say, a redhead because everyone in your family has red hair or a biracial donor if you're both biracial — the classifieds may be the way to go. Some centers have very few black donors; others have very few Asian donors. A good place to advertise is the campus newspaper or bulletin board in the student union at a large, diverse college campus.

Try some of the commercial donor matching companies, and do not assume that you have to restrict yourself to local ones. Many out-of-state companies are happy to have the donor travel to your fertility center. When you consider the cost of donor eggs (several thousand dollars), the additional cost of a flight and a couple of nights in a hotel is not that much of a premium.

Funding the donor egg cycle

The cost of using donor eggs can vary tremendously, depending on what you're looking for. Are you looking for a Harvard grad with blonde hair and blue eyes who stands 5 feet 7 inches tall, weighs 125 pounds, volunteers at the nursing home once a week, and bakes cookies for shut-ins in addition to running her law practice and taking care of her adorable twins, picture available upon request? You may be able to find her, but it will cost you. Some Grade-A egg donors are offering to donate eggs for a mere $5,000 *per egg*.

If you're looking for a normal person, like yourself, you'll probably pay between $5,000 and $10,000 to your donor to do an IVF cycle — with 10 to 15 eggs retrieved, one hopes. This covers the donor's fee for her services. Any testing is extra, as is the cost of the IVF cycle and medications for you and the egg donor.

The cost of the IVF cycle itself is around $10,000 in most clinics, and the medications are an additional $3,000 to $4,000.

A donor egg cycle at your average IVF clinic costs from $13,000 to $18,000, including medications, if you don't have insurance. If you're going the designer route, the cost may be much more.

Checking out your donor

Most centers send out donor lists every month or every six weeks. The donor's physical characteristics and family history are listed, as well as education level and current job. Also listed is her childbearing history. Most centers accept anonymous donors only if they're under 35 years old and have no major health issues or inherited family disease. Most centers also have the donor and her partner checked for all infectious diseases, such as HIV, hepatitis B and C, syphilis, and gonorrhea. Some also do psychological screenings to make sure that the donor fully understands the implications of egg donation and is mentally stable enough to handle donating.

If you're bringing a donor that you've found yourself to the clinic, she'll most likely be required to do all the same testing. If your donor is a relative, however, your clinic may allow you to waive some of the testing.

WARNING

The screening and testing required by the FDA is not something that can be waived as all clinics are required to perform this under federal law. If they don't, the clinic can be closed, so don't expect to get around these requirements.

Signing the documents: Lawyering up, again

You and your donor must sign legal consents. The donor signs that she's voluntarily donating her eggs and won't try to claim any parenting rights in the future. This consent is required even if the donor is someone you know.

You sign that you're voluntarily using donor eggs to create a child. You also sign that you and your partner (if you aren't a single parent) agree to be the sole legal parents of the child and assume all costs for bearing and raising the child.

At present, a child born from donor sperm, eggs, or embryos is automatically the child of the recipients and doesn't need to be legally adopted by either parent at birth.

Coordinating your Donor Oocyte Recipient "DOR" cycle

There are many ways to utilize the embryos from a cycle using donor eggs. The most common is to coordinate the two cycles. This requires controlling both the donor and recipient's cycle, which is usually done using oral contraceptives and Lupron. However, there are many ways to achieve this control. Once under control, the donor starts the stimulation and the recipient starts oral estrogen. The cycle is set by the donor's response to the stimulation. Once the donor receives the hCG trigger shot, the recipient adds progesterone to the estrogen. The oocytes are retrieved, sperm is added, and the embryos are cultured. After three to five days the embryos are examined, and an embryo is transferred to the recipient. Estrogen and progesterone are continued, and if you're pregnant, will continue into the late first trimester. After that your pregnancy is just like any other. Some cycles will have the retrieval and embryos created, but the embryos will be frozen and then used at a later time. Finally, eggs can be frozen and used at a later time.

Getting support

You can find numerous support groups on the internet, not only for egg recipients but also for donors. Go to your favorite search engine, type in "donor eggs," and see what you get! If you have any questions or doubts about donating eggs or receiving donor eggs, you should be able to find plenty of people on the bulletin boards who can help you with your decision.

TIP

If you want a more one-on-one approach, a mental health professional or a family counselor who specializes in reproductive medicine, adoptions, or other family situations may be very helpful. You can ask your fertility clinic for recommendations or contact Resolve for suggestions. (We discuss Resolve in more detail in Chapter 8.) Also, ASRM's mental health professional group lists those who specialize in donor situations.

Enlisting the Aid of a Surrogate

Asking someone for the use of her eggs is one thing; she only has to commit to a few weeks of time and discomfort. Asking someone to commit to your cause for nine whole months by being a *gestational carrier* (GC) is quite another.

The use of gestational carriers (or surrogates) has exploded with the advent of in vitro fertilization. Women with health issues, women who lack a uterus, and women with a history of recurrent miscarriage are among those who are using friends, family, or total strangers to carry and deliver their biological children.

TECHNICAL STUFF

Surrogacy is defined as a third-party reproductive arrangement in which a woman agrees to attempt a pregnancy and carry a child for another individual or couple. It can take several forms:

>> Traditional surrogacy involves a woman acting as a gestational carrier using her own eggs (and often the intended father's sperm) to create the pregnancy. At birth, she will give the child to another individual or couple to parent and — though she has a biological connection to the child — she does not intend to be involved in the child's life. Today, this can be very risky business as many states have banned this practice and GCs in traditional surrogacy arrangements have been known to change their minds and keep the babies, leading to tragic legal and emotional results.

>> Gestational surrogacy is an arrangement where a woman has an embryo that is not genetically related to her transferred to her uterus and she carries the pregnancy for another individual or couple.

Finding that special woman

Some people love to be pregnant, and other people love to be pregnant as long as they're getting paid for it. Either type may be suitable as a gestational carrier. Many women ask immediate family members first but remember that a "no" doesn't mean that person doesn't love you or want to help. Some women see pregnancy as a nine-month misery and wouldn't go through it if you begged them; others truly enjoy being pregnant and welcome the chance to help you out as well.

If your sister and best friend turn you down, you need to look a little further. What if your mom wants to do this for you? Would you feel funny about her giving birth to her grandchildren? How would you handle the local press? (You can assume that there may be some, because this type of human-interest story is very popular with the press.)

Using matching companies

The work of finding a gestational carrier has become much simpler with the introduction of numerous commercial businesses that help *intended parents* (IPs) — that's the person or couple wanting to be parents — find the right person to carry their child. Most fertility clinics have a roster of matching companies that they work with on a regular basis and are comfortable referring their patients to. Whether these commercial businesses are called coordinating programs or surrogacy companies, these programs generally recruit and prescreen the GCs so that you at least know that these woman have met the program's criteria (such as a basic background check, confirmation of previous pregnancy, and some medical information). One drawback to using commercial businesses is that there can often be a hefty fee for their administrative services, which is only part of the costs as you'll also have the GC's fee, as well as legal and medical costs.

Looking for your own surrogate

If all possible friends or relatives are out, you may want to look on the internet, where gestational carriers place ads and, of course, all sound like the salt of the earth. Again, some women love being pregnant and also don't mind the extra money. Others are just looking for the extra money.

If you take the initiative to search for a surrogate on your own, be aware that there are lots of websites, chat rooms, and internet listings that can help you connect, but not all are reliable. If you decide to go this route, you need to remember that you will need to take the appropriate steps to ensure that you get detailed and thorough information on any GC you are considering. This will take a lot of diligence on your part to get the right investigators, as well as legal and mental health professionals to help you navigate this potential arrangement.

WARNING

Don't sign up with the first wonderful-sounding candidate without doing *a lot* of research. Many women have even hired a private agent to check into the carrier's background. That's not a bad idea; it's easy on paper to say that you're something you're really not!

Traveling abroad for more options

Some patients have looked outside of their home countries for women to act as surrogates — due to the cost, privacy and access issues, or for convenience. There are numerous companies on the internet that advertise cross-border reproductive care (CBRC; traveling outside your country of domicile for reproductive treatment). While this may sound like a great alternative, as we caution in Chapter 22 and later in this chapter, U.S. law and practices will not follow you beyond U.S. borders, and there may be difficulties getting your baby home if you cannot prove parentage and citizenship. In addition, while treatment costs may be less, you need to factor in the travel and accommodation costs.

Sharing "your" pregnancy

You'll have to do in vitro fertilization to use a gestational carrier because you'll be transferring embryos to her uterus. The carrier will usually take Estrace, an estrogen pill, to thicken her uterine lining, for several weeks, followed by progesterone. The embryos are then transferred to her uterus. You and your carrier can do synchronized cycles so that the embryos can be transferred to her a few days after your egg retrieval without first being frozen. Or you can do an egg retrieval first and freeze the embryos to transfer to the carrier a month or even a year down the road. If you need an egg donor as well, the cycle will be coordinated by the clinic using the donor's eggs, your husband's sperm, and the surrogate's uterus.

Once the carrier gets pregnant, her pregnancy and delivery will proceed just like any other. Most couples are in fairly close contact with the carrier during the pregnancy, so that any problems that arise can be dealt with jointly. If you've hired a carrier rather than using a friend or relative, you should have a payment plan agreed on before doing the embryo transfer.

In most cases, the carrier agrees to let you be present for the delivery, so you can see the baby right away. You need to know your state's rules for putting your names on the birth certificate as the biological or intended parents of the baby. Your lawyer will be instrumental in getting the documents you'll need to verify that the baby is your child. (More on legal needs later in this chapter.) After a short hospital stay, you take the baby home with you.

Medical clearance of your surrogate

Anyone who is considering being a gestational carrier should be medically evaluated to ensure that it is safe for them to carry a pregnancy; otherwise, the risk to the gestational host outweighs any benefit. One issue that is frequently raised has to do with the fact that so many women are having children by C-section. So how many previous C-sections are safe for a woman before accepting her as a GH? This is not really known and needs to be addressed with the obstetrician providing OB care for the potential GC.

REMEMBER

No matter where you connect with a GC, expect to have your fertility clinic weigh in on whether she is "acceptable" as a GC. Most clinics have set criteria for GC selection, and ASRM has weighed in on this as well to help them make good decisions. This approval process is there to protect both you and the GC by ensuring that she is physically and mentally capable of carrying a pregnancy for you. Much of the pretesting (that may drive you absolutely crazy and will cost you extra dollars) is required under the FDA. This U.S. government agency set guidelines to prevent the transmission of infectious disease, and compliance applies to GCs as well as to egg donors and sperm donors.

Legal issues to follow to make sure your baby is really yours

On top of all the medical procedures that you need to deal with when you start contemplating surrogacy, you have to be aware of the applicable legal requirements or you may set a plan in motion that ends in you not being able to bring your baby home.

Laws regarding surrogacy arrangements vary greatly. The surrogacy laws where you (the intended parent) live, where the GC lives, and where the baby will be delivered all play a part in how you select a GC, have a legal agreement drafted, and get legal clearance that proves your baby is really yours. First and foremost, you need to know what the surrogacy laws are in your home state. Equally important, you need to know the surrogacy laws in the state where your GC will be delivering. Surprise! They may not be the same, or the states may have conflicting laws. If you choose a GC from overseas, you may have additional hurdles to jump as, depending upon where the GC delivers, you are looking at trying to get citizenship established for your baby — and a passport to bring that baby home.

Coauthor Lisa has heard many sad stories of babies being left behind in foreign countries because the parents couldn't secure a U.S. passport, parents who had to live for years between the United States and a foreign country, and the problems of securing a birth certificate with your name as the parent when there was a discrepancy in state laws. Her best advice is to learn all of the legal rules of establishing parentage *before* you start the ART cycle to create a pregnancy. There is no greater heartache than to have a child you can't bring home.

Several legal issues need to be addressed for all patients using a GC. Many clinics require that you have all the legal paperwork completed (and proven to them in writing) before they will start your ART cycle, whether it's a fresh donor egg/GC cycle or a frozen embryo/GC transfer cycle. Here is a short list of what you may be asked to complete:

>> Retain an attorney for you (the parents) and a separate attorney for the GC. You and your GC are on different sides of this agreement and each of you will need an advocate who represents you, individually. Sharing an attorney may seem like a great way to cut costs, but it runs the risk of creating conflicts of interest that can lead to problems down the road. All experts now agree that each party to a third-party reproductive arrangement needs their own attorney. By the way, it is expected that you as the intended parent will pay for all legal representation. The good news is that many ART attorneys charge by the transaction and not by the hour!

>> In some jurisdictions, you may need to have your fertility physician document the medical need for using a GC.

>> Sign a gestational surrogacy agreement (a legally binding contract) with the gestational carrier and provide the clinic with proof that this agreement has been completed. This agreement sets out your relationship with the woman who will carry your child and, among other items, spells out her responsibilities, where she will deliver, and the expenses and fees you will pay her.

>> Depending upon your state or the state where your baby will be delivered, you may need to have a pre-birth order filed with the court so that your name will appear on the child's birth certificate.

WARNING Be aware that legal requirements are going to take time and may lead to frustration, angst, and downright anger at not being able to get started on making your baby. Please understand that this is not intended as a blockade to moving forward but arises from the clinic's concern for you as the intended parent of any child it helps create.

TIP If you are looking at third-party reproduction using gestational surrogacy, you need to know all of the legal requirements involved. Yes, this costs extra in legal fees, but it's worth it. This is not the time to ask your cousin Vinny to do your agreements. With the increased complexity in surrogacy, birth record, and citizenship laws, you need an expert on your side. Lisa recommends finding an experienced ART attorney through the American Academy of Adoption and Assisted Reproductive Technology Attorneys (AAARTA). You can find an AAARTA attorney in your area by searching at www.aaarta.org/.

Embryo Donation

Some clinics maintain lists of couples who want to donate their embryos to another couple, usually because the donating couple has one or more children through IVF and doesn't want any more. Brokers also match unwanted embryos with prospective parents via the internet or through organizations dedicated to egg and embryo donation. Screening ranges from no more than infectious blood testing to a full-blown home study done by an adoption agency; you also receive information about the donating parents and usually some type of family genetic history.

Your name is on the birth certificate, and unless you give out the information, no one will know that you used donor embryos. Some couples find it easier emotionally to have a child who's not related to either one of them rather than using donor eggs or sperm.

WARNING

Of course, this method again brings up the possibility of legal questions, moral issues, and possible complications a few years down the road. At the time of this writing, no cases have been filed of embryo donors going to court to get their children back after their birth. But that doesn't mean that it couldn't happen in the future, despite the paperwork that parents sign when they donate their embryos.

Using donor embryos is fairly simple from a medical point of view. The procedure requires doing a frozen embryo transfer at an IVF clinic. This cycle requires minimal medication, usually just estrogen pills before the transfer and progesterone after the transfer to maintain the pregnancy. However, the legal issues associated with donor embryos can be quite complex; for example, if the child should be born with an abnormality, the potential for a lawsuit is considerable. For this reason, many fertility clinics have shied away from embryo donation.

Telling your Pregnancy Story (or Not)

Everyone agrees that how, when, and why you got pregnant is *your* story. You wrote it, so to speak, but getting to keep it to yourself can be a big question. Historically, adoption and third-party family building was a lot easier to keep a secret. In the past 20 years there has been a dramatic change in social and professional attitudes toward disclosure of gamete donor use, much like disclosure and openness in the adoption arena. With the advent of direct-to-consumer DNA testing (thank you, Ancestry and 23andMe), children born of donor gametes are discovering that there is no biology between them and their parents. This technology, and a much greater societal acceptance of donor pregnancies, has changed the options for sharing your story. Anonymity for donors and secrecy for parents can no longer be guaranteed, and most professionals believe that disclosure is in the best interest of the child. They learn their genetic identity, are not subject to the negativity of secrets, and can gain more access to medical information.

TIP

While your donor journey may no longer be a secret, you still have a say in when and how to tell your story.

Deciding whether family and friends really need to know

Will you tell your family? That depends on you, your family, and a host of other factors that only you know. Some people don't even tell their families that they're doing IVF, much less tell them that they're using donor eggs. Given the fact that anonymity is dying, it may be easier to explain your choice now than have to explain it when the email pops up saying that there is a half-sibling, half-grandchild out there somewhere. This scene is being played out in a convoluted case in an Oregon court after a woman found out through 23andMe that her son had been a sperm donor and there was a child with his DNA, and she does not want contact with the child, and the sperm bank filed a restraining order to enforce anonymity. As more parents share these third-party stories, we'll also get a better handle on how to describe donor-created relationships.

REMEMBER

Telling or not is ultimately your choice. In some cases, the there may be cultural or religious implications for not telling that outweigh the benefits. Only you can decide if your right to privacy is stronger than your child's right to genetic information, and when that balance may shift and your position changes.

Telling the child (or not): When and how to do this

It's possible — no, make that probable — that somewhere down the line, your child will find out that he or she is the product of donor eggs or sperm, even if you don't want him or her to know. It may happen in high school biology, where students often test their blood types. Or, more likely, when they decide to check their DNA. In rare instances, information has crept out when your child develops a rare inherited disease, and you need to go back to his biological family for information.

Keeping a secret like this is difficult, but dealing with negative family reactions, if there are any, is difficult too. There is plenty of data to show that secrets cause harm to the secret holder and all other stakeholders in the secret. But there is also data showing that being donor-conceived is not as detrimental as we used to believe. In fact, studies show that genetic relatedness has no impact on child-parent functioning, and parenting skills and a positive family environment are more important to a child's well-being than family structure.

That doesn't mean the telling will be easy. If you tell your child, you fear he'll cry, "You're not my *real* mother!" and if you don't tell, you'll cringe every time he says, "I wish I had a different mother!" All children say things like this, whether they're adopted, biological, or whatever; take it with a grain of salt!

TIP

Some experts suggest that telling your child about his donor conception around the age of six is optimal for acceptance. Regardless of how old your child is when/if you share your story, you may want to consider the following:

>> Keep it simple. The easiest language is the story of how your child came to be with the help of a kind man or woman. (Why the word "kind?" Experts say it implies a positive!)

>> Use available age-appropriate story books. These are easily found online.

>> Don't expect a big moment of awe — especially if your child is younger. Many kids react with "Okay but you're still my dad" and "Can we get dessert?"

>> If you choose not to tell, prepare yourself for the inadvertent disclosure when it comes.

Using a registry

You've seen the show one hundred times. Mothers, fathers, brothers, sisters meeting in a tearful on-air display of how technology can help locate and reunite long-lost relatives. Will this become commonplace in the case of donor eggs, sperm, and embryos in the future? Most gamete donors in the past had no intention of maintaining any contact with their future offspring, and most parents of children conceived through donor gametes weren't interested in future contact, either. The answer is that it's already happening. DNA testing is connecting the dots of donor offspring across the country — regardless of whether parents, children, or donors wanted it.

Today, you can find thousands of internet sites under sibling registry, parent registry, donor registry, and so on. Donors, parents, siblings, and children can be registered with agencies that will put interested parties together in the future. While these sites have traditionally been utilized mostly for adopted children and the biological parents, they are now being used to locate gamete donors, donors' families, donor siblings, and donor offspring.

THE DEBATE ABOUT DONOR-CONCEIVED ANONYMITY

A recent study (2017) asked French couples about whether they had told their children they were born using donor sperm. At the time of the study, about 40 percent had already told their children, and most of these had made that decision before proceeding with donor sperm. Of the 60 percent who had not told their child, 65 percent were planning on telling their child, but not just yet. Given the rapid change in the use of genetic testing, keeping donations anonymous will become very difficult. Some donor clinics now advertise that they have donors open to having some contact with any children born — some say after the child reaches age 18, and others are open to an ongoing relationship. Several recent court cases have questioned a sperm donor's right to remain anonymous. Analogies can easily be made for egg donors. It seems likely that some families won't talk about using donor eggs, either, although in a recent study, just over half the parents surveyed indicated that they planned to tell the child eventually.

The anonymity debate has been resolved differently in different places. But it is clear that it is not going to be left up to what the parents choose as it was historically. While some countries protect donor anonymity by law (for example, Spain, France, and Denmark), other countries have enacted laws allowing children access to identifying information after they attain a certain age (for example, Sweden, Austria, the Australian state of Victoria, Switzerland, the Netherlands, Norway, the United Kingdom, New Zealand, Germany, Ireland, and Finland). North America is slower to change donor anonymity rules: In Canada, a 2012 court decision overturned a ban on anonymous gamete donation, and the United States has no federal law on anonymity and only two states (Washington and California) have laws regulating donor anonymity.

For this reason, clinics, donor matching companies, and adoption agencies are crystal clear regarding the issue of disclosure. For example, sperm bank websites allow for exchange of medical information between parents and donors, explain how to reach out for specific information, and admonish you about *not* trying to locate donors without going through the bank. Most clinics also tell their patients that anonymity between donors and parents/children is not guaranteed, and they offer patients counseling on dealing with this issue.

Modern Families: Getting Pregnant

The definition of "family" has never been more diverse than it is today — and why not! There are many ways to parent and love a child, and the world of assisted reproductive medicine has made it easier for all manner of family to add a child.

When you're single or LBGTQIA

It's never been easier to have a child if you're a single parent or in a same-sex relationship, with sperm banks available to single or gay women and the use of gestational carriers and egg donors available to single or gay men. (See the section "Heading to the Bank — The Sperm or Egg "Cryo" Bank, That Is" for info on finding donor sperm.)

Finding sperm

If you're a single or gay woman, you're going to find it easier to have a baby than a single man — you've got the right equipment! All you need is the sperm, and sperm is something that's readily available, whether you want to use an anonymous donor or a close friend.

If you're considering using a friend as your donor, here are some of the benefits:

>> You're most likely aware of the person's personality traits.

>> You know what he looks like.

>> You probably like the person, or you wouldn't be asking him to do this for you.

Alas, where you find pros, you also find cons. Here are some of the potential complications that come from using a donor you know over one who remains anonymous:

>> How involved will he be in your child's life? No involvement, holiday visits, or heavy involvement?

>> If your parenting techniques differ, how much input will he have on how you raise your child?

>> If something happens to you, will he be the legal guardian?

If you're thinking of using an anonymous donor, consider the following pros:

>> You won't have to worry about the father wanting to be involved with the child.

>> You can be very picky about physical characteristics and other attributes.

On the con side, consider these issues:

>> You'll have to rely on what the catalog says about the donor, with no way of knowing how accurate the information really is.

>> You won't be able to tell your child much about his paternal heritage.

>> It may be difficult for your child to be able to contact his birth father, if he wants to.

TIP

Even if you don't foresee any complications down the road, writing up a legal document to cover your bases is always a wise idea.

WARNING

If you're using fresh sperm from a known donor, you need to be aware of the risk of contracting an infectious disease such as HIV or hepatitis. It's much wiser to use a frozen specimen after having your donor tested at the time the specimen is frozen, and then tested again six months later. If he's still negative, you can use the frozen specimen.

WARNING

Never try to do an intracervical or intrauterine insemination at home! You can place the sperm near the cervix but not inside it!

Finding eggs and a uterus

Things are certainly more complicated if you're a guy or gay couple trying to have a baby without a female partner. You just can't do it alone! If you want to be a dad, the first thing you need to find is a female. You may want to ask a friend, or you may want to hire a surrogate who'll carry the baby for you and then relinquish all parental rights to you. (See "Enlisting the Aid of a Surrogate" for more on surrogates.)

REMEMBER

Legal issues should be written up by a lawyer who's well versed in surrogacy in the state where the baby will be born, because that state's laws will govern your experience. Many of the laws that govern gay parent surrogacy also cover a single male's use of a surrogate or carrier, with California being the most liberal state.

Your lawyer will need to submit affidavits to the court from your clinic, your carrier or surrogate, and you to help establish paternity for the birth certificate. Some states require DNA testing to establish paternity; others don't.

Finding the right clinic

Fortunately, it has become far less common that a clinic will not work with singles or married patients from the LBGTQ community. If you live in a rural or particularly conservative area, you may have to travel to get the job done. ASRM has LGBTQIA resource information on its website (www.asrm.org).

REMEMBER

After you have your list of possibilities, mention your specific circumstances during your first phone call. You want to make sure that your doctor is supportive of your situation before you make an appointment.

Understanding the process

Patience is a virtue, but going through fertility treatment as a same-sex couple (especially male couples) can seem like it is taking forever! You are actually following the same processes as your hetero or single counterparts, plus or minus a counseling session or a legal review. Unmarried couples may be asked to consider/discuss co-parenting legal agreements so that they and any child they have are protected. As with all third-party reproductive treatments, choosing donors and gestational surrogates, completing medical testing (and FDA requirements), getting psychological clearance, and completing legal agreements all take time to organize — let alone accomplish.

Your goal is to have a baby, and the big "list of things to do" is really your best road map to reaching your goal.

Transgender fertility issues

Transgender is defined as a person whose gender identity is inconsistent with their gender assignment at birth. It is estimated that there are over a million transgender people in the United States. The gender assumed by the person can, but need not, include social, emotional, surgical, or medical aspects. A survey done in 2015 identified that about 50 percent of transgender people had utilized hormone therapies and 25 percent had undergone surgery. Over 50 percent of transgender people desire children, and one study showed that transwomen would have done sperm cryopreservation had it been offered to them.

For prepubertal transgender people, the use of long-acting GnRH agonists suppresses puberty, allowing more time to assess and transition to their gender choice. This therapy is reversible if the person chooses not to undergo identity reassignment. Transmen may choose to use testosterone. The long-term effect of this is unknown, and some studies, but not all, have demonstrated that this produced polycystic-like ovaries. For transwomen, the use of estrogen suppresses the release of FSH, and LH causes testosterone levels to drop. The reduced testosterone reduces sperm production. Like the situation for the transmen, the long-term effect of estrogen on sperm production is uncertain at this point.

For transmen contemplating removal of the ovaries, fertility options include oocyte or embryo cryopreservation. Transmen who have had their uterus removed can use a gestational host to create a pregnancy, much like single men. Transmen who retain their uterus can undergo a pregnancy, and in a study of 197 transmen, 60 pregnancies were reported — so it is possible. For transwomen, sperm banking is an option for fertility preservation. Some transwomen find it impossible to masturbate but can use testicular aspiration of sperm as an option. Uterine transplant is in its infancy but may someday make it possible for transwomen to carry and deliver a pregnancy.

As of the writing of this book, the field of fertility for transgender people is in its infancy. With more people acknowledging their gender identity and the increasing acceptance of transgender people, the field of reproductive medicine for transgender people should become more complete.

Chapter **21**

Moving On: Not Necessarily the End of The Road

How you get to this point isn't important. What matters is making decisions about what road to take next. You may choose to adopt, and after you make that decision, you need to make many more. Do you want to adopt internationally, interracially, through a public agency, or from a private source? Do you want a newborn or an older child?

You may choose instead to work with children as a teacher or social worker, or as a foster parent. Or you may decide that you can live a fulfilling life without children. In this chapter, we show you how to evaluate your choices and find the path that's right for you — when you're ready.

Letting Go of the Dream

Coauthor Jackie was sure that she had finally had enough. This realization came about three weeks prior to the start of the successful cycle that brought Jackie her beautiful daughter, Ava. Less than halfway through that cycle, which she referred to as a "goat rodeo" for all that went wrong, Jackie had decided that she *could not take another step.* She fought with her doctor, nurse, husband, and anyone else who would listen to her complain. She knew that she had reached her endpoint. Luckily, the light at the end of the tunnel wasn't a train. But then again, it generally never is.

Everyone reaches points in their lives when they instinctively know that they can't take another step. The process of infertility is no exception. The trick is knowing when you have reached the end of the line, or when a well-deserved break may be in order (we discuss ways to take a respite in Chapter 10).

But if you have truly gotten to that point of no return where you can't fathom another test, another shot, another phone call — regardless of the outcome, it's time to do something different.

REMEMBER

Letting go is never easy, and the higher the stakes, the more difficult the process.

When medicine can no longer help

Why is it so hard to determine when modern science can no longer help to achieve a pregnancy?

Coauthor Dr. R relates: After more years than I care to admit to, the saddest part of my commitment to my patients is to help them understand that the field of medicine has nothing remaining to help them conceive. How can a couple know that the questions: "What about just one more cycle of IVF; my friend said her friend got pregnant on her sixth cycle of IVF," and so on simply don't apply to them and in fact may prevent them from moving forward.

The core problem is that couples with the diagnosis of infertility are members of a group of patients who share the same diagnosis. The definition is based upon time as well as medical problem. This group of patients is actually composed of two groups: one can get pregnant (subfertile) and the other will never get pregnant (sterile). For the subfertile group, some will conceive without any help — it will just take more time — and the other group can conceive but only with medical intervention. At some point, there are no tests that will accurately identify which group a person belongs in. As time goes by, the subfertile group not requiring treatment will achieve a pregnancy and drop out of the remaining people. So the longer it takes without treatment, the more likely it is that they will not achieve a pregnancy. Likewise, where treatment is required to achieve a pregnancy, the longer treatment lasts, the less likely the treatment is to actually be effective. That means that at some point, those people remaining are sterile. But, the frustration is that often, there is no accurate way to define sterility. What can be defined more accurately is when treatment is no more effective than doing nothing.

For example, one study looked at women with PCOS. If they did Clomid therapy, after six attempts about 25 percent of the women had elevated male hormones and 50 percent were pregnant if the women had normal male hormones. (These were women under 40 years old.) If they then did three cycles of IVF, 58 percent of this group were pregnant. That's a lot of treatment, and at this point most patients would be encouraged to stop. But if they then added three cycles of FSH treatments, the overall pregnancy rate was 89 percent. Compare that to using treatment for age-related infertility. One study looked at the chance of achieving a pregnancy for women over age 42 using up to nine cycles of IVF. The per cycle pregnancy rate was 3–4 percent for each cycle for the first five cycles. For cycles six to nine, the rate was 0 except for the seventh cycle where two patients out of ten became pregnant. Did the IVF help them achieve a pregnancy or would they have conceived spontaneously? Frustratingly, there is absolutely no way to know.

There is also a phenomenon in medicine called the therapeutic illusion. This was described in 1978 by Dr. K.B. Thomas. The basis for this concept is the fact that some people will get better without treatment. If treatment was applied, then the conclusion is that the treatment worked. Both patients and physicians tend to overestimate the effectiveness of treatment. When treatment has not been successful, it is important to step back and ask, "What is the goal? Is the goal to just do IVF, is the goal to have a child, or is the goal to resolve issues that a person may have surrounding their fertility?" At some point, the goal of issue resolution takes center stage. How a person gets to that point is unique to each person. Sometimes, the hardest thing to do is to do nothing. Physicians are trained to do something, and most patients expect something to be done. But pursuing treatment that is no different than doing nothing will prevent the resolution of the greater issue of infertility.

Going through the grief process

Grief is one of life's most difficult emotions. Despite the fact that you may have many people around who are willing and able to help, grief can cause you to feel isolated, desperate, and hopeless. Either extreme of avoiding grief or immersing yourself in it can lead to depression, which actually stops you from moving through, and beyond, the grief process. As clichéd as it may sound, you can get through it, and time will help.

Perhaps the best way to deal with the morass of emotions brought on by the loss of the dream of a biological child is by looking at the grief process. Elisabeth Kubler-Ross, the author of *On Death and Dying*, identified the five stages of grief following the death of a loved one: denial, anger, bargaining, depression, and acceptance. The death of a dream is much the same. While using the death process may be helpful, it falls short when considering infertility. When a loved one dies there is a wake. There is a funeral. You can stand by the coffin and touch the deceased. You can go to the cemetery and see the grave. There is an easily defined, physical endpoint. That is not true for infertility. There is no physically definable endpoint that can be touched, buried, or seen. Infertility is based upon guessing (probability) that pregnancy will not occur, and using zero probability in medicine is very rarely done. How often have you heard that nothing is impossible? In fact, in the world of human physiology, some things are impossible.

REMEMBER

You may go through these stages of grief more than once. You may skip a stage or repeat it twice before you come to accept what has happened. Working through the grief process of not having a biological child takes time. And unfortunately, it's hard to hurry up the process no matter how much you want it to be over. The only way past grief is through it. But you don't have to do it alone.

Knowing when to get help (and what kind of help)

While grief is a process to move through, many people can get stuck in it as well. Figuring out whether you are stuck or not can be tricky and often requires the input of your friends, family, and even colleagues who may be more objective in offering you a reality check. Asking your partner or a trusted friend to help you figure out if you're dealing with your grief or dwelling on it too much can help give you clarity on what to do next. Friends, family, support groups, and books can help to buoy you through the process.

It's easy to isolate yourself when you're feeling the kind of pain brought on by grief. If you find that you can't even bring yourself to check in with those around you, you could probably use some guidance. If you are beset with the "Why me's?" that have you questioning yourself, your faith, and life as you know it, you would likely benefit from the wisdom that a pastor, priest, rabbi, or cleric may be able to provide. If your feelings of grief have become feelings of despair and hopelessness, particularly of the type that have you contemplating doing harm to yourself or someone else, you need help, and fast.

Professional help is a wonderful option for those whose hope switch is temporarily stuck in the off position. You can ask your family physician, fertility specialist, or nurse to recommend a therapist to help you work through your emotions. It's not about finding someone to tell you that your dreams can come true; it's working to re-tool those dreams to better fit your circumstances. Members of ASRM's mental health professional group are a wonderful resource. You can be happy again and you will, provided you deal with that which ails you. Don't be alarmed if a professional suggests antidepressants. This treatment, like your depression, may be a temporary situation. Whether through medication or talk therapy, you *can* find relief during this difficult time.

Opting to Adopt

A life without biological children doesn't mean a life without any children. Many children, both in the United States and abroad, need parents to love and care for them. Adoption is a tree with many branches, and you need to first decide what kind of child you're looking for. Are you open to adopting an older child or one with physical handicaps? Are you interested in a child of another race? Or are you willing to keep all your options open and try several different routes at one time?

More than 135,000 children are adopted each year in the United States. About 70 percent are adopted by stepparents or other relatives. Ninety percent of adoptions are domestic, and the other 10 percent come from foreign adoptions. Some adoptions are *open* adoptions, meaning that the adoptive and birth parents meet and continue to have some involvement in one another's lives. About 70 percent of domestic adoptions are open adoption. Other adoptions are arranged through established public agencies and usually don't include any contact between birth and adoptive families. Only 4 percent of adoptions are from unwanted pregnancies. Adoption can cost anywhere from a few dollars to thousands of dollars. We look briefly at different types of adoption.

Websites such as www.adoption.com also contain adoption forums, waiting children information, and ads for prospective adoptive parents. The Child Welfare Information Gateway (formerly, National Adoption Information Clearinghouse) can be found at https://sparkaction.org/content/national-adoption-information-clearinghous and also contains information on every aspect of adoption.

Considering traditional domestic adoption

When most people think about adoption, they think about traditional domestic adoption. An old movie, *Penny Serenade,* details the typical scenario: A couple is unable to have children, so they go through the process of adopting a Caucasian infant. The film contains the traditional themes — parents-to-be are evaluated by a strict social worker, and the baby is almost taken away because the hopeful father lost his job and income before the adoption was finalized. This type of adoption is becoming rarer today because more birth mothers are choosing to place their children through private adoption, which gives them more control over who will adopt their child (see the next section, "Looking into private domestic adoption" for more information on private adoptions). Some agencies still doing traditional adoptions are religious organizations and county and state adoption agencies.

In a traditional adoption, the adoptive parents usually have no contact with the birth parents. A social worker conducts a home study to make sure that you're financially and emotionally able to support a child. The children adopted are usually infants, although more older and special-needs children are starting to be adopted, especially through state and public agencies.

If you're older, have any type of criminal record, or aren't reasonably financially secure, the agency may turn you down. The number of people looking to adopt an infant far outweighs the number of infants available, so agencies can afford to be picky.

Looking into private domestic adoption

You've probably seen the ads, and maybe you've even written one: "Loving, financially secure couple wants to give your child a home." Newspapers and many websites contain these ads, written to appeal to young women looking to give their children up for adoption. If you really want a newborn, this method is probably your best route to adoption.

These adoptions are handled by a lawyer who may be your source for a baby in addition to being your legal adviser. You may also find an infant through an organization specializing in finding newborns. Your source for a baby may also be your pastor or your doctor.

Private adoption is expensive — according to current data you can pay on average $43,000 to adopt privately. Legitimate payable expenses in private adoption include lawyers' fees as well as the birth mom's living costs, pregnancy, delivery, and newborn care costs.

TIP

To be successful at a private adoption, tell everyone you know that you're looking. Write the most emotionally appealing ad you can, and send it to as many newspapers as you can afford. (Make sure the state in which you're advertising allows this type of ad — not all do.) Many prospective adoptive parents spend up to $7,000 in advertising costs alone. Also, create a website on the internet and make sure that you, your house, and your lifestyle are pictured in as appealing a manner as possible.

TIP

Get a good lawyer, even before you start looking. If you find a baby, you want to have all the legal issues taken care of as soon as possible.

After you find a possible candidate, keep your guard up all the time. Go slow and don't commit to anything right away. And, most importantly, don't give anyone money without having a lawyer review everything.

A private adoption can be as open as you want it to be. Some couples have the birth mother live with them before she delivers; others just have a few meetings at a neutral location. Some never meet the birth parents at all. You may be able to be at the delivery and take the baby home from the hospital, if the birth mother agrees. Many experts today argue that open adoption is better for the adopted child and his family because his origins are never hidden and are often well known. However, you must do what you feel is best for all involved.

WARNING

If you're normally a trusting person, you'd better learn to be wary and cautious during this process. We've heard of many cases of women pretending to be pregnant, taking money from more than one couple, or just reneging on the deal after the baby is born. You can't be too careful.

For information about the legalities of adoption, check the website of the Academy of Adoption and Assisted Reproductive Attorneys at https://adoptionart.org/.

Exploring international adoption

Harry Holt became an adoption pioneer when he and his wife headed off for Korea to help find families for the mixed-race children of the Korean War. Now, Holt is one of many agencies placing children from Korea, China, South America, and Vietnam, among others. (His website can be found at www.holtintl.org.)

While China, India, Ukraine, Colombia, South Korea, and Haiti are the main countries currently involved in adoptions, the rate of international adoption has dropped 72 percent between the years 2005–2015.

One reason that foreign countries have halted foreign adoptions claims that bans are in the "best interest" of the child. They cite cases of abuse after the foreign adoption. Russia passed a law banning U.S. adoptions and named it Yakovlev after a two-year-old adopted child who died in the U.S. from the heat of being left in a car. Ethiopia used similar logic in its ban, citing the death of a 13-year-old female who died from hypothermia and malnutrition. Fortunately, these tragic cases are rare, and the bans may actually reflect the role of politics as Russia purportedly ended adoptions after the U.S. imposed sanctions for unrelated corruption, and Romania adopted its ban in order to be allowed to enter the European Union.

Further, effective in 1995, the Hague Convention on International Adoption, which was supposed to address the issues of corruption and abuse raised by international adoption seems to actually have been responsible for a large part of the decline. The Convention requires documentation about the legal parentage, and this is just not present for a number of these kids. The Convention requires that efforts are made in their own country to see if they will be adopted domestically. This usually means an additional year in an orphanage, which reduces the chance that they will be adopted. Furthermore, poor countries could not meet the high standards set by the Convention. The rules raised the cost of adoption through fess imposed on agencies, parents, and adopting parents. Today, over 99 countries have signed on to the Hague Convention.

The trend in deceasing foreign adoptions seems to be continuing. There was an increase in adoptions from India and Columbia, but this was offset by a decrease in adoptions from China and Ethiopia. The U.S. has also suspended adoptions (temporarily or otherwise) from countries where Hague Convention criteria has not been met, such as Guatemala and Vietnam.

Not all foreign adoptions are done through agencies; some are private. The cost of adopting internationally is seldom less than a domestic adoption and, sometimes, is much more. Besides the costs for a home study, lawyers' fees, and agency services, there's the cost of travel and doing business in a foreign country.

Some parents feel more secure with a foreign adoption, because the chances of the birth parents showing up and asking to take their child back are perceived as lower than with a stateside adoption.

Some of the children up for adoption are younger than six months, but the red tape of international adoptions means that your baby may be closer to a year by the time you get him or her home. Some countries want you to stay in the country for several weeks; others let you pick your child up at the airport.

REMEMBER

Children adopted from foreign countries may be at greater risk for diseases and special needs related to their early childhood experiences than those adopted from the United States. Medical care abroad is not what it is in the U.S. and ranges from excellent to nearly nonexistent, depending on where your child came from. More countries are trying to place children in foster care rather than keep them in orphanages, to help their social and emotional development. Some children come with serious attachment disorders, and others may have undiagnosed medical conditions. It is important to have your child examined by a medical provider, even an adoption medical specialist, as soon as you bring them home.

Adopting a special-needs child

Plenty of children up for adoption, in this country and abroad, are classified as *special-needs children*. Usually, they have a physical handicap, but they may also have a mental or emotional handicap. Some children are classified as special-needs kids because they're not infants or toddlers, or because they're members of a racial minority.

Back in the heyday of adoption, before abortion was legal and having a child out of wedlock was a social stigma, children were plentiful, and older children (older being anyone over one year old back then), racially mixed children, and handicapped children were rarely adopted. Now, prospective parents are applying to adopt Down syndrome babies, children with serious emotional and physical disabilities, and children of a different race.

WARNING

Although it's easy to be caught up emotionally in the idea of raising a special-needs child, look realistically at your lifestyle and personalities before making a decision.

Social workers in the United States are still somewhat hesitant to place an African-American or Native American child in a family of a different race. Many Native American groups are vehemently opposed to their children being placed in white families, and many African-Americans feel the same way, saying the children won't develop a proper racial identity if they aren't raised by parents of the same race.

Starting as a foster parent

Some couples look at foster parenting as a way to get a foot in the door, so to speak. Although you may possibly be allowed to adopt a foster child, the majority of children in foster care aren't available for adoption.

However, some foster children are released for adoption. If they do become available for adoption, 64 percent will be adopted by their former foster family, so in some cases you may be able to adopt your foster child.

Foster parents usually need to take classes to qualify. They're also subject to home inspections and supervision from social workers. Foster parents receive a monthly stipend of anywhere from $1,200 to $3,700 a month, with the average being $1,989 per month, depending on where they live.

REMEMBER

Foster parenting can be very rewarding, but it can also be heartbreaking to see children you've come to care about go back to environments that were harmful to them in the first place. However, there's a real need for good foster parents, and if you want to be truly instrumental in the life of a child — or more than one — foster parenting can be a good place to start.

Deciding to be a "Family of Two" — Living Child-Free

So here you are. You've tried and tried to conceive your child, and you've run out of money, time, hope, or all of the above. Third-party reproduction (donor eggs or sperm) isn't an option for you. Adoption is neither financially nor emotionally feasible at this time. What do you do?

At this point, some couples decide not to parent and remain child-free. While this is a highly individual decision, it is something that is an option for all individuals facing fertility treatment and should be supported as a viable option for a healthy and happy lifestyle.

PERSONAL STORY

Coauthor Lisa recalls one of her favorite couples who went through multiple cycles of Clomid/IUI and IVF and were not successful in achieving a pregnancy. Lisa met with them to discuss "what's next," and was surprised to hear their decision. As Lisa explained another IVF cycle, the wife reached across the table and grabbed her hand. "Lisa," she said with a big smile on her face, "we have decided to be a family of two." She then went on to explain that they were stopping efforts to have a child of their own and wanted to put their energies into their two rambunctious nephews who lived near them and other interests such as their home, travel, and their jobs. When they hugged Lisa as they left the office, Lisa was reminded that not all successes mean a baby — some are defined by being happy with who you are.

REMEMBER

Keep in mind that not having children of your own doesn't mean that you have no children in your life whatsoever. You probably have nieces or nephews or friends' children to spoil and care for, or there are children's schools or organizations in your community that you can get involved in that would welcome your help — and your smiles!

Chapter **22**

The Future is Now! New Advances, New Concerns in Fertility

You probably remember hearing about Dolly, the famous cloned sheep. Now, if you believe the tabloids, cloned human babies are already a reality. Every week you see a story about one wealthy person or another harboring a little "Mini Me" created by scientists working secretly in some exotic place. More recently, there has been a buzz about "designer babies." The technological advance called CRISPR has the potential to allow modification of the genetic code and thus to alter the embryo. This is still in the arena of science fiction but is probably closer to reality than most people know.

Whether or not you believe the tabloids and all the hype, one thing is certain: Technology is a double-edged sword. Every scientific advance brings questions about what technology *can* do versus what it *should* do. IVF was highly controversial when it was introduced, resulting in restraining orders, debates, and public concern. Somewhat underappreciated is the fact that Dr. Edward and Dr. Steptoe fought for IVF and laid an enviable ethical base that resulted in the U.K. having a very ethical approach to IVF, which persists to this day.

In this chapter, we look at some of the hottest fertility debates, realizing that by the time this book is printed, there could well be a new "new technology" that dwarfs all others.

Looking into the Future: Long-Term Health Effects of Fertility Medication

Fertility medications, or *gonadotropins,* are natural hormones, normally produced by the body. And when you go through menopause, the blood levels of all of these hormones are going to be far higher than anything that can be attained by injecting fertility medication. However, when given to women of reproductive age, whose ovaries can and do respond, they are powerful stuff. Anyone who takes them through even one cycle can attest to the physical and emotional effects of having one's hormones surging at a much higher level than nature ever intended. Do people suffer long-term effects 2 or 20 years down the road? No one knows for sure, but here are the most recent conclusions on the safety of taking gonadotropins.

Effects on the mother

At this time, experts have no solid proof that taking gonadotropins has any long-term effect on women. Some studies have shown a possible link between fertility medications and ovarian cancer, but other studies have not supported these findings. The actual risk to the mother is short-term hyperstimulation, which occurs in about 1.5 percent of IVF cycles and occurs so severely that the mother needs to be admitted to a hospital 0.34 percent of IVF stimulation cycles. Infection, significant bleeding, and anesthetic complications occurred in less than 0.1 percent of the cycles. From 2000 to 2011, there were no maternal deaths due to IVF.

WARNING

One thing most studies have agreed upon is that the risk of ovarian cancer is higher in all women who've never become pregnant, regardless of whether or not they've taken fertility medications. So, if you've taken fertility drugs for any amount of time and never had a child, make sure to consult your gynecologist. Like many things, the recommendations about frequency of visits and what testing to do changes constantly as more is learned about heritability of disease. Your healthcare can be tailored to meet your set of circumstances, and thus global recommendations may not be appropriate for you. Only a close working relation-ship with your healthcare provider can make sure you have the optimal healthcare.

Effects on the baby

No one is sure whether ART procedures will have a long-term effect on the chil-dren conceived through their use — the children born through high-tech methods such as in vitro fertilization (IVF) aren't old enough yet. The oldest IVF baby, Louise Brown, was born in 1978. So, is there something that will show up when the IVF conceived children reach 60, or 80, or 100? Techniques such as ICSI (intra-cytoplasmic sperm injection) and assisted hatching are even newer; they've only been used extensively since the 1990s.

Because research is ongoing even as children are being born, high-tech treatment has an element of risk simply because the jury's still out on long-term effects. Given the limitation data, what do we know about those people who have been conceived through IVF? Trying to accurately determine if IVF is harmful to the children it creates is difficult. One complication is trying to understand whether any harm is due to the diagnosis of infertility itself or is related to the procedure of IVF. Most authors of the studies evaluating the effect of IVF suggest that some of the risk *is* due to the diagnosis of infertility. Some studies have suggested that high-tech babies have lower birth weight (33 grams [1.16 ounces] lighter) and earlier delivery (by half a day). A 2016 study concluded that many obstetric and neonatal risks were elevated in singleton IVF pregnancies, including such things as birth defects and neonatal death. While the increased risks were real, the actual chance of one of these risks is low because these complications occur infrequently (8.3 percent prevalence in IVF babies as opposed to 5.8 percent prevalence in spontaneously conceived babies).

More twins and triplets are born to moms using fertility meds, and multiples more commonly have low birth weight and developmental delays. Also, more babies are born to older mothers through high-tech treatment, and older women tend to have more complicated pregnancies than women under age 35.

It's important to note that up to this point, no effect of fertility medications themselves on the babies has been shown. Furthermore, fertility medications are natural hormones, normally present in the body. And even though they may be present at higher than normal values during the stimulation phase, they're all well out of your system by the time the embryo implants. So whatever effect these medications may have would have to be on the egg, and these effects are purely hypothetical. Still, only time will tell for sure.

Gathering Steam: The Genetics Tool Train

Ten years from today, will parents be routinely selecting the child of their choice, picking height, IQ, hair and eye color, and left- or right-handedness? Or will they even go one step further and have the potential to insert genes that they themselves don't possess into their children, with short parents having tall children, or brunettes having blondes, or vice versa?

Brushing up on the latest genetic capabilities

Right now, PGT (preimplantation genetic testing) is the testing of the embryo for genetic problems or for sex selection. (See Chapter 17 for more information about PGT and its uses.)

Currently, PGT can test for a wide variety of genetic diseases, including hemophilia, Huntington's, muscular dystrophy, sickle cell disease, and Tay-Sachs, as well as chromosomal defects, such as Down syndrome and Turner syndrome.

As genetic mapping advances, it's not hard to imagine parents screening embryos not only for sex or genetic diseases but also for hair and eye color, intelligence, and personality traits. Although it's possible that none of these traits will ever be able to be accurately determined by PGT, they may be. This possibility has ethicists concerned about where PGT is headed.

The potential for gene tinkering is limitless after certain traits have been mapped out and identified. The positive aspect of such manipulation may be the elimination of certain diseases or handicaps.

The negative side is that we could end up with populations skewed in one direction only, such as a nation full of tall, brunette, genius baseball players. Or we could find the male-to-female ratio off balance, as is happening in China with its now eliminated one-child-only rule.

Although the potential for using gene selection for good purposes is high, the potential for abuse is just as high. However, many experts feel that such fears are overstated. They point out that if people really wanted a tall, brown-eyed baby, they could already go to a sperm bank and get the sperm from a tall, brown-eyed sperm donor, and then match it with the egg of a tall, brown-eyed egg donor. The reality is that individuals are shaped by many factors, both genetic and environmental. Even identical twins, who have identical genes and were carried in their mother's womb at the same time, are not identical individuals. Forgotten in all the hype is that the genetic process is incredibly complicated. Many use simple

Mendelian genetics (think peas) to hypothesize about what might be able to be done. But the biology of characteristics or disease risk is immensely complicated, involving hundreds to thousands of genes and gene products. So it may never be able to accomplish the fine-tuning of human construction to accomplish parental goals — like the next Tom Brady or LeBron James.

Manipulating the human genome to improve humans is called *eugenics* and was developed by Francis Galton in 1883. Eugenics fell into disrepute due to the use of genetics by Nazi Germany. However, eugenics has been practiced in the animal industry since ancient times and continues today. Eugenics raises incredibly difficult ethical issues. As technology advances, very complex issues will arise based upon the concepts in eugenics. Societal ethics are enforced by the legal system, so the solution for the issues raised will eventually be played in the legislative bodies and courts. It promises to be an interesting future for future generations.

Sex selection: When you absolutely, positively want a boy (or a girl)

There are lots of old wives' tales about having a boy versus a girl — where to sleep, what to eat, what to wear, and so on. But if you already have five boys and would dearly love a girl, or if you carry a genetic link to a sex-determined disease, such as hemophilia, you're probably looking for something a little more scientific. None of the simple techniques or even more technical techniques for sex selection have proven successful. It is possible to select the sex of the child, but it requires IVF and preimplantation genetic testing to identify the sex of the embryo.

Transplanting Body Parts to Improve Fertility

While it seems a bit "sci-fi" to even consider new reproductive parts, if you can get a knee replacement, why couldn't you just get a new ovary, or uterus, or testes? Unfortunately, as advanced as medicine is, it is just not there yet, but there is some hope on the way.

"New" ovaries?

Other experimental techniques that may hold promise for freezing eggs for future use involve freezing a portion of the ovary and transplanting it back to the original owner or to another woman. This has been done for women undergoing chemotherapy; once the treatment is finished and the risk of recurrence is low, the tissue is transplanted either back to the pelvis or to the forearm. Follicles have developed in the ovary after it was transplanted.

The first baby was born after ovary transplantation from one identical twin to another in 2004; when this technique is refined, it could bring hope of delivering a genetic child to women who undergo chemotherapy.

Permanently "borrowing" a uterus

Currently, uterine transplantation is extremely new. As such, ASRM recommends that only centers working under the supervision of an *institutional review board* (IRB) should be offering uterine transplantation. The uterus can be either from a living woman or from a cadaver. The indication for uterine transplantation is a diagnosis of absolute *uterus-factor infertility* (UFI). The number of women with UFI is estimated to be 1–3 percent. Conditions causing UFI include being born without a uterus, hysterectomy, and conditions that cause the uterus to be nonfunctional, such as uterine scarring. Alternatives are adoption or using a gestational host. As of September 2018, 30 uterine transplantations had been performed worldwide with only 11 subsequent births. The average pregnancy went to 35 weeks (normal is 40 weeks) with no birth defects. Though still very rare, this procedure has potential to help select patients so it may become more frequent.

Putting Your Plans on Ice

Why has *fertility preservation*, the storage of eggs, sperm, or embryos through cryopreservation, become such a hot topic today? Maybe it's because society is becoming more aware of efficacy of freezing gametes and the success of IVF and other forms of *assisted reproductive technologies* (ART). More likely, it's because we have learned how to manage otherwise devastating diseases and people are living to have children.

CAN TRANSPLANTATION HELP TESTES?

Currently, and sadly, no reports (or hints of experiments) on transplanting testicular tissue from one person to another have been reported. Work is progressing on stem cell use for male factor infertility. Stay tuned!

Giving hope to patients with diseases that threaten their fertility

The major reason that diseases create a situation where gamete freezing is recommended arises when the gonads will be exposed to some process that will irreparably damage them. Cancer is the primary disease where gamete preservation is advisable, but other diseases, such as some connective tissue diseases being treated with gonad-toxic chemotherapy, are conditions where freezing eggs or sperm are indicated.

Frequently, when cancer is diagnosed, time becomes a major issue. Males can produce specimens for freezing almost immediately. Centers vary in how they freeze the sperm, but many will freeze so that there are enough sperm for intrauterine insemination or more commonly for IVF. Far fewer sperm are needed for IVF, so a single specimen can be used for numerous cycles of IVF. Intrauterine insemination requires considerably more sperm, and thus fewer cycles can be obtained from each ejaculate. Success rates are approximately 10–15 percent per attempt using intrauterine insemination and 40 percent using IVF with ICSI. Female factors, especially age, decease these success rates. Overall pregnancy rates depend upon a number of factors, but when the female is under the age of 35 with no fertility factors, the overall rate approaches 85 percent within six inseminations and similar rates with three cycles of IVF. Treatments that can cause sterility include chemotherapy, radiation to the testis, and surgery. For men treated with chemotherapy, not all will become sterile and remain without sperm. Research suggests that men with previous exposure to chemotherapy can safely father children after the chemotherapy from freshly ejaculated sperm.

The story for women is vastly different, less successful, more costly, and more complicated. The reasons for fertility preservation for women are similar to those for men, including surgery, radiation, and chemotherapy. Chemotherapy has a variable effect on female fertility, with some having no effect and other types of chemotherapy almost always causing menopause and loss of fertility. Fertility preservation can include freezing ovarian tissue, which has been used successfully only in a very limited number of situations. The most common form of fertility preservation uses IVF where the woman undergoes treatment with FSH for a number of days and then a retrieval where the eggs are removed and then frozen. This raises a number of issues, with time being a prime factor. For most women only one cycle will be possible and thus a very limited number of eggs can be stored. Yet for younger women with normal fertility, if they have at least 12 eggs, their chance of conceiving is approximately 80 percent. Many women do fertility preservation for breast cancer and are usually older, so fewer eggs ae retrieved and the overall chance of success is lower. For breast cancer patients whose tumor is estrogen, progesterone receptor positive, the fact that IVF increases the levels of these hormones has raised concerns that the IVF will accelerate the cancer. Newer stimulation protocols can use estrogen-blocking compounds to limit the overall amount of estrogen. Finally, time usually requires that the stimulation be started immediately and cannot wait for the normal cycling of the woman's menstrual cycle. The protocols can be adjusted so that the stimulation can begin within a few days of the diagnosis, but it still takes about three weeks before the eggs are retrieved.

While sperm freezing is relatively inexpensive (roughly $200 per sperm specimen), the cost for egg freezing can be about $10,000 (including medication) as it requires doing an egg retrieval. So many patients cannot afford fertility preservation for egg freezing unless they are able to find donated cycles or nonprofit groups that pay for these services. Fortunately, several states have passed laws that provide insurance coverage for patients needing fertility preservation. Most of these laws cover patients who are faced with medical treatment that will render future fertility difficult, if not impossible. Illinois recently passed a law mandating coverage. In addition, institutions have started to look at protecting fertility for those with hazardous jobs, such as military personnel in combat zones. In 2016, the Obama administration suggested offering freezing of eggs and sperm to soldiers going to combat zones. Late in 2019, a bill was introduced in Congress to mandate this benefit, but the outcome is unknown at this time.

Social freezing: Stalling parenting until you are "ready"

Advances in technology have permitted the successful freezing of eggs. The technical term for this is oocyte cryopreservation or OC. Women who want to delay pregnancy can choose to undergo IVF and have the eggs retrieved before they are fertilized. These will keep for years so that the woman has the option of using them at a later date. Egg for egg, frozen eggs are almost as good as fresh eggs. For younger women, if they can freeze more than 12 to 15 eggs, their overall chance of having one child approaches 80 percent — not 100 percent. The process involves a number of days of injection of the hormone FSH and an egg retrieval. The cost with medication is close to $10,000 for one retrieval. There are yearly storage fees that can be from $400 to $600 per year. The actual use of these frozen eggs is not that great. Most women never develop a need to use them. However, they do provide a hedge against the natural age-related decline in female fertility. The ability to freeze eggs has opened another source of revenue, and this has not gone unnoticed. There is considerable media hype for egg freezing, and some employers have offered egg freezing as a benefit.

Deciding the future: Disposition documents are a must

Whenever you decide to save (freeze) eggs, sperm, or embryos for future use, you will be asked to sign one or more documents for the holding company (whoever is holding your frozen property). These documents are important as they do the following:

>> Give the clinic permission to freeze your eggs, sperm, or embryos

>> Give the holding company permission to store your embryos (and specify your agreement to pay for storage)

>> Direct final disposition of your eggs, sperm, or embryos in the event you are unavailable, divorce, or die

These situations include using them to create a pregnancy (perhaps through donation to another person or couple), donating them for approved research, or discarding them in the current ethically accepted procedure.

TIP

When presented with these documents, you need to take time to decide what you want done with your eggs, sperm, or embryos if your situation changes (you are no longer single or suddenly single), or you can no longer make these decisions (you cannot be found — it happens! — or you are dead). You will have to make these decisions and document your wishes for who gets your eggs, sperm, or embryos in a variety of situations, or if you want them discarded.

REMEMBER

Your initial decisions at the time your eggs, sperm, or embryos were frozen will carry a lot of weight with any court that may be faced with deciding the fate of these eggs, sperm, or embryos. So take your time and make this a well-thought-out decision. Also, by agreeing to store your gametes or embryos, you agree to pay for the storage and allow storage facilities to dispose of your material if you fail to pay for the storage.

Getting Up to Speed on Reproductive Law

The field of reproductive law is a growing area that has been struggling to keep up with the rapid advances in fertility medicine and genetics. While assisted reproductive technology remains a largely unregulated business in the United States (at both the federal and state level) professional guidelines and court cases have given us some parameters for best practices and dispute resolution. This section looks at some of the areas of reproductive law that have captured headlines recently.

Posthumous conception: When your family wants to have your baby

It's not difficult or expensive to do. It creates a child. It usually helps heal wounds that come from the death of a loved one. So why is there so much controversy over posthumous conception?

Posthumous collection of sperm — removing sperm from the testes after a man has died — has been done on just about every continent. The legal issues have been discussed almost as much as the ethical issues. And there's still little legal or moral consensus about using a deceased man's sperm to create a child.

The person using the sperm is usually the spouse or partner of the dead man. Sometimes, but not always, she has advance written permission to collect and use the sperm at the time of his death. Legal issues have revolved around inheritance of the dead man's property and the payment of Social Security to the children who are born after a man's death — more than 300 days after his death.

The waters become murkier when the man has given no written permission for the sperm extraction. Can a spouse or partner legally request this be done? How does she know that it's what the man would have wanted done? Does it matter?

Today, many jurisdictions require that surviving family members provide some sort of proof that the deceased family member wanted to have children even if they were not alive to parent the children before they can use frozen eggs, sperm, or embryos to create a pregnancy. For example, one widow used a videotape in which her husband, who had been killed in a car accident, expressed a desire to have children someday as support for her request to have sperm removed at the time of his death. In another situation, a single man left his sperm to his girlfriend to "have a family," and she was allowed to do so over the objections of his adult children.

With sperm and egg freezing becoming more available for fertility preservation (in the face of medically necessary treatment) and reproductive management (gamete freezing to voluntarily postpone reproduction), cases like these and even more complex ones will be popping up in courts all over the world in the next few years. As discussed earlier, whenever you cryopreserve gametes or embryos, it is essential that you get to decide what will happen to them if you are no longer able to make decisions about their use or disposition.

Make sure that you have signed current disposition documents about your frozen eggs, sperm, or embryos so that everyone knows what you want done.

A few years ago, England found itself with more than 300,000 embryos in storage tanks that weren't being used or paid for by the people who created them. Because English law stipulated that frozen embryos must be used within five years, unless the parents were granted an extension, the embryos were destroyed.

In the United States, hundreds of thousands of embryos are frozen in storage tanks. Some will be used for another pregnancy attempt by their parents, but others will be left frozen, unpaid for, and unused. In the United States, clinics who have documented proof that they tried to contact parents can destroy embryos that are deemed "abandoned" after five years, according to guidelines from the American Society for Reproductive Medicine (ASRM).

REMEMBER

The United States still has no hard and fast rules for frozen embryos. Each state rules differently when the cases go to court.

Infertility centers try to prevent these types of lawsuits by having couples sign a form at the time of egg retrieval stating what they want done with their embryos if they die or are divorced. However, courts differ as to whether these decisions are binding or are merely an indication of what you wanted at the time the embryos were created.

Even if parents don't divorce or die, the decision of what to do with frozen embryos is a tough one because the choices are limited. Parents can donate the embryos to research, donate them to another couple, or have them destroyed. Not liking any of the choices, many parents just keep the embryos in storage, postponing any decision on what to do with them.

Frozen embryos have survived and created healthy children after a ten-year freezing period, so most centers aren't anxious to destroy embryos after five years. (Theoretically, gametes and embryos can survive frozen for centuries.)

Divvying up leftover embryos after the "Big D"

In an ideal world, couples would use up all their embryos, having one baby initially and then one or more a few years later. However, for various reasons, that often doesn't happen. Leftover embryos then become a huge emotional and legal headache for most IVF centers. It takes space to store them and costs money to maintain the storage tanks. Few centers want to make decisions about potential human beings without some input from their parents, even if the parents haven't been seen or heard from in years.

When parents separate or divorce with embryos still in storage, frozen embryos can become a bitter battleground. In more than one case, divorcing couples have fought publicly over what should be done with their unused embryos. One ex-husband wanted to implant the embryos in his new wife! Other cases are faced with deciding if a divorcing spouse with cancer (who has no remaining eggs) should get the embryos because they provide her only chance to be a biologic parent. And these disputes are not limited to divorce situations, as the Sofia Vergara-Nick Loeb drama has shown us.

REMEMBER

Your disposition documents can be a help here as to who gets the embryos, but they are not a guarantee. Your state court will have the final say in any embryo dispute. As an alternative, many couples now look to freezing oocytes instead of embryos (and creating embryos as they need them) to avoid these issues — just a thought!

Ethics and extra embryos

The controversy over using "leftover embryos" for stem cell research has created heated debates among ethicists. Is it ethically justifiable to destroy embryos — that many argue will be destroyed anyway — to potentially save other people? Or is the destruction of human embryos — potential people in their own right — wrong even if it's done for a good cause? Whose life takes precedence? These are hard questions with hard answers that many ethicists are still debating, and that many IVF patients agonize over on a personal level. While all of the debate is intellectually fascinating, the resolution of difficult social issues is left to the legal system. What is ethical may not always be legal and vice versa. So, the resolution of many of these issues is done at both the state and federal legislative level and in the courts. That takes time and in the end is usually complicated.

Getting your baby home: Passports, parents, and government interference

A growing area of concern for patients who seek to use gestational surrogates in countries outside their home country is how to get their baby home after its born. Many countries require proof that the child is biologically related to the parent in order to get citizenship. For example, the U.S. government will grant U.S. citizenship to a child born abroad if the U.S. citizen father is the genetic parent of the child or the U.S. citizen mother is the genetic and/or the gestational and legal mother of the child at the time and place of the child's birth and meets all other statutory requirements to transmit U.S. citizenship to the child at birth. In these cases, it is possible to get a U.S. passport for the child. However, in cases of donor egg and/or donor sperm use, obtaining a passport or other travel documents becomes much more problematic. There have been numerous stories of couples having children abroad and then having no legal way to establish citizenship, which leaves the babies where they were born and the "family" very divided.

TIP

It is essential to consult a reproductive law attorney well-versed in immigration law *before* you attempt to create a pregnancy and deliver your child in another country. While you cannot get a passport or travel documents until the child is born, knowing the process and any potential hang-ups before you start can save you a lot of grief later on.

Saving Stem Cells for Research: Raising Ethical Concerns

Stem cells are cells that can be grown into any type of tissue or organ. In other words, they're not specific.

Human embryos are a good source of stem cells, and it could be possible to substitute DNA from a living person into a human egg after the egg's DNA was removed. The egg could then be "shocked" to get it to grow, and after two weeks or so, the stem cells would be removed. Of course, in the process, the embryo would cease to exist.

The stem cells would then be grown into whatever the adult needed — organs, skin, or other tissue. Because the genetic match would be exact, the person's body wouldn't reject the new organ or tissue. People needing organ transplants or new skin after a burn may find this type of science valuable.

Some doctors feel that the surplus of embryos destroyed every year should be used for stem cell development. Others feel that the potential life of the embryo shouldn't be sacrificed to save an already living person. Many people with frozen embryos would like to see something positive done with embryos that they donate for research and would rather have them used for stem cell development than just be destroyed.

Parents with sick children have already been in the news for trying to create embryos for the specific purpose of donating stem cells to their living child. Others have had a baby specifically for the purpose of donating blood or tissue to a sick child. Whether it's morally and ethically acceptable to give birth to a child so that that child can save another's life is a question that's still under debate.

CUTTING THE CORD — BUT SAVING IT

Stem cells can be obtained from other places besides human embryos. Many parents are now banking blood from their child's umbilical cord in case the child needs stem cells at a later date. Unfortunately, the utility and/or cost-effectiveness of such an approach has not yet been evaluated. One possible strategy would collect all of the umbilical blood in a given community, with the idea of setting up a stem cell bank. It has been estimated that 10,000 specimens would be required to have a sample of every possible combination of HLA genes. When someone needed stem cells, say for a bone marrow transplant, such stem cells would then be available. As with so many aspects of this new science, only time will tell.

Animal cloning from an adult hasn't been very successful, but separating cells at an early embryonic stage has worked fairly well. The trouble with this technique is that it doesn't have much practicality in humans. Although identical twins, triplets, or more could be created, few families are looking to have an army of identical children.

Cloning and Human Concerns

People talk about cloning as if all cloning were the same thing. In reality, there are three different types of cloning: those that have been successful, those that have been partially successful, and those that haven't been done at all yet as far as we know. We discuss the first two in this section (as we don't know about the third!).

The cloning causing the most controversy is the type that produced Dolly the sheep. It involves taking a healthy embryo, removing its DNA, and putting the DNA from another person into the embryo. Any cell contains DNA, so obtaining DNA isn't difficult. If the embryo continues growing normally, it can be placed into a host uterus to grow for nine months.

There are numerous concerns about cloning. Many of the offspring cloned so far have had serious abnormalities. There is also concern that cloned individuals might age much faster than normal because their DNA was obtained from a mature adult.

TECHNICAL STUFF

People wanting an exact copy of themselves may be disappointed because cloned animals aren't totally identical. Environmental influences can change certain characteristics and alter appearance.

THE CREATION OF DOLLY

The cloning technique that created Dolly, the well-known cloned sheep, involved taking a cell from another sheep and putting it into a sheep embryo. The genetic material was removed from the embryo so that the only DNA was from the donor sheep, which was about six years old at the time. Dolly was the only successful clone born out of about 300 original attempts. Dolly started to develop arthritis when she was almost six years old, causing concern that she was aging faster than normal. In early 2003, Dolly had to be euthanized at the age of six after being diagnosed with a progressive lung disease. Sheep usually live to be 12 to 14 years old. Calf cloning has been mildly successful; 73 percent of pregnancies end in miscarriage, and 20 percent die soon after birth. Some are born oversized, with enlarged tongues, with immune deficiencies, or with diseases such as diabetes.

Another type of cloning that could be used to create human beings has been done pretty successfully in animals. It involves taking a cell from an embryo and allowing it to grow into a second, identical embryo. This is how identical twins occur in nature.

It would be possible to give birth to identical twins several years apart by using this technique, which is done frequently in farming. It would also be possible to do genetic testing on the "cloned" embryo while freezing the original. If the clone passed the genetic tests, the "original" could then be thawed and implanted.

Forcing Clinics to Decide Who's Fit to Parent

If you're fertile, you can become a parent anytime you want. No one is in your bedroom rating your ability to raise children. And after children are born, they're taken only from parents who've crossed far over the line of normal parenting behavior.

People who do IVF are no better or worse as parents than anyone else; the potential for child abuse or neglect exists just as it does in any other population. Some clinics require psychological screening for their patients, trying to weed out those who are psychologically unprepared to raise children; others do not.

Not long ago, a father was arrested for beating his infant son to death. The father had used IVF with donor eggs and a gestational carrier to create his son. This case raised questions about how aggressive clinics should be in evaluating patients for parenthood. Should potential parents be turned away because they don't fit a typical social mold? In Australia, for example, gay women aren't allowed to do IVF. Should IVF parents be required to have a certain income level or be of a certain intelligence level?

At this time, most clinics set their own rules for evaluating patients. One prime example is the use of donor eggs or embryos for older women — older as in over 55. Many centers use 55 as an arbitrary cutoff age. Why 55 and not 65? Some centers do strict testing on patients over 40 to make sure that they're healthy enough to carry a pregnancy. Yet some 45-year-olds are much healthier than some 25-year-olds.

IVF (just like choosing to have a child) isn't well regulated in the United States. Although most centers follow guidelines set by ASRM and the Society of Assisted Reproductive Technology (SART), guidelines are only that. A patient denied treatment at one center may be accepted at another. Currently, IVF clinics are held to the same standard as many businesses. There are federal and state laws about discrimination. For a person who feels they have been denied their legal rights, the courts can intervene and direct a clinic as to how to proceed.

Realizing that Machines and People are Fallible

Black children born to white couples. Embryos, eggs, and sperm lost to freezer failures. A clinic in California charged with more than 100 cases of taking one woman's eggs and giving them to another and of selling embryos left in storage. These are just a few of the mistakes that fertility clinics have made. Ethical guidelines and now certain laws have dealt with misconduct (which should never be tolerated!), and self-imposed internal processes have reduced many risky behaviors.

Most clinics are extremely careful not to work on eggs or embryos belonging to two different people at the same time. They label everything that they're working on to prevent mix-ups (some clinic even use electronic labels on all gametes), yet mix-ups do sometimes occur.

When a clinic makes these kinds of mistakes, saying sorry isn't nearly good enough. Most of the highly publicized cases of parents ending up with the wrong children have come to light only because the parents and children were of different races. It's hard to say whether similar errors have been made and not discovered because parents and children were all of the same race.

In one instance involving black children and white parents, the error was made in the andrology lab; sperm from a black man was used instead of the sperm from the Caucasian spouse. In this case, the birth mother was also the biological mother, making the children genetically hers.

In a recent case, embryos from two Caucasian couples were implanted in an Asian couple. Tragically, the Asian couple gave birth to twins and then had to turn them over to their biological parents.

TIP

It's hard to safeguard yourself against errors like these. The errors aren't made purposely; they're the result of fallible human beings making mistakes or mechanical errors in machinery. You can help keep mistakes to a minimum by reading everything you're given to sign and making sure that your name is properly spelled on everything. When you leave a semen specimen, make sure that it's labeled properly. When the embryologist hands your embryos over for transfer, make sure that she says your proper name. It may seem pedantic for a clinic to require a number of identity proofs, but the purpose is to limit the risk of error.

REMEMBER

If you have questions at any point about your eggs or embryos, ask them at that time. If there's any question of error, getting to the bottom of it right then is much easier than getting to the bottom of it nine months later.

Looking Beyond IVF

The field of reproductive endocrinology has seen incredible advances — things never imagined. Trying to divine the future of IVF will surely be inadequate and inaccurate. However, it does seem that in the future, the issues will be genetic engineering and personalized medicine using artificial intelligence. The process will become easier with the elimination of injections. The REI specialist may be replaced by the gynecologist, and the small practice could become extinct as larger healthcare systems buy the independent, small practitioner. Age may become a non-issue if stem cell research can create eggs.

6

Part of Tens

Chapter **23**

Ten "Fake News" Stories about Fertility

We hear so much today about "fake news." Is it real or isn't it? Surprisingly enough, this phenomenon has existed in the field of science and medicine for . . . ever. From the early "snake oil salesmen" to the pills and potions of self-proclaimed shamans to the latest news bulletin claiming that immortality is just around the corner, medical professionals often find themselves trying to separate the glitter from the goods.

Infertility is no exception to this. How many of these tidbits have you heard — or believed?

News for Rodents

While technically not in the "fake news" category, a new (pick one) drug, procedure, treatment has been found to reverse *anything* when tested in mice. As a news producer once told co-author Jackie, "Great news for rodents!"

It's crucial to remember that testing in animals, while an important step in determining the effectiveness and safety of a medical treatment, is only the *first step*. Most of these do not make it past the first step — and remain a good option only for rodents. The scientific chain of proof before a treatment can be considered for use in humans (or even more complex mammals!) is a long one. Those in the medical community generally reserve judgment on these tidbits, which may very well stop at being rodent food for thought!

Reading about Medical Miracles

Everyone wants to jump on the bandwagon when it comes to reporting stories of medical miracles. Keep in mind that most (or make that *all*) medical journals avoid the use of the word "miracle" at all costs! Medicine and science are long and painstaking processes and rarely come across a "gimme" (or a simple, great cure) that appears out of nowhere, also known as a miracle.

WARNING

Actually, ASRM cautions infertility specialists against ever using the world miracle, as it is a setup for disappointment and doesn't meet the burden of proof required. But, miraculous stories of women giving birth at (pick one) 50, 60, 70, or 80 without (considerable) assistance is the kind of story that *sells.* Whether a celebrity-based magazine about people (we're not naming any names here!) or an outright tabloid, consider the source.

Celebrity Fecundity (also known as Fertility)

Hollywood would like us to believe that celebrities are aging without any of the ill side effects that we humans encounter including weight gain, wrinkles, and loss of fertility. Photoshop or CGI (computer-generated imagery) goes a long way in helping to sustain this myth. So does leaving out just a "little bit" of crucial information. For example, the 55-year-old female celebrity who has "miraculously" (there's that word again!) given birth to her first child with just a glass of wine and a prayer was more likely utilizing the best that ART has to offer, including donor eggs or egg freezing. Really, how else can celebrities maintain the pedestal that we often put them on without appearing to be better than the rest of us at defying all odds? They can't.

Cell Phones Decrease Male Fertility

A literature search on PubMed for cell phones and male infertility turned up almost 50 articles, with some articles showing a difference and some not showing a difference. Many of the articles focused on the semen analysis but not the actual chance of achieving a pregnancy. Since the amount of time a man uses his cell phone varies considerably, there are a number of other things that may influence the semen analysis. For example, is the student, coffee-house devotee using his phone the same as the 95th-floor, high-powered executive? A representative study published in 2015 found no difference in semen results based upon cell phone usage.

There was a reduced sperm count based upon internet usage with those using the internet more frequently having lower sperm counts. That raises the contentious issue of whether sitting and thus increasing testicular temperature can reduce the sperm counts.

A 2018 study looked at cell phone usage with 4G for rats. Who knew rats had cell phones? These poor little fellows were exposed to varying lengths of exposure to 4G LTE cell phones and — if that weren't enough, egad — their testicles were assessed for number of sperm cells. The longer the exposure, the lower the number of sperm cells. Not the best study to volunteer for if you are a male rat.

But wait: Cell phones aren't the only source of non-ionizing radiations. What about laptops, Wi-Fi, microwave ovens, and on and on. After an extensive review of the currently available research, the authors of a 2018 review concluded that non-ionizing radiation may decrease sperm parameters. They could not conclusively say this was so nor did they say the evidence conclusively demonstrated that cell phone usage causes infertility. So again — maybe!

Increased Longevity Means a Larger Fertility Window

Not so much. The increased longevity (humans living longer) arises from things like antibiotics, anesthesia, pharmaceuticals, immunization, and sanitary conditions, to mention a few.

The effect of these advances in the 19th and especially the 20th century increased the worldwide life expectancy of women from 54 years in1900 to 75 years in 2019. (U.S. rates are even higher at 81 years!) The average life expectancy in 1800 was between 30 and 40. So the increase in life expectancy derived from something that could be corrected. For example, women becoming infected after childbirth died at an alarming rate until antibiotics were developed that cured the infection.

In 1900, for every 1,000 births, seven women died and 40 percent were due to infections. By 1997, the maternal mortality decreased to less than 0.1 per 1,000 deliveries. But nothing has changed the underlying problem with age-related infertility. No medication has been developed that allows women to make eggs after she is born. No medication nor intervention has been devised that prevents the ovary from destroying the pool of eggs.

So, while life expectancy has increased because of problems that have solutions, living longer has not translated into longer fertility potential because nothing fixes the issue of limited egg number and rapid egg usage and wastage.

Men Don't Undergo Menopause

Hah! The first thing to understand is that male menopause is not the same as male fertility. The debate about age and male infertility rages, but in general, males can father children well into their 70s and maybe even 80s if they are capable of ejaculating.

But males experience a decline in their testosterone levels as they age. Colloquially, this is called "low T." The symptoms include fatigue, depression, sexual dysfunction, weakness, and loss of muscle mass, just to name a few of the symptoms.

Not all doctors agree that low T, as male menopause, actually exists, but if you ask men, they will tell you that it does. Measuring the testosterone levels may define a cause of male menopause. For men symptomatic with low T, testosterone replacement may be a solution.

Looking Good Means Your Fertility Is Good

Just because you can pass for 30 something, be aware that your ovaries have a mind of their own! So, you look great, feel well, eat healthy, and exercise often — congratulations! These are all excellent lifestyle choices that can help you maintain good health, to some degree, in the short and long term. They can certainly give you a great base for gestating a child and raising one with healthy habits. But, if you are 40 something, your ovaries are not in on the secret. Your ovaries will always reflect your biologic age no matter how good you look and feel.

You Can Glue Your Embryos to Your Uterus

While this may appear to be the peak of fake news, hold on, maybe you can, sometimes. Have we confused you yet?

In 2012 a study was published that found no increased pregnancy rate when embryo glue was used. A Cochrane database report in 2014 said it might improve pregnancy rate. So, where do we stand? First of all, is embryo glue actually glue? Is it like that white pasty glue we (well, apparently not coauthor Lisa) ate when we were in the third and fourth grade? Mmmmm, delicious! No! Embryo glue is not glue at all.

Embryo glue is a solution that contains hyaluronic acid. Hyaluronic acid is a naturally occurring substance in the secretions in the female reproductive tract. It tends to make things sticky. So dipping an embryo into the solution may make the embryo sticky and thus help with implantation.

A study published in 2018 used a solution of hyaluronic acid–enhanced media for frozen embryo transfers. They found that for the first transfer, the pregnancy rate was less than when not using the solution. When the patient had a second frozen embryo transfer and the solution was used, there was no difference seen. If the patient returned for a third frozen embryo transfer, then the use of the solution did improve the pregnancy rate. If a person has had two normal appearing embryos transferred and has no evidence that they implanted, she may have recurrent implantation failure (RIF). Some physicians have suggested that for this group of patients (those with RIF), the embryo glue may help.

Procreation Vacations Work

Vacations are great, but do they increase the chance for a pregnancy? Sorry guys, not so much. Before you book a multi-thousand-dollar vacation hoping it will help you get pregnant, you may want to reflect on what is keeping you from getting pregnant in the first place.

Males with very low counts, women with blocked tubes, women who don't ovulate on their own, women with endometriosis, age-related infertility — these and other diagnostic categories for infertility will not be helped by going on a vacation. It's hard to imagine how lying in the sun in Tahiti can magically unblock tubes. So why even make the suggestion?

But, does this work for those patients with unexplained infertility? The reasoning is that coping with infertility increases stress. Vacations are supposed to reduce stress, ergo, taking a vacation will help you get pregnant. There are heated debates about the importance of stress in causing infertility. There is little debate as to whether infertility causes stress. And if you don't know the answer to this debate, you haven't really had infertility.

Infertility causes stress! Under normal circumstances, taking a vacation can reduce stress. However, taking a vacation to improve the chance of pregnancy may actually increase the stress level — there is no credible evidence looking at this possibility.

TIP

Taking a vacation to get a vacation from fertility treatments makes more sense. Breaking the daily grind of fertility treatment can be much needed and the expense is more than worth it.

Adopt and You'll Get Pregnant

Maybe, but the adoption does not increase the normal treatment independent pregnancy rate (the rate of pregnancy without treatment). There is a chance that any person who has stopped fertility treatments and does nothing will get pregnant without any further treatment.

If you evaluate a large number of patients who have adopted, some of them achieved a pregnancy on their own. But the chance is the same as for those who did not adopt. An interesting study from 2018 looked at what happened five years after patients had undergone IVF. The majority did no more IVF. For those who had adopted, almost 7–8 percent had a spontaneous pregnancy.

Overall, five years after IVF over 90 percent of the patients were living with children in the family. Some were from more IVF, some from spontaneous pregnancies, some as stepparents, and some from adoption. For this study almost 10 percent had a spontaneous pregnancy after stopping IVF and having not been successful with the IVF they had done.

REMEMBER

Various studies will have somewhat different figures, but the overall point is that most people can have children in their family — just not as easily as they had expected.

Chapter **24**

Ten Things to Know in Early Pregnancy

Yay! Can you believe it? You made it out of the Infertility Club, and you are now part of the Pregnant Club. We knew you could do it! So, no worries, right? Well, maybe not so much. You may have just replaced one set of worries with another. No sweat! In this chapter, we offer some help as you "graduate" from your fertility clinic to your obstetrician's office.

Good Pregnancy or Not?

So, the pregnancy test is positive — now what? The hormone that is measured for pregnancy is human chorionic gonadotropin. Specifically, it's one of the components of the beta chain and is thus called beta hCG. For the most part, only the pregnancy — the trophectoderm, specifically — makes hCG, so any amount of hCG is a sign of an implantation of an embryo and shows in the blood roughly ten days after ovulation. As the pregnancy grows, more hCG is produced. A normal pregnancy will secrete a normal amount of hCG, which is a rise of more than 60 percent in 48 hours. Frequently, the rise is said to double every 48 hours, but that's not always true, and a normal pregnancy may not have a doubling of the hCG every 48 hours.

What does low progesterone mean if you are pregnant? The issue of low progesterone when you are pregnant is whether the low progesterone is a sign of an abnormal pregnancy or whether the low progesterone is causing an abnormal pregnancy. With very few exceptions, an abnormal pregnancy will cause low progesterone. This is especially true if the pregnancy has an abnormal number of chromosomes. Considering that this is the cause of the low progesterone, treating a low progesterone with progesterone makes little sense. That having been said, many physicians prescribe progesterone and there seems to be no adverse effects of doing so.

What is a biochemical pregnancy? Somewhat aggravatingly, the term "biochemical" has crept into the lexicon of infertility. It implies that somehow a biochemical pregnancy is unique. The reality is that a biochemical pregnancy is a pregnancy that fails to grow to a size that can be seen on ultrasound or diagnosed if the pregnancy tissue is passed vaginally and assayed by pathology. Most biochemical pregnancies fail to progress because they are genetically abnormal with an abnormal number of chromosomes.

What is a pregnancy of unknown location? A normal pregnancy will grow to a size where it can be seen on ultrasound somewhere in the fifth week of pregnancy (calculated from the first day of the last menstrual period). By the sixth week, a normal pregnancy will be seen on ultrasound as a gestational sac (GS) — the pregnancy unit. If the GS is in the uterus, it is termed a clinical pregnancy even if it is not normal and ends as a miscarriage. If the pregnancy is in the tubes and can be seen on ultrasound, it is called an ectopic pregnancy. Sometimes there is a pregnancy that is developing abnormally in the uterus or in the tube and cannot be seen. This is a pregnancy of unknown location and is usually treated as an ectopic pregnancy.

Bleeding Is Bad, Right?

What about first trimester bleeding? Bleeding early in a pregnancy is a scary and concerning problem. Sometimes, it is the first sign that something is terribly wrong with the pregnancy and the pregnancy will end as a first trimester loss. Other times the bleeding has no significant correlation to the outcome of the pregnancy.

First trimester bleeding is common. Over 25 percent of pregnant patients experience vaginal bleeding sometime before week twelve of a pregnancy. Of those women who bleed in the first trimester, a little over half miscarry. However, not all bleeding is the same. Some women will have a small amount of bleeding with no cramping while other women will experience heavy bleeding and cramping.

Women who have heavy bleeding are three times more likely to miscarry. Those women with light bleeding, no cramping, and bleeding less than two days have no increased chance of miscarriage when compared to women without bleeding.

If you are spotting or bleeding, contact your physician. Most probably, she will draw blood to measure the hCG and or perform an ultrasound. The thing to remember is that no amount of measuring the pregnancy by the hCG or ultrasound will alter the course of the pregnancy. At best, the information can distinguish a normal pregnancy from an abnormal pregnancy and help determine what action to take.

What About Exercise?

Regular exercise has been associated with a number of health benefits. ACOG recommends that a pregnant woman, at a minimum, should maintain her pre-pregnancy level of exercise. So, if you are one of those fortunate people who have a healthy lifestyle, being pregnant is no excuse to stop. However, for the rest of the world, the pre-pregnant and pregnant period are a good time to develop a healthy lifestyle incorporating sound eating habits and exercise.

In 2008, the U.S. Department of Health and Human Services issued guidelines for physical activity. The guidelines suggest that healthy pregnant and postpartum women should do at least 150 minutes of moderate-intensity exercise, such as brisk walking, spread over the week. If a woman has a very high prepregnant level of activity, it is okay to continue that when pregnant after a discussion with your obstetrician to make sure there are no reasons for reducing her exercise level.

There are obvious pre-pregnant conditions that are absolute contraindications when pregnant, such as significant heart disease, severe lung disease, incompetent cervix, abnormal placement of placenta (previa), multiple gestations, or severe anemia. But most women are aware of these conditions and should be under the care of their OB prior to conceiving. A number of less severe conditions may suggest the need to restrict a woman's level of aerobic exercise, but these can be discussed with the OB. Not all types of exercise carry the same risk, so the type of exercise matters. For example, walking, swimming, stationary cycling, and yoga are safe. Exercises such as contact sports, those activities with a high risk of falling, sky or scuba diving, or "Hot Yoga" should be avoided. If you are exercising and you feel anything unusual that suggests you should stop exercising (think bleeding or significant pain), then stop exercising. This is definitely *not* a no pain, no gain situation.

Can I Fly When I'm Pregnant?

Coauthor Dr. R recalls, "Once when I was a young, mouthy adolescent, my mother asked if she could fly somewhere and I asked if she had a broom — only once did I make that mistake." So, can you fly when pregnant? Yes — just use an airplane. Air travel is safe when a woman is pregnant, especially in early pregnancy. Turbulence can't be predicted, so the seatbelt should be used at all times. Most people do not fly frequently enough to be harmed by the increased cosmic radiation, but flight attendants and pilots may be. Pilots and flight attendants need to contact their employer for further information and company policy regarding flying when pregnant.

Should I Quit My Job?

According to the ACOG practice bulletin, working during pregnancy is generally safe. As of 2015, 70 percent of women with children under the age of 18 were in the labor force. Of these, 56 percent of pregnant women worked full time during the pregnancy.

Jobs where it may not be safe to work while pregnant require individual investigation. For example, what about jobs where there are toxic chemicals? While thousands of chemicals are used in industry today, very few have been documented to be harmful to a pregnant woman. However, some chemicals are considered to increase risks for fetal anomalies and miscarriage. These include heavy metals like lead, mercury, or arsenic; some pesticides and herbicides; some solvents; ionizing radiation; and chemotherapeutic medicines. OSHA regulates exposure to some of these potential hazards, but if you are concerned about the risk, you can consult the chemical's data safety sheet, CDC-NIOSH (https://www.cdc.gov/niosh/index.htm), and your employer. Sometimes, accommodations can be made to make sure you are comfortable with any potential risk.

The information available on night shift work or extensive occupational lifting is mixed, but there may be a slight increased risk for miscarriage. Studies did show a slight increase in the risk for preterm birth for some work conditions, such as work where the person was standing for more than three hours or carrying more than 11 pounds. Physically demanding work has been shown to increase low back pain and musculoskeletal problems. For these conditions, accommodations have been shown to reduce the risk. For example, where the work involves standing for prolonged periods of time, things like floor mats, sit-stand workstations, support hose, and appropriate shoes have been shown to help. Jobs requiring lifting do pose a risk of back pain and musculoskeletal injuries. The National Institute of Occupational Safety and Health has made recommendations for pregnant women for weight limits. An excellent summary of these recommendations published by ACOG can be found at www.ncbi.nlm.nih.gov/pmc/articles/PMC4552317/pdf/nihms717922.pdf.

Should I Get a Flu Shot?

The answer to this is easy: Yes! Unfortunately, vaccination has become a hot topic with fears of risks like autism from being vaccinated. These undue fears have already needlessly cost lives.

In recent years, there have been 24,000 deaths in the United States per year due to influenza. In the 2009 influenza pandemic (an infection that is prevalent over an entire nation or worldwide), pregnant women between the ages of 18 and 29 accounted for 16 percent of deaths from the influenza infection. A study done by the FDA's Vaccine Adverse Event Reporting System reported no or mild adverse outcomes in over 2 million people vaccinated. There were no adverse effects on the infants. This is one example of how bad science, fake news, and conspiracy theories have caused needless deaths.

When Should I See My Ob/Gyn?

You have a positive pregnancy test. *Yay!* Then another one. *Double-yay!* But you are still at the fertility clinic. There will come a time when you need to move from the care of your REI to the care of an obstetrician (OB). There is no set standard. Some REIs like to monitor patients and manage their early obstetric care. Other REIs do a single ultrasound to document that the pregnancy is in the uterus and that the fetus has fetal heart motion. When your REI tells you it's time to move on, as coauthor Lisa likes to say, "You have now graduated!"

It is a very good idea to have chosen an obstetrician, the physician who will manage your pregnancy and deliver your baby, prior to treatment for infertility so that when the good news comes, the OB is already on the team. Occasionally, there may be a question or problem that is more appropriately handled by your OB rather than by the REI. So, having an established relationship with an OB will avoid the problem of whose patient you are. Also, OBs differ in how they handle certain problems, and since that is the person who will manage you to the finish line, it is helpful to already have that doctor on board.

Do I Have to Stay on My Medication?

Sometimes women feel that they are not pregnant and will stop their medications. Whether this can cause a pregnancy to fail is up for debate, but a good rule of thumb is to stay on your medications until your REI has told you exactly what to do with your meds. Also, this is probably not the best time to start meds that you were not on unless you clear this with your REI.

On the other end of the spectrum, if the pregnancy test was positive, you may figure you are pregnant so, what the heck, you can stop all those injections and other meds from the fertility office. *No!* There was a reason that the fertility clinic prescribed the medications, and you are most often sent on to see your OB with a list of instructions on what meds to stay on and when to stop. Even though you are an IVF "glad grad," you still need the drugs. So, don't change anything until you talk to your OB.

Dealing with a UTI

Urinary tract infections (UTIs) are the second most common problem for pregnant women behind anemia. Left unattended to, they can cause severe infections of the kidneys *(pyelonephritis)*, which can be harmful to the pregnancy. So, do you start by downing a gallon of cranberry juice and hope that cures the problem, or is it time to consult your physician? The most common treatment for UTIs is oral antibiotics, which properly prescribed and taken, are safe in early pregnancy. When in doubt, consult your physician.

What Is Happening to My Skin?

Skin changes are common in pregnancy. Common changes include dark spots on the breasts, nipples, or inner thighs and sometimes brown patches on the face *(melasma)*. Other changes include *linea nigra* (a dark line running from the belly button to the pubic hair line), stretch marks, acne, varicose veins, and changes in hair and nail growth.

Some of these changes are due to the hormones that are present during pregnancy, and some, such as varicose veins, are due to the physical presence of the fetus as it gets bigger. Over-the-counter medications that can be used during pregnancy include topical benzoyl peroxide, azelaic acid, and glycolic acid. Some prescription medications should not be used during pregnancy, and these include isotretinoin, oral tetracyclines, and topical retinoids.

Many women experience increased hair growth, perhaps in places where there had been very little hair. These changes usually return to normal by six months postpartum (after the child's birth), but many women experience hair loss in the first three months postpartum.

Varicose veins are common in pregnancy due to the weight of the pregnancy as it grows and places pressure upon the veins that return the blood from the legs. Varicose veins are almost impossible to prevent, but certain physical accommodations can be made to lessen swelling and discomfort. These include not sitting with your legs crossed, moving around, elevating your legs as often as you can, considering support hose (consult your OB first), and avoiding (good luck) constipation by eating high-fiber foods and adequate liquids.

Index

assisted hatching (AH), 318–319

Assisted Reproductive Technologies (ART), 210, 259, 396

atresia, in ovaries, 26

atretic eggs, 308

autism, 120–121

autosomal dominant, 45–46

azithromycin, 60

azoospermia, 213, 354

azospermic factor (AZF), 45

B

baby showers, 179–180

bacteria, viruses vs., 60

bargaining stage of grief, 340

basal body temperature (BBT), 99–101

beats per minute (BPM), 335

beta hCG (human chorionic gonadotropin), 223, 227, 332, 417–418

bicycling, 223

biochemical pregnancy, 333

birth control pills, 30, 153, 286

birth defects, 264–265

black cohosh, 156

blastocyst, 311

blastocyst embryos, 313

blastocyst formation, 150

blastomeres, 311

bleeding, 32, 204–206, 418–419

blighted ovum, 229–230

blood

drawing, cost of, 18

forced into fallopian tubes, 23

irritating tissues around ovary, 102

medical tests for, 73, 187–192

blood callbacks, 288

blood relatives, 12

blood tests, 218–219, 226

blue cohosh, 158

board certified, 136

board eligible, 136

body mass index (BMI), 148–149, 254

body parts, transplanting to improve fertility, 395–396

body temperature

affecting chances of pregnancy, 68–69

of scrotum, 36

timing sex and, 99–101

borders, crossing, 278–279

BRCA 1 and 2, 12

breastfeeding, 87

breasts

cancer in, 12, 129

overview, 27

sore, 330

brokers, 364

bromocriptine, 190

Brown, Louise, 10

bulletin boards, 141–142

C

cabergoline, 190

callbacks, 291–292

canalization defects, 24

cancer

choriocarcinoma, 112

effects on fertility, 397–398

in family tree, 12

in females, 129–130

fertility and, 128–131

human papilloma virus (HPV) and, 58

in males, 130

in testicles, 130

carrier screening, 50

Centers for Disease Control (CDC), 141, 267

cerclage, 23

cervical cancer, 130

cervical conization, 130

cervical infections, 32

cervical motion tenderness (CMT), 253

cervical mucus, 36, 101–102

cervix, 23, 102

cesarean section (C-section), 25, 63

chancre, 62

chemical exposure, 223

chemical pregnancy, 226–227

chemistry panel, 73

chemotherapy, 129, 130, 131

Chinese medicine, 163–164

chlamydia, 59–60, 67

chlamydial pneumonia, 60

choriocarcinoma, 112, 230

chorionic villus sampling (CVS), 337

chromosomes
  abnormalities in, 12, 236
  defects in, 394
  in eggs, 26–27
  evaluating, 306
  genetics and, 42
  testing in parents, 231–232

cleavage stage embryo, 311

clinics
  choosing, 266–269
  mistakes made from, 406–407
  for single parents, 378

Clomid, 18, 245–248

clomiphene citrate, 245–246

cloning, 404–405

cocaine, 56, 223

codons, 42

Coenzyme Q10 (CoQ10), 162, 163

coffee, 55–56

coloring hair, 327

compounded capsules, 302

conceiving, 8

conception, 237–238
  posthumous, 400–401
  statistics on, 8–9

condom collection, 252

confirmation bias, 347

consent forms, 295–296

controlled ovarian hyperstimulation (COH), 253–256, 264

copulation. *See* sex

corona radiate, 26

corpus luteum, 29, 227

costs
  donating eggs to reduce, 276–277
  infertility, 16–19
  insurance plan coverage, 269–270
  IVF, 259–261

overview, 269
  pregnancy, 143–144

cramping, 331

Crinone, 301, 302

CRISPR (CRISPRCas9), 51, 391

cross-border reproduction, 280, 357

cross-border reproductive care (CBRC), 370

crossing borders, 278–279

cryobiology, 131

cryptorchidism, 34–35

cumulus layer, 26

cycles. *See* menstruation

cystic fibrosis, 12, 46

cysts, 187

cytomegalovirus (CMV), 60–61

cytosine (C), 42

D

day of assessment, 312–313

day of embryo, 311

defects, genetics and, 49–50

dehydroepiandrosterone sulfate (DHEA-S) hormone, 191

denial stage of grief, 340

Department of Health and Human Services (HHS), 80

depression stage of grief, 340

diabetes, 125–126

diet, 10, 148–152

dilate, defined, 228

dilation and curettage (D&C), 25, 130, 229

diseases
  affecting fertility, 121–128
  chlamydial pneumonia, 60
  diagnosing, 12
  genetic, 355, 394
  infectious, 358
  inheriting, 12, 45–46
  listeria, 151
  recessive genes and, 12
  single-nucleotide polymorphisms (SNPs) and, 44
  systemic lupus erythematosus (SLE), 192
  that threaten fertility, giving hope to patients with, 397

factors affecting, 115–131

increasing chances of, 95–113, 119–120, 148–169

lifestyle and, 53–57, 68–71

preventing, 108

resources for, 141–143

symptoms of, 330–332

pre-implantation genetic diagnosis (PGD), 116, 266

preimplantation genetic testing, for aneuploid, 48–49

preimplantation genetic testing (PGT), 316–317, 318, 338, 394

premature ovarian failure (POF), 104

premature ovarian insufficiency (POI), 129

prenatal vitamin, 155

prescription medications, 74–75

previewing egg retrieval, 297

primary care physician (PCP), 72

primary dysmenorrhea, 32

primrose oil, 157

privacy, 16, 146

private adoption, 386

private domestic adoption, 386–387

processed sugar, 151

products of conception (PCC), 231

progesterone, 29, 189, 227, 301

prolactin, 73, 189–190, 219

prolactinoma, 189

proliferative phase, 29

Prometrium capsules, 302

prostate, examining, 216

prostate cancer, 12

proteins, 29, 43

protocol, 285–288

proximal occlusion, 201

pyelonephritis, 422

Q

qi, 164

R

radiographic embolization, 217

recessive genes, 12

recovery, from IVF, 299

recurrent implantation failure (RIF), 238, 415

recurrent miscarriage (RPL), 235–238

red clover, 157

red raspberry leaves, 157

referrals, of doctors, 140

reflex ovulators, 98

registries, 375–376

regrouping, 342

relationships, 16–17. *See also* mates

relaxation response, 167

religion, 168

reproductive endocrinologist and infertility specialist (REI), 77, 136, 244

reproductive law

ethics and leftover embryos, 402

leftover embryos, 401

overview, 399

passports, parents, and government interference and, 402–403

posthumous conception, 400–401

requirements, reviewing for donors, 361

Resolve website, 140–141

results, receiving, 332–333

retrieval team, meeting, 296–297

retrograde ejaculation (RE), 74, 126, 221–222

rheumatoid arthritis (RA), 127

rodents, studies on, 411–412

Rotterdam criteria, 122

S

sales, shopping for, 279–280

saline infused hysterosonogram (SIS), 202

saliva test, 106–108

scanning uteruses, 226

scar tissue

caused by dilation and curettage (D&C), 87–88

in female anatomy, 196–197

preventing implantation of fetus, 25

schedules, for egg retrieval, 295

schizophrenia, 121

scholarship program from drug companies, 279

scientific method, 345

screening test, 186

About the Authors

Dr. John Rinehart holds many degrees but is at the core a clinician physician — taking care of patients on a daily basis. Dr. Rinehart has an MD, PhD (physiology), JD, and two master's degrees (zoology and, most recently, predictive analytics). Dr. Rinehart has practiced in the area of reproductive endocrinology in the Chicago area since 1986 and is actively involved with medical resident education and pursing the application of AI (artificial intelligence) to improve the field of reproductive endocrinology.

Dr. Rinehart spends much of his non-clinical time reading about diverse topics from mathematics to politics. Recently, the addition of two grandchildren to his life is happily occupying more of his time. Finally, Dr. Rinehart is an avid fan of college football (Go Buckeyes!).

Lisa Rinehart is a nurse and an attorney who currently works as a risk management consultant in her own firm, LegalCare Consulting, Inc., working in areas of risk identification and resolution, as well as medical practice development, regulatory compliance, contract review, and physician representation.

Being a definite people-person, Lisa is a frequent speaker at professional meetings and enjoys being a mentor and coach to other healthcare providers, and a support system to the patients she serves.

In her spare time, Lisa's passion is her family — especially being a proud "Mom" to her daughter, Beth, and "Nana" to her precious grandchildren Adela and Vinny. She enjoys cooking (particularly old family recipes) and spending time with family and friends. Lisa is also an avid reader who can't be without her e-book and fills her downtime by crocheting baby blankets for many of the "little ones" in her life.

Jackie Thompson is an account director for Hirons/Chicago, working in all areas of public and media relations and marketing. She is also a partner in JD Thompson Communications.

Writing, however, is her first love and what she considers her strongest skill. Fortunately, she is able to pursue this love as her vocation whether developing content for clients, creating stories to pitch to the media, or sharing her experiences of having been a fertility patient.

In her spare time, Jackie spends her time living, loving, and learning with her husband, Darren, and their fertility miracle children, Ava Rose (16) and Eli Leonard (13), along with a parade of basset hounds and other pets.

Dedications

From Dr. Rinehart: My effort for the creation of this book is dedicated to Lisa, who by being the very special person she is has made me a much better person, physician, and — I hope — husband. Thank you, Lisa.

From Lisa: This book is dedicated to my husband, John. Because of you, I became a much better me, and am eternally grateful for having "us" — our very special place.

From Jackie: This book is dedicated to Darren Thompson, the best friend, husband, and father I could have ever wanted, and to Ava Rose and Eli Leonard, the children of my dreams. You are my present and my future. And to my past; my loving parents who are always with me in spirit, Larissa and Leonard Meyers.

Authors' Acknowledgments

From Dr. Rinehart: Being a card-carrying "boomer" has allowed me to experience some of the most amazing human accomplishments. Neil Armstrong, first man on the moon, is from my hometown. The digital revolution has given me new excitement for research. But none has been more amazing than the advent of IVF. I was an intern at Hopkins learning to be a micro-surgeon dedicated to reconstructing a damaged female pelvis when a fellow resident announce the birth of Louis Brown. Almost to a person, we said that IVF was a fluke and would never work. How wrong we were. Literally thousands of children later, it is still thrilling when a woman's pregnancy test is positive. The excitement throughout all of this the opportunity to learn. Daily, patients expand my life experience by teaching me something I never knew. But the love of learning originated from my mother, a teacher, who instilled in me a true love of learning. For that I am truly grateful. However, IVF is technical, and it is easy to get lost in the data. But the most rewarding aspect of being a physician is the humanity of the profession. For that, I learned from Lisa, my wife and co-author, who has exposed me to the reward of experiencing life with patients, teaching me the value of nursing, and with her amazing family, has accepted me as a member of a large, caring family. I am grateful that Jackie (co-author) suggested we do this book and to Lisa (co-author) for the work she has done to bring the book to fruition.

From Lisa: Little did I know that my 1989 interview for a nursing position with a brand-new fertility center would create a whole new life path for me. What started as a dream (my boss's as she came into work all excited that she had found me the "perfect" job) soon became my passion when I got the job and later married my new boss, John Rinehart. Thirty years later I credit him and this wonderful, inventive, and oh-so-people-driven field of fertility medicine for helping me become who I am today. Fertility medicine not only gave me my husband and my dear friend Jackie, it allowed me a springboard to blend my nursing and legal backgrounds to help further an evolving field. This book is my attempt to share what I have learned from John, all of my colleagues in the field, and all of the patients who have let me into their lives, with patients who are still in the thick of their fertility journey. Thank you and a big hug to all of my patients, mentors, co-workers, employees, colleagues, and friends — I have learned so much from each of you. I am so very grateful to my co-authors, John (who champions me through all of my projects), Jackie (who made me believe I could do this), and Sharon (whose previous work gave us a rock solid foundation), and to everyone at Wiley, especially my encouraging editors, for allowing me to get my thoughts on paper. My hope is that this book will find its way to anyone faced with having to ask for help to have a baby. It is a journey you didn't seek but a goal you can reach with today's medicine. May this book bring you the information you might not have had, and maybe even a little encouragement to keep going. Growing up as one of nine children, and now as a mother and grandmother, family means everything to me — the family that is blood and those I have chosen to be a part of my life. Hopefully, dear reader, you will find your way to a family, and if my words have helped even a little bit, I will consider myself so very blessed.

From Jackie: Despite being a Pollyanna at heart, few statements get my goat more than "what doesn't kill you makes you stronger." I, for one, would opt for an easy life at the expense of a little less strength! That said, NOTHING could be a greater truth than this, as it applied to my struggle with infertility. No doubt, it made my sweet and supportive husband, Darren, and I that much closer. It ultimately resulted in our two amazing children, Ava and Eli, both (gulp!) teenagers at the time of this book's printing. It brought me colleagues and friends that I would never have otherwise met, gotten to know, and today count as near and dear to my heart and integral to my life, particularly my co-authors, John, Lisa, and Sharon. It also brought a new mission to my life, in writing these books (this being the third to date) to share information and help to educate others who are walking the same path that I did 20 years ago. I will be forever grateful to an amazing group of patient and hardworking editors at Wiley who allowed this to happen.

I would love to say that I have not been challenged ever again since those days of infertility. Alas, this is not true. But, I believe that infertility gave me a template and a stronger support system for facing other challenges in life. Infertility and the initial 1 percent chance I was given of conceiving a child (let alone two!) has instilled in me an unshakeable faith that anything is possible, and an immeasurable gratitude of things that I don't understand but yet believe.

Today, I look in awe at the miracles that life has brought me despite the hardships. These lessons learned began by going through infertility in the first place. While I don't "wish" infertility on anyone, I am profoundly grateful for what it has brought and taught me in my life. Dear Reader, I wish for you the same.

Publisher's Acknowledgments

Senior Acquisitions Editor: Tracy Boggier

Editorial Project Manager and Development Editor: Christina N. Guthrie

Copy Editor: Christine Pingleton

Production Editor: Mohammed Zafar Ali

Illustrator: Kathryn Born

Cover Image: © Birte Möller/EyeEm/ Getty Images